COMPLIMENTARY
COPY

PHARMACOKINETIC ANALYSIS

PHARMACOKINETIC ANALYSIS

A PRACTICAL APPROACH

Peter I. D. Lee, Ph.D.
Janssen Research Foundation
Titusville, New Jersey

Gordon L. Amidon, Ph.D.
College of Pharmacy
University of Michigan
Ann Arbor, Michigan

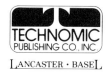

TECHNOMIC
PUBLISHING CO., INC.
LANCASTER · BASEL

Pharmacokinetic Analysis
a **TECHNOMIC**®publication

Published in the Western Hemisphere by
Technomic Publishing Company, Inc.
851 New Holland Avenue, Box 3535
Lancaster, Pennsylvania 17604 U.S.A.

Distributed in the Rest of the World by
Technomic Publishing AG
Missionsstrasse 44
CH-4055 Basel, Switzerland

Printed in the United States of America
10 9 8 7 6 5 4 3 2 1

Main entry under title:
  Pharmacokinetic Analysis: A Practical Approach

A Technomic Publishing Company book
Bibliography: p.
Includes index p. 543

Library of Congress Catalog Card No. 96-60272
ISBN No. 1-56676-425-4

This book was written to provide an accessible introduction to the very large and important field of pharmacokinetics. There are many approaches to pharmacokinetics, for example, approaches based on compartmental models, clearance, or residence time. While these views are of considerable importance to the specialist, the prerequisite physiological or mathematical knowledge often impedes the new student. The "Time Constant Approach" has been selected as a unifying view within which to present the important application areas of pharmacokinetics. In addition to providing a consistent view for all of the application areas, this approach provides the novice with an intuitive time view that is meaningful from the beginning. The Time Constant Approach allows one to get a "feel" for the data and to relate it to other data in a direct and accessible manner. In addition, because of the robustness, reproducibility, simplicity, and flexibility of its implementation, the Time Constant Approach is suitable for routine pharmacokinetic analysis.

The many advantages of the Time Constant Approach can be summarized as follows. For the novice in the pharmacokinetic field, such as pharmacy undergraduate students, and for those from other disciplines, such as biologists, chemists, and medical doctors:

- The Time Constant Approach gives a unifying view of many application areas in pharmacokinetics, including absorption, distribution, metabolism, drug interactions, special populations, and modification of pharmacokinetics by diseases.
- "Time" is a sensible unit. When pharmacokinetics are discussed from the point of view of "time," it makes the subjects easy to understand. For example, it is more comprehensible to say, "It takes

3 hours for a drug to be absorbed," than to say, "The absorption rate constant of a drug is 0.333 hr^{-1}."

- The Time Constant Approach facilitates intuitive interpretation of concentration profiles. Useful information about pharmacokinetics can be extracted by visual inspection of the concentration-time curve.
- The estimation method for time constants is simple, which involves, most of the time, only the area under the concentration curve (AUC) and the area under the first moment of the concentration curve (AUMC). One can estimate all the time constants using a spreadsheet software program.
- The Time Constant Approach provides additional information about pharmacokinetics of a drug, compared with the noncompartmental method. For example, the Time Constant Approach characterizes absorption, distribution, renal excretion, and metabolism in detail.

For the specialist in the pharmacokinetic field, such as pharmacy graduate students, pharmacokineticists, pharmacologists, and other pharmaceutical researchers and scientists:

- The Time Constant Approach provides much more information than the noncompartmental method; therefore, it allows a more detailed pharmacokinetic analysis.
- The estimation method for time constants is simple, robust, and reproducible because the estimation involves only the calculation of AUC and AUMC but no regression procedure. Therefore, the Time Constant Approach can be reliably used in routine pharmacokinetic analyses.
- The estimated values of a time constant is independent of the complexity of a model. The pharmacokinetic model of a drug may gradually become complicated as more pharmacokinetic information is gathered throughout the drug development process. However, the estimated values of time constants are consistent while the pharmacokinetic model is being built up.
- Time constants are correlated to physiological time scales, such as blood perfusion time through organs. This correlation provides a rationale for scaling up the time constants among different animal species.

This book covers most of the important areas in the pharmacokinetic field and is organized into five sections. Section I consists of four chapters: Chapter 1 gives a general introduction to the Time Constant Approach, and Chapters 2 to 4 present the Time Constant Approach, elaborating on the physiological meaning, the method of estimation, applications to pharma-cokinetics such as interspecies scaling, and observation of time constants from concentration-time profiles. Sections II to V organize the applications of the Time Constant Approach into four areas in the pharmacokinetic field. Section II discusses the influence of formulation on pharma-cokinetics; Section III scrutinizes some of the basic pharmacokinetic pro-cesses: absorption, distribution, metabolism, and pharmacodynamics; Section IV examines the interactions of concurrent medication and food with pharmacokinetics; and Section IV covers the pharmacokinetics in spe-cial populations, such as those stratified by age, gender, and diseases.

Each chapter in Sections II to V focuses on one clinical factor that affects the pharmacokinetics of a drug, for example, dosage, metabolism, food ef-fects, or renal impairment. Each chapter begins by identifying the pharma-cokinetic processes and the key time constants potentially affected by the clinical factor. Common themes are developed, by virtue of the Time Con-stant Approach, that link observations made under the condition discussed in the chapter to other clinical conditions. These common themes are simi-lar patterns of variations in time constants, which can be attributed to the same underlying mechanisms, in response to the changes in different clini-cal factors. In this way, the Time Constant Approach gives the reader an in-tegrated view to the various areas in pharmacokinetics. Following that, three to six pharmacokinetic models are presented to describe possible sce-narios that may occur under the influence of the clinical factor. Subse-quently, the Time Constant Approach is applied to at least three simulated case studies (to validate the approach) and to at least three literature ex-amples (to illustrate the utility of the approach). The presentation of Time Constant Approach in the examples is consistent throughout the book using the Time Constant Plot to give the reader a unifying view of all pharma-cokinetic areas. Additional references in the specific pharmacokinetic area can be found at the end of each chapter.

Software, in the form of an EXCEL® Macro spreadsheet for WINDOWS® will be available to assist with developing and understanding of the examples given in the book. This software is meant as a teaching tool to supplement the text. Computer software for use in pharmacokinetic anal-ysis, in addition to the commonly available statistical software packages is reviewed in Reference [1].

REFERENCE

1. Gex-Farbry M. and Balant L. P. in *Pharmacokinetics of Drugs,* P. G. Welling and L. P. Balant, eds. Springer-Verlag, New York, Chapter 18, 1994, p. 507.

BASICS AND METHODS

CHAPTER 1

Introduction

This text presents a unifying view of pharmacokinetics, which is called the Time Constant Approach. This approach is analogous to the noncompartmental, the compartmental, and the statistical moment approaches, the three most frequently used methods in analyzing pharmacokinetic data; therefore, the Time Constant Approach used in this text to solve pharmacokinetic problems should not be totally unfamiliar to those who have used any of the other approaches. As a result of a synergistical synthesis from the three other approaches, the Time Constant Approach possesses the following advantages: (1) the estimation of time constants is simple, robust, and reproducible; (2) the Time Constant Approach provides a consistent view across different types of clinical studies, regardless of the complexity of models or amount of data; (3) the Time Constant Approach provides detailed information about the pharmacokinetics of drugs; and (4) the pharmacokinetic time constants are correlated to the physiological time scales, which provides a rationale for scaling up pharmacokinetic information from animals to human. These advantages of the Time Constant Approach will be demonstrated in Chapters 1 to 4 and illustrated by extensive examples throughout Chapters 5 to 19.

To introduce the Time Constant View of pharmacokinetics, we have to define the way we look at the pharmacokinetics of drug disposition. The Time Constant Approach shares some of the same foundations as the compartmental modeling approach. The pharmacokinetics of drugs can be looked at as a combination of physiological compartments and pharmacokinetic processes (Figure 1.1). The compartments are places where a drug may reside. These places can be specified by physical spaces (such as the stomach, intestine, blood, various tissues, and organs) and, for metabolized drugs, by different chemical forms derived from the drug. For exam-

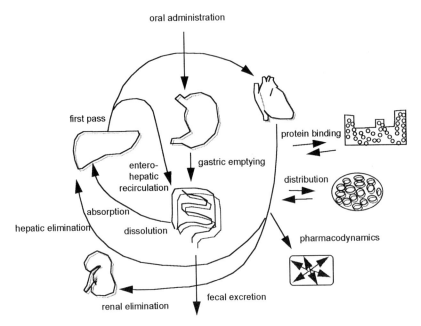

FIGURE 1.1. The pharmacokinetics of drugs can be looked at as a combination of physiological compartments and pharmacokinetic processes. The function of pharmacokinetic processes is to move drugs from one compartment to another, and each of the processes occur for a various time length.

ple, by this definition, metabolite M1 is recognized as a compartment. The action of a pharmacokinetic process is to move the drug from one compartment to another; for example, the intestinal absorption process moves the drug from intestine to blood. These compartments and processes are interwoven to create the whole pharmacokinetic model.

With the way we look at pharmacokinetics, we can now establish the concept of time constant. First of all, each of the pharmacokinetic processes does not occur instantaneously; it takes time. For example, gastric emptying, which moves a drug from stomach to intestine, typically takes 10 to 90 minutes, and the absorption of a drug typically takes less than a few hours, depending on the physicochemical properties of the drug, the formulation, the physiology of the intestine, and other factors. Therefore, each pharmacokinetic process is associated with a characteristic time, which specifies how fast the process occurs. The time constant of a process is defined as the average time it would take for the process to move the equivalent of the total amount of a drug in one compartment to another. Therefore, pharmacokinetics can be viewed as a number of processes that move drugs between places, each occurring with a characteristic length of time (Figure 1.1).

The implementation of Time Constant Approach is straightforward. The estimation of time constants, most of the time, only involves the calculation of area under the concentration curve and area under the first moment curve. Numerical model fitting is not required. Thus, the results are robust and reproducible. In addition, individual time constants can be estimated separately with limited concentration information. For example, the hepatic elimination time can be estimated without calculating renal elimination time or absorption time concurrently. Therefore, the Time Constant Approach is suitable for routine pharmacokinetic analysis because of its robustness, simplicity, and flexibility.

The Time Constant Approach can provide a consistent view of pharmacokinetics for a drug throughout the drug development process. The pharmacokinetic model established for a drug may be modified from time to time throughout the course of the drug development process as more information becomes available. For example, as soon as a metabolite is identified and its assay methodology becomes available, a new compartment corresponding to the metabolite can be added to the model. Importantly, the time constants estimated according to the simpler models will be consistent with those from the more complicated models. This consistency allows an accurate and reliable estimation of time constants from the early stage of the drug development. The details of model building in the Time Constant Approach will be discussed in Chapter 2.

The Time Constant Approach is especially useful in analyzing pharmacokinetic data obtained at comparative conditions. For example, AUC may change at comparative conditions of age, gender, hepatic function, renal function, food, drug interaction, or formulation via very different mechanisms under each condition. The strength of the Time Constant Approach lies in its capability to identify the mechanism (processes) responsible for the change in the descriptive parameters (AUC) under each clinical condition. The time constants that are influenced most by a clinical factor are called the key time constants under the clinical condition. The key time constants can be estimated separately from the other time constants, requiring only limited pharmacokinetic information. For example, the hepatic elimination time can be estimated from metabolite and parent drug concentration profiles without calculating renal elimination time or absorption time concurrently, both of which may require additional information such as urine and intravenous data.

The identification of the key time constants under various clinical conditions effectively facilitates the determination of dosing regimens in patients by providing insightful information about pharmacokinetic processes. For example, if the AUC of a drug increases under a clinical condition due to an increase in hepatic or renal elimination time, then the recommended dosing regimen may be a decrease in frequency with the same dose. On the other hand, if the AUC of a drug increases due to an increase in the extent of absorption, then the recommended dosing regimen may be a decrease in dose with the same frequency.

Once a set of time constants is determined in a pharmacokinetic study, the information derived from the time constants is valuable in predicting the results and helping the design of future studies. The following are some examples of useful information that may be derived from a study: (1) Does the renal elimination time or the hepatic elimination time limit the total elimination? If the renal elimination time limits the total elimination, factors affecting liver functions, such as hepatic diseases, age, gender, and drug interaction, will have a relatively small effect on the drug concentration. (2) Is the first pass metabolism significant and does it affect the mean residence time? If the first pass effect is significant, one can predict that concentration may change with food and conditions affecting the hepatic function. (3) Is the tissue distribution extensive enough to dominate the decay time of the concentration curve? If so, conditions that may change tissue distribution (such as competitors to protein binding sites, renal impairment, and age) require attention since they are likely to affect the decay time. (4) Does a change in the protein binding affect the renal elimination time and volume of distribution? If so, factors affecting protein binding may produce change in concentration profile. (5) Are the absorption time, hepatic elimination time, or renal elimination time nonlinear with dose or concentration? If yes, a nonlinear relationship may be expected in a sustained release versus immediate release formulations study, a pharmacokinetic/pharmacodynamic study, and a tissue distribution study. (6) Is the absorption time greater than the elimination time (this is referred to as a flip-flop)? If so, factors affecting elimination time may not result in change in the decay time.

Most importantly, the Time Constant Approach integrates the results from various pharmacokinetic studies and presents an overall picture of the pharmacokinetics of a drug. Very often, the same contributing factors may produce similar effects on the descriptive parameters in different studies. Some good examples of these contributing factors are those listed in the previous paragraph. The Time Constant Approach can identify the common themes among studies with very different objectives. Therefore, a consistent story can be told about the pharmacokinetics of a drug across studies. For example, change in renal elimination time can be a common theme in renal impairment, hepatic impairment, age, and gender studies. These common themes can help us summarize and understand the characteristics of drug disposition, and allow us to make rational decisions on the dosing regimens in complicated clinical situations.

An important characteristic of the pharmacokinetic time constants is that they are correlated with physiological time constants (e.g., transport, diffusion, binding, dissociation, and enzyme time constants). The most useful physiological time constant is the organ perfusion time, the time required for the total blood volume to pass through an organ. The pharmacokinetic time constant of a process is proportional to the perfusion time of the associated organ. For example, the metabolic elimination time (a pharmacokinetic time constant) is equal to the hepatic perfusion time (a physiological time constant) multiplied by the inverse of the hepatic extraction ratio (a proportionality constant). Therefore, the pharmacokinetics of drugs can also be viewed as a result of the perfusion of blood through various compartments, carrying drugs from one place to another.

Since the pharmacokinetic time constants are proportional to the physiological time scales, the time constants are readily scaled between different species. Before the administration of a novel drug to human subjects, it is imperative to predict the disposition of the drug in humans from animal data. The Time Constant Approach provides a rationale to scale time constants of pharmacokinetic processes from animals to men based on blood volume and organ perfusion rate. For example, as long as the renal extraction ratio is constant, the renal elimination time can be scaled among species as a function of glomerular perfusion time.

The Time Constant Approach also provides the rationale to predict and quantify the influence of clinical factors on drug disposition, since pharmacokinetic time constants are correlated with physiological time scales. For example, the hepatic elimination time is equal to the hepatic perfusion time multiplied by the inverse of hepatic extraction ratio. Consequently, any factor affecting hepatic perfusion time (hepatic blood flow) or extraction ratio (hepatic enzyme activity) may alter the elimination time.

The Time Constant Approach enables physiological meaningful analyses to interpret pharmacokinetic observation. One of the basic observations of the pharmacokinetics of a drug is the plasma concentration time profile. A number of descriptive parameters are designed to describe the concentration profile: examples are the maximum concentration (C_{max}), the terminal slope (λ_z), and the area under the curve (AUC). These descriptive pharmacokinetic parameters determine primarily the shape of the concentration profile and the amount of the drug in plasma. The temporal change of a drug concentration in a compartment can be determined by the time constants associated with the transfer of the drug into and out of the compartment. Therefore, the Time Constant Approach deals with information about individual pharmacokinetic processes that contribute to producing the shape of the concentration profile.

SOLVING THE PHARMACOKINETIC PUZZLE

Following administration, a drug is subjected to an array of physicochemical and physiological processes, such as disintegration, dissolution, absorption, distribution, and elimination (Figure 1.1). Each of these processes can be described by linear or nonlinear rate kinetics. The main objective of pharmacokinetic studies is to quantify the drug disposition kinetics and to correlate the drug plasma concentration and pharmacological effect time profiles with the drug disposition kinetics. Therefore, a class of clinical studies is designed to collect information about the basic kinetics of drug disposition processes. These "information studies" include metabolism, pharmacokinetics/pharmacodynamics, and tissue penetration studies. In addition, many clinical factors influence the rate kinetics of the pharmacokinetic processes; examples of these clinical factors are food, dose, diseases, and age. Therefore, another class of clinical studies are designed to compare the pharmacokinetics of drugs under comparative conditions. Examples of these "comparison studies" are food study, dose proportionality study, renal impairment study, and young versus elderly study.

The analysis of the "information" and "comparison" pharmacokinetic studies are similar to solving a puzzle (Figure 1.2). Each study examines some pieces of the whole drug disposition processes. For example, a metabolism study examines the metabolic pathways, a food study examines the absorption, and a renal impairment study examines the elimination and distribution; therefore, each clinical study can provide detailed information about some specific pharmacokinetic processes but very little about the other processes. Accordingly, a good methodology for pharmacokinetic analysis should have the capability, first, to identify the key pharma-

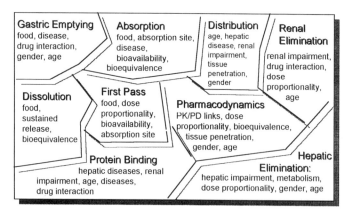

FIGURE 1.2. Pharmacokinetic analysis is similar to solving a puzzle consisting of physicochemical and physiological processes. Each clinical study provides information about several pieces of the puzzle. For example, a food study provides information about gastric emptying, dissolution, absorption, and first pass effect.

TABLE 1.1. *The Key Time Constants Associated with Individual Pharmacokinetic Processes.*

Physicochemical and Physiological Processes	Key Time Constants
Gastric emptying	T_{emp}
Dissolution	T_{dis}
Absorption	T_a
Distribution	T_{12}
Redistribution	T_{21}
Pharmacodynamics	T_{eo}
Renal elimination	T_{el}
Metabolism	T_m

cokinetic processes that are affected by the conditions designed in a clinical study, and then to quantify the rate kinetics of these key processes (Table 1.1).

Currently, the analyses of pharmacokinetic and pharmacodynamic data are often limited to two methodologies—noncompartmental approach and compartmental approach. The noncompartmental method provides simple descriptive pharmacokinetic parameters, such as the area under the plasma drug concentration curve, the maximum plasma concentration, the time to reach the maximum concentration, half-life, and apparent volume of distribution. However, the drawbacks of the noncompartmental approach are that the results are not physiologically insightful and the model can be oversimplified. For example, the area under the metabolite concentration curve (AUC_M) may change with dose, food, age, or disease for different reasons. However, the noncompartmental method cannot identify the mechanism of change in AUC_M in each individual case. The drawbacks of the noncompartmental method become significant when multiple compartment models are necessary to describe the pharmacokinetics, such as those involving metabolism, tissue distribution, pharmacokinetic/pharmacodynamic, first pass effects, and slow dissolution.

In a compartmental method, the serum drug concentrations and pharmacodynamic effects are fitted to multi-parameter models. This method describes detailed pharmacokinetic processes and provides insightful information; however, some drawbacks are that (1) the regression process does not always converge; (2) the solution for a regression may be a local minimum; (3) the estimated parameters are not always reproducible, depending on numerical algorithm, convergent criteria, weighting scheme, and initial values of the parameters; (4) the concentration profiles must be reasonably smooth; and (5) good fits to the data are sometimes obtained by adding extra parameters to the models to increase their degrees of freedom. For exam-

ple, concentration profiles may exhibit multiple peaks due to gastric emptying or enterohepatic recirculation and become difficult to be fitted to a simple model, or the absorption or distribution phase may be too fast to be
captured by widely scattered time points and the insufficient concentration
information cannot be fitted to a reasonable model.

The Time Constant Approach presented in this book is a synthesis of the
noncompartmental and compartmental methods and thus has the advantages of both. The Time Constant Approach starts by defining a physiologically meaningful model based on the pharmacokinetic processes involved.
The calculation of time constants is straightforward and, most of the time,
only involves the estimation of areas under the curves and the areas under
the first moment curves. The advantages of the Time Constant Approach
are as follows:

- physiologically insightful—Selection of the most appropriate model
  is possible.
- general—Pharmacokinetics involving multiple compartments can be
  handled.
- focused on key parameters—The key pharmacokinetic parameters
  can be estimated without simultaneously estimating nonkey
  parameters.
- simple calculation—Numerical model fitting is not required.
- able to handle nonsmooth data—The parameter estimation is robust
  and reproducible.

CHARACTERIZING CONCENTRATION PROFILES
BY THE TIME CONSTANT APPROACH

Once a drug is absorbed into the body, the pharmacological effects of the
drug are, in most of the cases, positively correlated with the concentrations
of the drug or its metabolites in the blood, tissues, or the targeted organs. Therefore, two basic questions concerning the drug concentrations
must be answered from a pharmacokinetic analysis: (1) How high is the
drug concentration? (Is it within the therapeutic window?) (2) How long
can the concentration be maintained? The two key parameters characterizing the concentration profiles in a physiological compartment, the
maximum concentration and the mean residence time, are dependent on the
time constants at which rates the drug enters and exits the compartment.
Let's take one piece of the pharmacokinetic puzzle—metabolism—as an
example. Four simple scenarios of metabolism are illustrated in Figures 1.3
and 1.4.

Figure 1.3 shows an example of a two-compartment model arranged in series; the first compartment represents the parent drug, and the second compartment represents the metabolite. On the left panel of Figure 1.3, the formation time of the metabolite is shorter than its elimination time. Once the drug (C) is absorbed, it is rapidly converted to the metabolite (M), which then accumulates in the body for a long time. As a result, the metabolite exhibits a higher concentration and longer mean residence time than the parent drug.

On the right panel of Figure 1.3, the formation time of the metabolite is longer than its elimination time. Once the drug is absorbed, it is slowly converted to the metabolite, and the metabolite is quickly eliminated from the body. As a result, the parent drug exhibits a higher concentration than the metabolite, but the mean residence times of the drug and its metabolite are similar.

Figure 1.4 shows an example of two metabolite compartments arranged in parallel. On the left panel, the formation time of metabolite M1 is longer than the formation time of M2, while the elimination time of M1 is shorter than the elimination time of M2. Once it is abosrbed into the body, a large fraction of the drug is quickly converted into metabolite M2, which accumulates in the body due to a slow elimination. Only a small fraction of the absorbed drug is converted into metabolite M1, which is quickly eliminated from the body. As a result, metabolite M2 exhibits a higher concentration and a longer mean residence time than metaoblite M1.

On the right panel of Figure 1.4, the formation and elimination time of

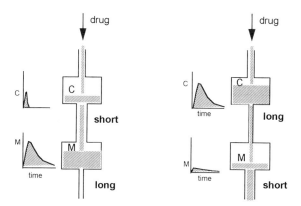

FIGURE 1.3. Two compartments arranged in series. On the left panel, the formation time of the metabolite is shorter than its elimination time. On the right panel, the formation time of the metabolite is longer than its elimination time.

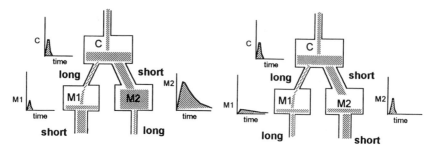

FIGURE 1.4. Two compartments arranged in parallel. On the left panel, the formation time of metabolite M1 is longer than the formation time of M2, while the elimination time of M1 is shorter than the elimination time of M2. On the right panel of Figure 1.4, the formation and elimination time of M1 are longer than those of M2.

M1 are longer than those of M2. Once the drug is absorbed, most of the drug is rapidly converted into metabolite M2, which is then rapidly eliminated. A small fraction of the drug is converted into metabolite M1, which accumulates in the body for a long period of time. As a result, both metabolites exhibit low concentrations, but metabolite M1 has a longer mean residence time than metabolite M2. From the illustrations in Figure 1.4, it is clear that the temporal change in the concentrations of a drug and its metabolite in the body is a function of the time constants of the relevant pharmacokinetic processes.

To summarize, the Time Constant Approach recognizes pharmacokinetics as a number of processes that move drugs between physiological compartments, each process occurring at its own characteristic length of time. The Time Constant Approach is a methodology used to correlate descriptive pharmacokinetic events with time constants of pharmacokinetic processes. The descriptive pharmacokinetic events include change in the maximum concentration (C_{max}), the time to reach the maximum concentration (T_{max}), the area under the concentration curve (AUC), and the terminal half-life $(t_{1/2})$. The pharmacokinetic processes include gastric emptying, dissolution, absorption, renal elimination, hepatic elimination, distribution to peripheral compartment, distribution to the effect site, elimination from the effect site, elimination of the metabolite, and any rate limited process that involves the drug and its metabolite. The time constants of pharmacokinetics processes can be estimated from the area under the concentration curve, the area under the first moment of the concentration curve, the partial area under the concentration curve, and the curve stripping technique.

The Time Constant Approach involves the following five steps:

(1) Define the question to be answered in a clinical study and review the concentration profiles.

(2) Identify the key time constants.

(3) Establish the appropriate compartmental model.

(4) Estimate the time constants of the key pharmacokinetic processes.

(5) Correlate the descriptive pharmacokinetic events with the time constants.

This book consists of nineteen chapters. The next three chapters, Chapters 2–4, give the theoretical background of the Time Constant Approach that is applied throughout the book. Each of the remaining fifteen chapters discusses one of the following topics: bioavailability, bioequivalence, dose proportionality, diseases, drug interaction, food effects, gastrointestinal absorption sites, hepatic impairment, male versus female, metabolism, pharmacokinetic/pharmacodynamic links, renal impairment, sustained release versus immediate release, tissue penetration, and young versus elderly. Each chapter starts with a discussion of the key pharmacokinetic parameters in the specific clinical study. Then several models are presented, and the key pharmacokinetic parameters are derived based on the models. To illustrate the validity of the Time Constant Approach, case studies simulating the conditions (for example, food, age, and diseases) in each type of clinical study using the models are discussed. At the end of each chapter, several examples from the literature are presented to demonstrate the utility of the Time Constant Approach.

CHAPTER 2

Time Constant Approach

This chapter presents the basic concepts and theories of the Time Constant Approach. The first section of this chapter describes intuitively the meanings of time constants and mean residence time. The second section discusses the physiological meanings and clinical applications of time constants. The next section defines time constants and mean residence time mathematically. In the fourth section, the fundamental relationship between mean residence time and time constants is illustrated with several models. The fifth section gives a simple example of a model containing time constants. In the sixth section, the time constant plot is introduced as a comprehensive way of presenting Time Constant Approach of pharmacokinetics. The seventh section discusses the relationship between time constants and the rate limiting step of drug disposition processes. In the eighth section, more complex models are discussed, and the advantage of the Time Constant Approach in model building during drug development is examined. In the ninth section, the advantages of the Time Constant Approach compared with the compartmental modeling is given using an example. In the tenth section, the concept of "drug-defined model" is introduced and illustrated with examples. In the eleventh section, the model-independent nature in the estimation of time constants is discussed.

TIME CONSTANTS AND MEAN RESIDENCE TIMES

In this section, we will attempt to present an intuitive description of the physiological meanings of time constants and mean residence time. Both time scales are useful measures of pharmacokinetics of drug disposition in the human body. As mentioned in Chapter 1, the pharmacokinetics of drugs

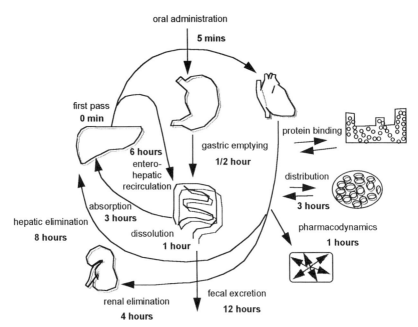

FIGURE 2.1. Each pharmacokinetic process during drug disposition takes time. In this example, a tablet is administered orally with a small amount of water in a 5-minute period. Suppose the drug does not dissolve under the acidic condition in the stomach. Then it will take the tablet one-half hour to enter the intestinal tract due to the gastric emptying. The tablet dissolves in the intestine in about 1 hour, and at the same time, the dissolved drug is absorbed into the blood within 3 hours. So far, it has taken an average of 4 hours and 35 minutes for the drug to reach the systemic circulation after it is swallowed. The drug in the blood can be eliminated renally or hepatically within 4 and 8 hours, respectively. Therefore, the drug will appear in the urine within approximately 7.5 hours on an average. The tissue distribution will delay the appearance of the drug in urine, since the drug spends some time residing in the tissue. In this example, it takes an average of 3 hours for the drug to penetrate into the tissue. It also takes 1 hour for the drug in the blood to reach the pharmacodynamic effect sites (1-hour lag time between pharmacological effect-time and plasma concentration-time profiles); therefore, the drug is effective in about 4.5 hours (average) after dosing.

16

can be viewed as a combination of compartments and processes. Pharmacokinetic processes transfer drug molecules from compartment to compartment until the drug molecules are removed from the body. The transferring processes take time so that the drug does not disappear instantaneously from the body but spend some time in the compartments (Figure 2.1). Consequently, there are two types of characteristic time scales describing the pharmacokinetics: one measures how fast the drug is transferred between compartments, and another measures how long the drug stays in the compartments.

Let's now consider the first type of characteristic time scale for measuring how fast a drug molecule is transferred from one compartment to another – the time constant. The measure of time constant is an average value because there are many molecules transferred between two compartments, and it takes different lengths of time to transfer each molecule. In other words, if we can examine the molecules individually, some of them will move faster between compartments than the others do. The time constant is then defined as the concentration-average time required to transfer the drug molecules from one compartment to another. Next, we will illustrate the pharmacokinetic meanings of time constants using the following examples. Each of these examples examines a part of the drug disposition process illustrated in Figure 2.1.

Example 1

Consider the following example: a drug tablet is dissolved in the stomach during the quiescent phase of gastric motility cycle. The schematic diagram of the dissolution process and the resulting concentration profile are shown below:

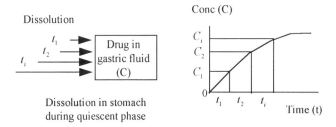

During the dissolution process, some of the drug molecules will dissolve faster and have shorter dissolution times than the other molecules. For example, a small amount of the drug equal to $C_1 * V$, where V is the volume of distribution, dissolves within time t_1; therefore, these molecules have a dissolution time of t_1. A second group of molecules, of which the amount is equal to $(C_2 - C_1)*V$, dissolves within time t_2 and has a dissolution time of t_2. Therefore, some molecules dissolve within time t_1, some within t_2, some within t_i; and so on. The average dissolution time is the concentration-average time for all the molecules to dissolve. This example can be generalized to any case where a drug enters a compartment without exiting.

Example 2

Let's now examine the situation opposite to Example 1, where a drug is given as a bolus and eliminated solely from the blood compartment. The schematic diagram of the elimination process and the typical concentration profile are shown below:

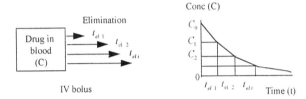

The drug is given instantaneously to produce an initial concentration in the blood (C_0). Immediately following the administration, within time t_{ell}, a small amount of the drug molecules, equal to $(C_0 - C_1)*V$, is removed from the blood; then a second group of molecules, equal to $(C_1 - C_2)*V$, is removed within time t_{el2}, and so on. This results in a distribution of removal times of the molecules. Then the average elimination time constant is the concentration-average time for all the molecules to be removed from the blood.

Example 3

In the above examples, we have examined two cases, each involving only one process transferring a drug molecule either into or out of a compartment. In most of the real world cases, multiple processes are often involved in a pharmacokinetic compartment. The following is an example, where a drug is orally absorbed into the blood and then eliminated from the blood:

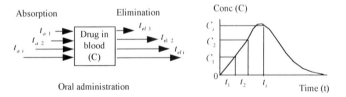

In this example, two processes are involved: absorption and elimination; therefore, the drug molecules will have a distribution of absorption time and a distribution of elimination time. As a result, drug molecules may spend various lengths of time to enter the blood and then stay in the blood for various lengths of time before they are removed from the blood. The average time of drug molecules residing in a compartment is defined as the mean residence time. Clearly, the elimination time will affect the mean residence time, since the longer the elimination time, the longer the drug will reside in the compartment. The absorption time will also affect the mean residence time in the following ways. If it takes a drug molecule a time length of t_{al} to be absorbed into the blood, when the molecule gets in the blood the time is already t_{al}. If it takes the same molecule another time length of t_{ell} to leave the blood, when it exits the compartment, the time will be $t_{al} + t_{ell}$; therefore the apparent residence time for this molecule, when it exits from the blood, is $t_{al} + t_{ell}$. Each molecule will have a different residence time; therefore, there is a distribution of residence time of all molecules. In this example, the mean residence time of the drug ($\bar{t}_c$) is equal to summation of the average absorption time (T_a) and the average elimination time (T_{el}). In general, the mean residence time in a compartment is the summation of mean input time and mean output time of the compartment.

$$\text{Mean residence time } (\bar{t}) = \text{Mean input time } (T_{in})$$

$$+ \text{ Mean output time } (T_{out}) \qquad (2.1)$$

where the mean input time is the average of all input times and the mean output time is the average of all output times. Equation (2.1) is one fundamental equation from which the relationships between mean residence times and time constants of all linear compartmental models can be derived. The derivations of these relationships for several useful models are discussed in a later section of this chapter.

Example 4

So far in this section, examples involving only irreversible processes have been discussed. When reversible processes are involved, the relationship between time constants and mean residence time is more complex. The following is an example where a drug is absorbed into the blood, reversibly distributed to the tissue, and eliminated from the blood:

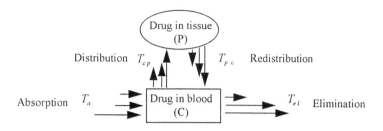

Peripheral distribution

In this example, the drug molecules enter the blood with a mean absorption time of T_a. After the drug enters the blood, two things may happen; it may be either eliminated from the blood or distributed into the tissue. If the molecule is eliminated from the blood without being distributed to the tissue, the residence time of the molecule will be the sum of the corresponding absorption and elimination times, $t_{ai} + t_{elj}$, where i and j represent the i-th and j-th absorption and elimination times, respectively. If a drug molecule is distributed to the tissue once before being eliminated from the blood, the residence time of the molecule will be the sum of the time constants of all processes involved, i.e., $t_{ai} + t_{cpj} + t_{pck} + t_{elm}$, where i, j, k, and m represent the corresponding absorption, distribution, redistribution, and elimination times. If a molecule is circulated between the blood and the tissue compartments several times before it is eliminated from the body, the residence time of the molecule will be much longer, as a sum of all the processes involved. The mean residence time of the drug in this case is the concentration-average residence time of all molecules, which is equal to $T_a + T_{el} + [(T_{el}T_{pc})/T_{cp}]$ for linear systems. The derivation of this mean residence time is based on Equation (2.1) and is presented in a later section of this chapter.

Example 5

Next, we will examine a case where two parallel processes are involved in the removal of a drug from the blood compartment as shown in the schematic diagram below:

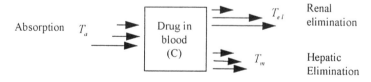

Hepatic and renal eliminations in parallel

In this example, it takes an average time of T_a for the drug molecules to be absorbed into the blood compartment. Once a molecule is in the blood, the molecule can be eliminated through two routes: hepatic or renal. If the hepatic elimination is inhibited (e.g., hepatic impairment), then the mean residence time of the drug molecule is $T_a + T_{el}$. On the other hand, if the renal elimination is inhibited (e.g., renal impairment), then the mean residence time of the drug molecules is $T_a + T_m$. However, in normal healthy subjects, as a result of the combined hepatic and renal eliminations, the mean residence time of the drug molecules becomes $T_a + [(T_m T_{el})/(T_m + T_{el})]$ for linear systems. The derivation of this mean residence time is also discussed in a later section of this chapter.

Example 6

In many cases, pharmacokinetic processes are arranged in series as shown in the following example of a metabolic pathway:

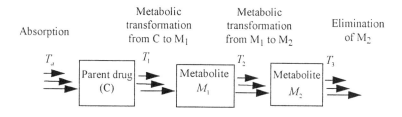

Metabolic pathway in series

In this example, each drug molecule will go through four processes from entering the blood as the parent drug C to leaving the blood as a metabolite M_2. Therefore, the residence time of a molecule is $t_{ai} + t_{1j}$ in compartment C, $t_{ai} + t_{1j} + t_{2k}$ in compartment M_1, and $t_{ai} + t_{1j} + t_{2k} + t_{3m}$ in compartment M_2, where i, j, k, and m represent the corresponding time constants in each metabolic transformation process. Obviously, the mean residence time of the drug in compartment C is $T_a + T_1$, in M_1 is $T_a + T_1 + T_2$, and in M_2 is $T_a + T_1 + T_2 + T_3$.

From the above examples, there is an intuitive description of the meanings of pharmacokinetic time constants and mean residence time. The detailed derivation of the relationships between the mean residence times and the time constants for the above models will be discussed in a later section in this chapter. Before we define the time constants and mean residence time in mathematical terms, more physiological meanings and clinical applications of time constants will be discussed.

PHYSIOLOGICAL MEANINGS AND CLINICAL APPLICATIONS OF TIME CONSTANTS

As illustrated in the previous section, time constants are associated with individual pharmacokinetic processes involved in the disposition of drugs, such as absorption, elimination, and distribution. On the other hand, the descriptive pharmacokinetic parameters, such as C_{max}, T_{max}, and AUC, are direct observations from the blood concentration-time profiles of drugs. Therefore, time constants are the underlying parameters that control drug disposition processes and dictate the shape of the concentration-time profiles (and thus determine the descriptive parameters). Many clinical factors, such as diseases and food intake, may affect specific time constants and consequently result in a change in observed descriptive parameters. The following are some important time constants frequently useful in the Time Constant Approach.

Absorption Time

The absorption time (T_a) represents the concentration-average time required for the absorption of the drug. There are other time constants and parameters used to characterize the absorption process. These include gastric emptying time (T_{emp}), the release time from sustained release formulation (T_r), the fraction absorbed (f), and the first pass bioavailability (F). The clinical factors affecting the absorption time include formulation, food, drug interaction, age, gender, and Crohn's disease. The absorption time does not affect the area under the concentration curve but may affect the maximum concentration, the time to reach the maximum concentration, and the terminal half-life. If the absorption time increases under a clinical condition, the maximum concentration will decrease, and the time to reach the maximum concentration will be prolonged. If the absorption time becomes longer than the elimination time, a flip-flop of the blood concentration profile will occur, and the decay time of terminal phase becomes equal to the absorption time.

Renal Elimination Time

The renal elimination time (T_{el}) represents the concentration-average time required for the kidney to excrete the drug. The clinical factors affecting the renal elimination time include age, renal diseases, hepatic impairment, change in protein binding, drug interaction, and nonlinear renal elimination. The renal elimination time may affect the area under the curve, the terminal half-life, and the renal clearance. When the renal elimination time increases under some clinical conditions, the area under the curve and the terminal half-life increase, and the renal clearance decreases; however, renal clearance, area under the concentration curve, and terminal half-life also depend on the volume of distribution, and many clinical factors may affect both renal elimination time and volume of distribution simultaneously, for examples, renal impairment, age, pregnancy, and protein binding.

Hepatic Elimination Time

The hepatic elimination time (T_m) represents the concentration-average time required for the liver to eliminate the drug. The clinical factors affecting the hepatic elimination time include nonlinear metabolism, drug interaction, hepatic impairment, renal impairment, thyroidism, congestive heart failure, age, and gender. The hepatic elimination time affects the area under the concentration curve, the maximum concentration, the elimination half-life, and the hepatic clearance. If the hepatic elimination time increases under certain clinical conditions, the area under the concentration curve, the maximum concentration, and the terminal half-life increase, while the hepatic clearance decreases.

Total Elimination Time

The total elimination time ($T_{el,t}$) is equal to $1/(1/T_{el} + 1/T_m)$. It is therefore the elimination time as a combined result of the renal and hepatic elimination. Clinical factors affecting the renal elimination time or the hepatic elimination time will also affect the total elimination time.

Renal Clearance Time and Hepatic Clearance Time

The renal clearance time (T_{el}/V_c) is the time required for the kidney to clear the drug in one unit volume of blood, and the hepatic clearance time (T_m/V_c) is the time required for the liver to clear the drug in one unit volume of blood. The clinical factors that affect the renal elimination time or the volume of distribution will also affect the renal clearance time. Similarly, the clinical factors that affect the hepatic elimination time will also affect the hepatic clearance time. Therefore, clinical factors affecting volume of distribution, such as protein binding and hepatic impairment, may also affect the extraction ratio and, consequently, the clearance times.

Distribution Time

The distribution and redistribution times (T_{12} and T_{21}) are the concentration-average time for distributing the drug between the central and peripheral compartments. The clinical factors affecting the distribution times include protein binding, drug interaction, age, pregnancy, and renal impairment. When no elimination occurs in the tissue, the distribution time itself does not affect the AUC but will affect the terminal half-life. However, the clinical factors affecting the distribution time will also affect the volume of distribution and, consequently, the AUC.

Decay Time

The decay time (T_z) is equal to the inverse of the terminal slope $(1/\lambda_z)$ of the semilogarithm blood concentration curve. The decay time is not associated with any specific pharmacokinetic process. It is usually a combination of elimination time and distribution times and, sometimes, is equal to the absorption time if a flip-flop occurs. Clinical factors affecting the decay time include nonlinear metabolism, age, gender, hepatic impairment, renal diseases, thyroidism, and congestive heart failure.

Effect Site Elimination Time

The effect site elimination time (T_{eo}) represents the concentration-average time required for removing the drug from the pharmacological effect site. The effect site elimination time is an important parameter in pharmacokinetic/pharmacodynamic studies. The value of T_{eo} determines the lag time between the effect and concentration profile and dominates the terminal half-life of the effect curve. Clinical factors that may affect the effect site elimination time include age, gender, and diseases.

MATHEMATICAL DEFINITIONS OF TIME CONSTANTS AND MEAN RESIDENCE TIME

In the previous two sections, the meanings of time constants and their clinical applications were described. Here, the time constants and the mean residence time will be defined mathematically. As discussed earlier, a residence time is a measure of how long a drug substance resides in a compartment. Let us examine a compartment with multiple processes, transferring a drug into and out of the compartment:

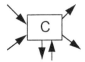

A compartment with multiple inputs and outputs

There are numerous drug molecules that reside in the compartment at a given time, each entering the compartment through one of the inputs and leaving through one of the outputs. Each molecule may spend a different length of time in the compartment because of the distribution of input and output times; therefore, there also exists a distribution of time length with which the drug molecules stay in the compartment. The mean residence time $\bar{t}$ of the drug molecules in the compartment is defined as the concentration-average time with which the drug stays in the compartment

$$\text{Mean residence time } (\bar{t}) = \frac{\int_0^\infty Ctdt}{\int_0^\infty Cdt}$$

$$= \frac{\text{Area under the first moment curve (AUMC)}}{\text{Area under the curve (AUC)}} \qquad (2.2)$$

Therefore, the mean residence time can be estimated simply from the ratio of area under the first moment curve to the area under the curve.

Next, the time constant is defined: it is a measure of how fast a drug substance is transferred from one physicochemical/physiological compartment to another. In the above example, the time constant T_n of the n-th process is defined as the concentration-average time required for the n-th process "alone" to remove the drug away from the compartment. This can be illustrated by the following schematic diagram:

The n-th process

Notice that the model is simplified to contain only one process of interest, according to the above definition of time constant. Intuitively, the amount of time required to remove the drug is equal to the time the drug stays in the compartment. For example, if it takes 3 hours for the intestine to absorb (remove) a drug, then the drug will stay in the intestine for 3 hours before it is completely absorbed (removed). The time constant (T_n) of the n-th process can then be defined as follows:

$$\text{Time constant of the } n\text{-th process } (T_n) = \left. \frac{\int_0^\infty Ctdt}{\int_0^\infty Cdt} \right|_{n\text{-th process}}$$

$$= \frac{\text{Area under the first moment curve (AUMC)}}{\text{Area under the curve (AUC)}} \Bigg|_{n\text{-th process}} \qquad (2.3)$$

which is equal to the mean residence time of the drug in the compartment when the n-th process "alone" is removing the drug. If the n-th process is the only removal process involved and the removal rate follows linear first-order kinetics, then $C = C_0 e^{-K_n t}$, where K_n is the rate constant and C_0 is the initial concentration at time 0. In this case, the time constant becomes

$$
\begin{aligned}
&\text{The time constant of the } n\text{-th} \\
&\text{process with linear kinetics } (T_n)
\end{aligned}
= \frac{\displaystyle\int_0^\infty Ctdt}{\displaystyle\int_0^\infty Cdt} \Bigg|_{n\text{-th process}}
$$

$$= \frac{\displaystyle\int_0^\infty C_0 e^{-K_n t} t dt}{\displaystyle\int_0^\infty C_0 e^{-K_n t} dt} \qquad \frac{1}{\text{Rate constant } (K_n)} \qquad (2.4)$$

From this definition, a residence time is associated with a physico-chemical or physiological compartment, and a time constant is associated with a physicochemical or physiological process. The time constant is a more sensible way of describing pharmacokinetic processes than the rate constant. For example, the absorption of a drug can be described as a process either requiring an average time (time constant) of 3 hours or exhibiting a rate constant of 0.33 hr^{-1}. The time constant gives a direct and clear sense of how fast the absorption occurs, while the rate constant is indirect.

There is a large body of literature discussing mean residence times in compartments, while very few investigate time constants of pharmacokinetic processes. Yamaoka et al. [63] and Cutler [28] introduced, in 1978, the application of statistical moment theory for the estimation of mean residence time in pharmacokinetics. Since then, mean residence time has been defined in many ways: an alternative estimation procedure for mean residence time following intravenous (iv) administration was proposed by Chanter [8]; Cutler [29] defined mean residence time in linear and nonlinear systems following iv administration; Veng-Pedersen et al. [53] and Kasuya [37] defined different types of mean residence times following iv administration; and Benet [2] and Wagner [57] defined different types of mean residence times following both iv and oral (po) administrations. The estimation of mean residence time was also discussed using noncompartmental approach following iv administration [6,39], using the one-compartment model following iv and po dosings [44], and using a two-compartment model following iv administration [38]. The mean residence times for reversible metabolism models following iv administration were studied extensively [1,9,10,17–19,21,25,26,30,43]. The mean residence time for models considering a first pass effect following po dosing were derived for irreversible metabolism [7,42,60], reversible metabolism [20,22], and a model-independent approach [3]. The mean residence times of drugs in the body and tissue were derived following iv administration [32,54,55] and po administration [52]. The mean residence time of metabolites in the body and tissue following iv administrations were derived [12–14,51,56]. The mean residence times following multiple administrations of iv [24] and po [45,49,59] doses were defined using noncompartmental or model-independent approaches. The mean residence times of pharmacokinetic systems with nonlinear kinetics were estimated using the Michaelis-Menten equation following iv administrations [15,23]. The mean residence times of tracers following iv administration were estimated using a non-compartmental approach [48], a two connected compartment model [46], and various multi-compartment models with reversible kinetics [27]. The mean residence times in recirculatory models following iv administration were derived [58,62,64]. The mean residence times of stochastic models following iv administrations were also derived for various models [31,40]. Apparently, most of the theories in mean residence times were derived for intravenous administration.

There is less literature discussing pharmacokinetic time constants, and most of them are focused on the absorption of drugs. The dissolution time was derived for in vitro studies using one- and two-compartment models [47] and for in vivo studies using a noncompartmental approach [50]. The absorption time was derived using a noncompartmental approach [2, 33,41,61], one- and two-compartment models [11], and a reversible metabolism model with first pass effect [22]. The elimination times of metabolites with an irreversible metabolism following an iv administration were derived using partial area under the concentration-time curves [16]. The elimination times of metabolites were also derived for one- and two-compartment models following iv administration [4]. The transfer time of tracers between two connected compartments following iv administration were derived using a stochastic method [46]. The elimination times in local perfusion models were derived following constant perfusion [34–36]. The time constants in chemical kinetics were derived for various models [5].

Apparently, the literature discussions on elimination times were limited to iv administrations.

There seems to be a lack of literature discussion in many other time constants in pharmacokinetics, such as hepatic elimination time, renal elimination time, tissue distribution time, metabolic formation times for sequential and parallel metabolism, elimination time of effect site compartment, and time constants for more complicated multi-compartment models. In this text, we will discuss the time constants and mean residence times of compartmental models with various complexity following both po and iv administrations. In addition to the theories, the discussion will be focused on the applications of the Time Constant Approach to clinical pharmacokinetic studies by using real and simulated data as illustrating examples.

In this section, mathematically, the time constants and the mean residence time have been defined. We will see next how they are related quantitatively.

DERIVATION OF MEAN RESIDENCE TIME FROM INPUT AND OUTPUT TIMES

In complicated pharmacokinetic models describing real-life data, there can be multiple inputs and outputs transferring a drug into and out of a compartment. Both the mean input time (T_{in}) and the mean output time (T_{out}) will affect the mean residence time $(\bar{t}_C)$ of the drug molecules in the compartment. Intuitively, the longer the mean output time, the longer the molecules will reside in the compartment. On the other hand, if a drug has a mean input time of T_{in} into a compartment, when the drug molecules enter the compartment, the time is already T_{in}; therefore, the input time also contributes to the apparent mean residence time of the drug when it exits the compartment. This section presents one fundamental equation [Equation (2.5)] describing the relationship between the mean residence time, the mean input time, and the mean output time. From this fundamental equation, the relationship between mean residence time and time constants in all linear models can be derived. To illustrate this relationship, a schematic plot of a compartment with multiple inputs and outputs is shown below:

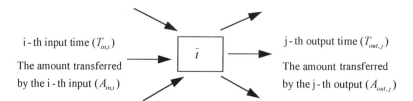

i - th input time $(T_{in,i})$

The amount transferred by the i - th input $(A_{in,i})$

j - th output time $(T_{out,j})$

The amount transferred by the j - th output $(A_{out,j})$

In this model, the input time and amount transferred by the i-th input process are represented by $T_{in,i}$ and $A_{in,i}$, while the output time constant and amount transferred by the j-th output process are represented by $T_{out,j}$ and $A_{out,j}$. An input time ($T_{in,i}$) is equal to either the mean residence time of the prior compartment, or to the input time when the drug is administered directly into the compartment through the i-th input process [Equation (2.8)]. On the other hand, an output time constant ($T_{out,j}$) is the time that is required for the j-th process "alone" to transfer the drug from one compartment to another, as discussed earlier in this chapter. The fundamental relationship between the mean residence time of drug molecules in a compartment, the mean input time, and the mean output time is

$$\text{Mean residence time } (\bar{t}) \ = \ \text{Mean input time } (T_{in})$$

$$+ \ \text{Mean output time } (T_{out}) \qquad (2.5)$$

For a system with linear kinetics, the mean input time is the amount-average of all input times, and the mean output time is the amount-average of all output times

$$\text{Mean input time } (T_{in}) \ = \ \frac{\text{Sum of (input time} \times \text{amount input)}}{\text{Total amount input}}$$

$$= \ \frac{\sum\limits_{i} T_{in,i} \cdot A_{in,i}}{A_{in,tot}} \qquad (2.6)$$

$$\text{Mean output time } (T_{out}) \ = \ \frac{\begin{array}{c}\text{Sum of (output time constant}\\ \times \text{ amount removed}^2)\end{array}}{\text{Total amount removed}^2}$$

$$= \ \frac{\sum\limits_{j} T_{out,j} \cdot A_{out,j}^2}{A_{out,tot}^2} \qquad (2.7)$$

where

$$\text{Input time } (T_{in,i}) \ = \ \begin{cases} 0 & \text{iv bolus} \\ T/2 & \text{iv infusion} \\ T_a & \text{Absorption} \\ t_{in,i} & \text{Mean residence time of prior compartment} \end{cases}$$

$$(2.8)$$

Output time constant $(T_{out,j})$ = Time constant defined in Equation (2.3)

$$(2.9)$$

and $A_{in,tot}$ and $A_{out,tot}$ are the total amounts of inputs and outputs, respectively. Equation (2.6) defines an amount-average input time. Equation (2.7) defines an amount-average output time based on the following derivation. The output time constant of the j-th process $(T_{out,j})$ is the time required for the process "alone" to remove the total amount of the drug from the compartment. Then for the j-process to remove an amount of $A_{out,j}$ with the existence of other parallel output processes, the time required is proportional to the amount removed [actual output time = $T_{out,j}\,(A_{out,j}/A_{out,tot})$] as illustrated in Figure 2.2.

Consequently the amount-average output time is

$$\text{Mean output time } (T_{out}) = \frac{\text{Sum of (actual output time}\ \times\ \text{amount removed)}}{\text{Total amount removed}}$$

$$= \frac{\displaystyle\sum_{j} \frac{T_{out,j} \cdot A_{out,j}}{A_{out,tot}} \cdot A_{out,j}}{A_{out,tot}} \qquad (2.10)$$

which turns out to be Equation (2.7).

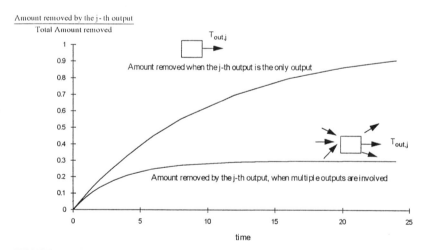

FIGURE 2.2.   The cumulative amount removed by the j-th process under two cases: (1) the j-th process is the only output, and (2) multiple outputs are involved. The ratio of the actual output times for the j-th process between the two cases is equal to the ratio of amounts removed between the two for a linear system.

For a linear system with first-order kinetics, the amount removed by the j-th process is proportional to the rate constants $K_{out,j} = 1/T_{out,j}$, as described in the following equation:

$$\frac{A_{j,out}}{A_{out,tot}} = \frac{1/T_{out,j}}{\sum_j 1/T_{out,j}} \tag{2.11}$$

Substituting Equation (2.11) into (2.7) gives

$$\text{Mean output time } (T_{out}) = \frac{1}{\sum_j 1/T_{out,j}} \tag{2.12}$$

Equations (2.5), (2.6), and (2.12) are the fundamental equations from which the relationships between mean residence times and time constants of linear compartmental models can be derived. The following are the derivations of the relationship between time constants and mean residence times for several frequently used models.

Model 1

This is a simple one-compartment model. It is clear from Equation (2.5) that, for this model,

$$\text{Mean residence time } (\bar{t}) = T_a + T_{el} \tag{2.13}$$

Model 2

This model illustrates parallel elimination processes. For a linear system, it can be derived from Equations (2.5) and (2.12) that

$$\text{Mean residence time } (\bar{t}) = \text{Mean input time } (T_{in})$$

$$+ \text{ Mean output time } (T_{out})$$

$$= T_a + \frac{1}{1/T_m + 1/T_{el}} \tag{2.14}$$

Model 3

$$\xrightarrow{T_a \ A_a} \boxed{\bar{t}_c} \xrightarrow{T_m \ A_m} \boxed{\bar{t}_m} \xrightarrow{T_{mel} \ A_{mel}}$$

This model represents elimination processes in series. From Equation (2.5) it is evident that

$$\text{Mean residence time of C } (\bar{t}_C) = T_a + T_m \qquad (2.15)$$

$$\text{Mean residence time of M } (\bar{t}_M) = \bar{t}_C + T_{mel} \qquad (2.16)$$

Model 4

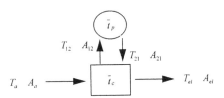

This is a two-compartment tissue distribution model. From Equations (2.5) and (2.12), it can be derived that

$$\text{Mean residence time of C } (\bar{t}_C) = \text{Mean input time } (T_{c,in})$$

$$+ \text{ Mean output time } (T_{c,out})$$

$$= \left(T_a \frac{A_a}{A_a + A_{21}} + \bar{t}_P \frac{A_{21}}{A_a + A_{21}} \right)$$

$$+ \frac{1}{1/T_{12} + 1/T_{el}} \qquad (2.17)$$

$$\text{Mean residence time of P } (\bar{t}_P) = \bar{t}_C + T_{21} \qquad (2.18)$$

The values of amount absorbed (A_a) and amount redistributed (A_{21}) must be determined next, so that the mean residence time can be estimated. Assuming that the amount absorbed and amount eliminated are equal to FD,

$$\text{Amount absorbed } (A_a) = \text{Amount eliminated } (A_{el}) = FD \qquad (2.19)$$

where F is the bioavailability and D is the dose. It can be deduced from Equation (2.11) that

Amount distributed (A_{12}) = Amount redistributed (A_{21}) = $\dfrac{T_{el}}{T_{12}}FD$ (2.20)

Then from Equation (2.17), knowing A_a and A_{21} from Equations (2.19) and (2.20), it can be derived that

$$\bar{t}_C = T_a\frac{FD}{FD + FD \cdot T_{el}/T_{12}} + \bar{t}_P\frac{FD \cdot T_{el}/T_{12}}{FD + FD \cdot T_{el}/T_{12}} + \frac{1}{1/T_{12} + 1/T_{el}}$$

(2.21)

Substituting Equation (2.18) into (2.21) gives

$$\bar{t}_C = T_a\frac{1}{1 + T_{el}/T_{12}} + (\bar{t}_C + T_{21})\frac{T_{el}/T_{12}}{1 + T_{el}/T_{12}} + \frac{1}{1/T_{12} + 1/T_{el}}$$

(2.22)

Multiplying both sides of Equation (2.22) by $1/(1 + T_{el}/T_{12})$ and rearranging terms obtains

$$\text{Mean residence time of C } (\bar{t}_C) = T_a + T_{21}\frac{T_{el}}{T_{12}} + T_{el}$$

(2.23)

The examples given in this section describe simple but frequently encountered pharmacokinetics. For more complicated models shown in Appendix 1, the relationship between mean residence times and time constants can also be derived based on Equation (2.5).

A SIMPLE EXAMPLE

The simplest example, shown below, is one compartment with two irreversible first-order processes in series. The actions of the two processes are (1) absorption of the drug into the compartment and (2) elimination of the drug from the compartment.

The time constants of this model are as follows:

T_a the process time constant associated with absorption

T_{el} the process time constant associated with elimination
$\bar{t}$ the mean residence time of the drug in the compartment
T_{el}/V the clearance time from the compartment (where V is the volume of distribution)
T_z the decay time of the drug concentration in the compartment

In the next section, the way to clearly present the time constants in a bar graph format to optimally extract information from the constants will be discussed.

TIME CONSTANT PLOT

Time constant plots are used throughout the book to facilitate the comparison of time constants of various pharmacokinetic processes under different clinical conditions, since the comparison of time constants is the key objective of all the clinical studies.

In general, clinical trials can be grouped into two categories based on their purposes: (1) comparison studies and (2) information studies. Comparison studies involve conducting trials with different conditions, for example, bioequivalence, food effects, young versus elderly, drug interaction, healthy versus hepatic impairment, dose proportionality, male versus female, and bioavailability studies. Information studies usually involve measuring drug concentrations in more than one compartment, for example, tissue distribution, metabolism, and pharmacokinetic/pharmacodynamic links studies.

In a comparison study, one or more key time constants are identified, which are most likely to be affected by the clinical conditions of interest, for example, absorption time in a bioequivalence study. Then the key time constants estimated under different conditions are assessed to determine the significance of the difference. In an information study, the key time constants are those defining the rate between the compartments of interest, for example, distribution time constants in the tissue penetration study. The objective of an information study is then to determine how fast the drug substance distributes from one compartment to another and how long the drug stays in a compartment.

The estimated time constants of various pharmacokinetic processes under different clinical conditions can be presented in time constant plots. An example of such a plot is shown in Figure 2.3. Time constants of a pharmacokinetic process at different dose levels are presented side by side as a group as indicated in the x-axis label, and different dose levels are represented by different patterns of the bar as indicated in the legend. It is clear

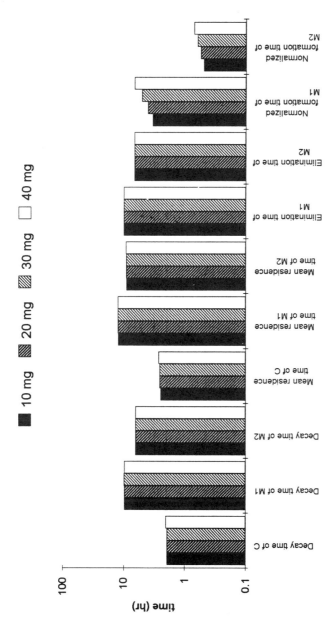

FIGURE 2.3. An example of a time constant plot. The time constants are estimated at various dose levels in a simulated dose proportionality study. The dose level only affects the hepatic elimination time $T_{m1} * V_{m1}/V_c$ and $T_{m2} * V_{m2}/V_c$.

from this time constant plot that the dose level only affects the hepatic elimination times T_{m1} and T_{m2}.

The time constants have now been defined and the relationship between time constants and mean residence times derived. Next, the impact of the time constants on the object of attention in pharmacokinetics, the concentration profile, will be examined.

THE RELATIONSHIP OF RATE LIMITING TIME CONSTANTS TO THE CONCENTRATION PROFILE

In this section, the important role of time constants in dictating the concentration-time profiles of drugs is discovered. The pharmacokinetics/ pharmacodynamics of a drug often involve more than one physicochemical/ physiological compartment arranged in series. The magnitude of time constants will determine the concentration in each compartment. The following shows an example of a multi-compartmental model in which three compartments in series describe the pharmacokinetics of a drug:

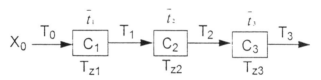

The elimination time constants T_0, T_1, T_2, and T_3 represent the average time required to transfer the drug from one compartment to another, the mean residence times $\bar{t}_1$, $\bar{t}_2$, and $\bar{t}_3$ represent the average time with which the drug stays in each compartment, and the decay times T_{z1}, T_{z2} and T_{z3} describe the time required for the decay of the concentration profiles. The rate limiting step of this compartmental model will be the process that exhibits the longest elimination time constant. Let's consider two cases, where either T_1 or T_2 is the rate limiting time constant.

Case 1

Assuming that the time constant T_2 is much greater than the other elimination times as presented by the following time constant plot (Figure 2.4), then the rate limiting step is the process associated with the time constant T_2.

As a result of T_2 being the limiting time constant, the drug substance accumulates in the second compartment to a greater extent than in the first compartment, as shown in the simulated concentration-time profile of Figure 2.5.

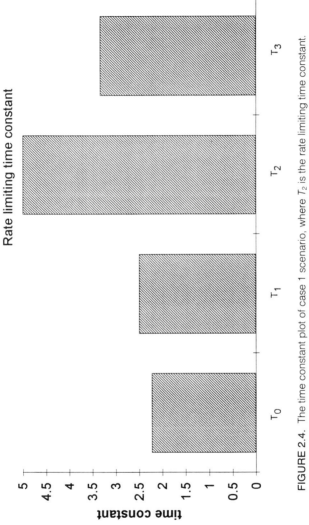

FIGURE 2.4. The time constant plot of case 1 scenario, where T_2 is the rate limiting time constant.

37

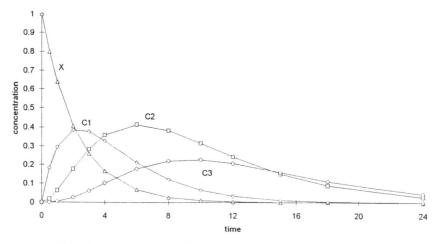

FIGURE 2.5. The concentration profiles in case 1, with T_2 as the rate limiting time constant.

In this case, there are four decay times (T_z values) associated with the decays of the concentrations (of drug or metabolites) in the four compartments. The decay times of those compartments prior to the rate limiting step are equal to the corresponding elimination time, while the decay times of those compartments later than the rate limiting step are dominated by the rate limiting time constants T_2. Therefore, the rate limiting step in a series of compartments can be identified by examining the decay times of concentration-time profiles in all compartments. The decay times of C_2 and C_3 are about the same, but the decay times of X and C_1 are different from those of C_2 and C_3 because T_2 is the rate limiting step and it only affects the concentrations in the compartments later than the second compartment. Therefore, in this example, for those compartments prior to the rate limiting step, the decay time is equal to the elimination time

$$T_{z0} = T_0 \tag{2.24}$$

$$T_{z1} = T_1 \tag{2.25}$$

$$T_{z2} = T_2 \tag{2.26}$$

For those compartments later than the rate limiting steps

$$T_{z3} = T_{z2} = T_2 \tag{2.27}$$

As a general rule, the decay times of concentration profiles in compartments before the rate limiting step are shorter than those after the rate limiting step. This rule relates the observed decay times (given by the terminal slopes) to the underlying process time constants (elimination time). This suggests that the measurement of some observed time constants may aid us in the estimation of other underlying time constants.

Case 2

The important role of time constants in determining concentration-time profile can be illustrated by changing the rate limiting step in the above example. In this case, let us increase T_1 so that it becomes the rate limiting step. The time constant plot after such an increase in T_1 is shown in Figure 2.6. Since T_1 becomes the rate limiting step, the drug accumulates in the first compartment as shown in Figure 2.7. As a result, the decay time in the first compartment T_{z1} is longer than the decay time T_{z0}, while the decay times in those compartments later than the rate limiting step are similar. The relationship between the decay times and the elimination time is as follows:

$$T_{z0} = T_0 \tag{2.28}$$

$$T_{z3} = T_{z2} = T_{z1} = T_1 \tag{2.29}$$

This change (case 2 versus case 1) in rate limiting step is not unrealistic. For example, patients with liver dysfunction may have an impaired metabolism to the drug. In the model, this impairment is represented by an increase in T_1. As a result of the liver impairment, the parent drug may be accumulated in the body, and the characteristics of the concentration profiles will be modified. In this case, the utility of estimating T_1 from the concentration-time curves is clear. (It is clear if the model reflects the real world. The issue of model building will be addressed later in this chapter.)

MODEL BUILDING IN TIME CONSTANT APPROACH

In the early stages of a drug development process, the pharmacokinetics of the drug may be incompletely understood. The initial pharmacokinetic model describing the disposition of the drug may be fairly simple. As more information about the drug is gathered, more complicated models can be established. This model-building process, based on limited available information, is inevitable since the knowledge of the drug is accumulated with time.

40

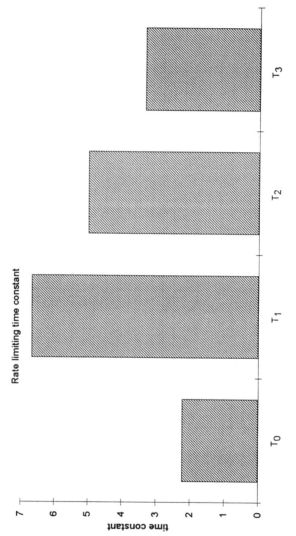

FIGURE 2.6. The time constant plot of case 2 scenario, where T_1 is the rate limiting time constant.

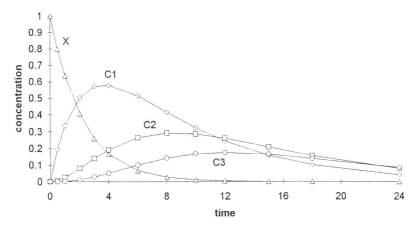

FIGURE 2.7. The concentration profiles in case 2, with T_1 as the rate limiting time constant.

One of the great advantages of the Time Constant Approach in the model-building process is that the time constants estimated from the simpler models in the early stage are applicable to the more complicated models established later. This allows (1) a consistent view of the pharmacokinetics of a drug throughout its development, (2) accumulation of useful information on the pharmacokinetics from the very beginning, and (3) a combination of information from different pharmacokinetic studies. A hypothetical example of a model-building process using the Time Constant Approach is shown in Table 2.1. A one-compartmental model is assumed for the pharmacokinetics in stage 1, and additional compartments are added to the model when metabolites are discovered or tissue concentrations are measured. The time constants estimated from different models at various stages are applicable to each other, since the equations for estimating the time constants do not change with models. For example, the equation for estimating the hepatic clearance time toward M1 is the same in stage 2 as in stages 3–5. Therefore, one does not have to reanalyze the data from the early stages when more complicated models have been developed. This means the information obtained from the Time Constant Approach can be accumulated along the drug development process. In other words, the time constants estimated from any model are always equal to their unique values, regardless of the complexity of the models.

It is worth mentioning that the pharmacokinetic information can be accumulated from simple models to complicated models only if the compartments are connected by the same processes in all models. For example,

TABLE 2.1. *In the Time Constant Approach, Complicated Models Can Be Built on the Simpler Models, and the Time Constants Estimated from the Simple Models Are Applicable to the Complicated Ones.*

Stage	Event	Model	Time Constants
1	The first PK study, where only the drug concentration is measured		$$\frac{T_{el}}{V_c} = \frac{AUC_c}{X_c}$$ $$\bar{t}_c = \frac{AUMC_c}{AUC_c}$$
2	Discover a metabolite		$$\frac{T_{mel1}}{V_{m1}} = \frac{AUC_{m1}}{X_{m1}}$$ $$T_{m1}\frac{V_{m1}}{V_c} = \frac{AUC_c}{AUC_{m1}}\left(\frac{AUMC_{m1}}{AUC_{m1}} - \frac{AUMC_c}{AUC_c}\right)$$ $$\bar{t}_{m1} = \frac{AUMC_{m1}}{AUC_{m1}}$$
3	Discover a second metabolite		$$\frac{T_{mel2}}{V_{m2}} = \frac{AUC_{m2}}{X_{m2}}$$ $$T_{m2}\frac{V_{m2}}{V_c} = \frac{AUC_c}{AUC_{m2}}\left(\frac{AUMC_{m2}}{AUC_{m2}} - \frac{AUMC_c}{AUC_c}\right)$$ $$\bar{t}_{m2} = \frac{AUMC_{m2}}{AUC_{m2}}$$

TABLE 2.1. (continued).

Stage	Event	Model	Time Constants
4	Measure tissue concentration	Compartments: C_p, C, $M1$, $M2$; constants T_{12}, T_{21}, T_{el}, T_{m1}, T_{m2}, T_{mel1}, T_{mel2}; outputs X_c, X_{m1}, X_{m2}	$$T_{21} = \frac{AUMC_p}{AUC_p} - \frac{AUMC_c}{AUC_c}$$ $$T_{12}\frac{V_p}{V_c} = \frac{AUC_c}{AUC_p}\left(\frac{AUMC_p}{AUC_p} - \frac{AUMC_c}{AUC_c}\right)$$ $$\bar{t}_p = \frac{AUMC_p}{AUC_p}$$
5	Discover a third metabolite, which is converted from metabolite M2	Compartments: C_p, C, $M1$, $M2$, $M3$; constants T_{12}, T_{21}, T_{el}, T_{m1}, T_{m2}, T_{m3}, T_{mel1}, T_{mel2}, T_{mel3}; outputs X_c, X_{m1}, X_{m2}, X_{m3}	$$\frac{T_{mel3}}{V_{m3}} = \frac{AUC_{m3}}{X_{m3}}$$ $$T_{m3}\frac{V_{m3}}{V_{m2}} = \frac{AUC_{m2}}{AUC_{m3}}\left(\frac{AUMC_{m3}}{AUC_{m3}} - \frac{AUMC_{m2}}{AUC_{m2}}\right)$$ $$\bar{t}_{m3} = \frac{AUMC_{m3}}{AUC_{m3}}$$

compartments M2 and C are connected by the same process characterized by time constants T_{m2} in stages 3–5. However, if in stage 5 metabolite M2 is found to be converted from metabolite M1 instead of C, the value of T_{m2} estimated in stages 3 and 4 is not applicable to stage 5. In this case, the incomplete data (M3 not measured) obtained in stages 3 and 4 are still useful and can be reanalyzed based on the new model established in stage 5. The incomplete data will still give the unique values of some, but not all, of the time constants.

To summarize, model building is a continuous process during the drug development. New models can be built on or modified based on the simple ones. In all cases, by using the Time Constant Approach, the information derived from the incomplete data and simple models in the early stages are applicable to the more complicated models established later. The Time Constant Approach provides a consistent view of the pharmacokinetics to link information obtained in various stages throughout the drug development.

AN EXAMPLE COMPARING TIME CONSTANT APPROACH AND COMPARTMENTAL MODELING

Both Time Constant Approach and compartmental modeling are based on well-defined pharmacokinetic models. Therefore, both approaches provide detailed information about individual drug disposition processes, i.e., time constants in the Time Constant Approach and rate constants in the compartmental modeling; however, the main difference between these two approaches lies in their fundamental views on pharmacokinetics and the methodologies used for parameter estimation. This difference between the two approaches results in apparent advantages of the Time Constant Approach over the compartmental modeling in terms of the robustness, reproducibility, flexibility, and simplicity in parameter estimation. These advantages of the Time Constant Approach are illustrated by comparing the two methods using the example shown in Table 2.1.

Let's examine the following scenarios as described in Table 2.1. Assume the drug has two metabolites, and the model of stage 4 in the table is the most representative model describing the pharmacokinetics. To summarize the model, the concentration profile of the drug demonstrates biexponential decay, and the two metabolites are direct products of the parent drug. Figure 2.8 shows simulated concentration profiles of the drug and metabolites according to the model in stage 4. In order to mimic the real-life data, a 15% variability is added to all the time points 6 hours postdose. In stage 1 of the drug development, only the parent drug concentration profile is available,

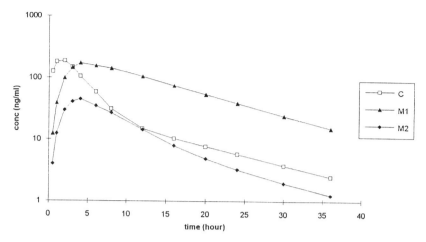

FIGURE 2.8. Simulated concentration profiles of the drug and metabolites according to the model in stage 4 of Table 2.1. In order to mimic the real-life data, a 15% variability is added to all the time points 6 hours postdose. The time constants estimated using the Time Constant Approach are listed in Table 2.2, comparing with the theoretical values. The rate constants estimated from compartment modeling are listed in Table 2.3.

in stage 2 the concentration profile of metabolite 1 is available as well, and in stage 3 concentration profiles of all three compounds are available. It can be shown from this example whether the Time Constant Approach and the compartmental modeling can provide reproducible and reliable results, regardless of the models and amount of information available in various stages of the drug development. The results from the two approaches are discussed below.

Time Constant Approach

The formulas used to estimate the time constants are shown in Table 2.1, and the estimated time constants are listed in Table 2.2, in comparison with the theoretical values. The estimated time constants always correspond well to the theoretical values, regardless of the models in various stages described in Table 2.1. In stage 2, where only one metabolite is discovered, the time constants T_{el}/V_c, T_{mel1}/V_{m1}, T_{mel1}, T_{m1}/V_c and $T_{m1}*V_{m1}/V_c$ can be correctly estimated. In stage 3, both metabolites are discovered but no tissue distribution is assumed, and, again, all the estimated time constants are close to the theoretical values. As a matter of fact, all the time constants in Table 2.2 can be correctly estimated before stage 4. Therefore, the estimated parameters by the Time Constant Approach are consistent and

TABLE 2.2. *The Estimated Time Constants Based on the Time Constant Approach, Compared with the Theoretical Values.*

Parameter	Earliest Stage the Parameter Can Be Correctly Estimated	Time Constant Approach (% deviation from theoretical value)	Theoretical Value
$\bar{t}_c$	1	7.56 (6.1%)	7.12
$\bar{t}_{m1}$	2	14.83 (−5%)	15.45
$\bar{t}_{m2}$	3	10.21 (−11.7%)	11.56
$T_{m1}*V_{m1}/V_c$	2	3.04 (9.5%)	2.77
$T_{m2}*V_{m2}/V_c$	3	7.25 (−12.9%)	8.33
T_{m1}/V_c	2	0.335 (0.6%)	0.337
T_{m2}/V_c	3	0.983 (−1.6%)	1.0
T_{el}/V_c	2	0.58 (5.0%)	0.56
T_{mel1}/V_{m1}	2	0.87 (5.0%)	0.83
T_{mel2}/V_{m2}	3	0.42 (5%)	0.4
T_{mel1}	2	7.56 (−9.2%)	8.33
T_{mel2}	3	2.94 (26.3%)	4.0

reliable, even from the early stages of the drug development, when the information about the drug is limited and the pharmacokinetic models are simple. Another advantage of the Time Constant Approach is that all the time constants can be estimated separately. The equations listed in Table 2.1 are independent from each other. Therefore, if only partial information is available, certain parameters can still be estimated. For example, the time constants associated with metabolite 2 can be correctly estimated without the information concerning metabolite 1. The model-independent nature in the estimation of time constants is discussed in a later section of this chapter.

COMPARTMENTAL MODELING

Next, let's consider the compartmental modeling. First of all, the equations describing the concentration profiles must be established before applying the compartmental modeling. The equations describing the model in stage 2 are

$$C = \frac{K_a f F X_0}{V_c} \left[\frac{1}{K_{el} + K_{m1} + K_{m2} - K_a} e^{-K_a t} \right.$$

$$\left. + \frac{1}{K_a - K_{el} - K_{m1} - K_{m2}} e^{-(K_{el} + K_{m1} + K_{m2})t} \right] \quad (2.30)$$

$$M_1 = \frac{K_a K_{m1} f F X_0}{V_{m1}} \left[\frac{1}{(K_{el} + K_{m1} - K_a)(K_{mel1} - K_a)} e^{-K_a t} \right.$$

$$+ \frac{1}{(K_a - K_{el} - K_{m1})(K_{mel1} - K_{el} - K_{m1})} e^{-(K_{el} + K_{m1})t}$$

$$\left. + \frac{1}{(K_{el} + K_{m1} - K_{mel1})(K_a - K_{mel1})} e^{-K_{mel1} t} \right] \quad (2.31)$$

The equations describing the model in stage 3 are

$$C = \frac{K_a f F X_0}{V_c} \left[\frac{1}{K_{el} + K_{m1} + K_{m2} - K_a} e^{-K_a t} \right.$$

$$\left. + \frac{1}{K_a - K_{el} - K_{m1} - K_{m2}} e^{-(K_{el} + K_{m1} + K_{m2})t} \right] \quad (2.32)$$

$$M_1 = \frac{K_a K_{m1} f F X_0}{V_{m1}} \left[\frac{1}{(K_{el} + K_{m1} + K_{m2} - K_a)(K_{mel1} - K_a)} e^{-K_a t} \right.$$

$$+ \frac{1}{(K_a - K_{el} - K_{m1} - K_{m2})(K_{mel1} - K_{el} - K_{m1} - K_{m2})} e^{-(K_{el} + K_{m1} + K_{m2})t}$$

$$\left. + \frac{1}{(K_{el} + K_{m1} + K_{m2} - K_{mel1})(K_a - K_{mel1})} e^{-K_{mel1} t} \right] \tag{2.33}$$

$$M_2 = \frac{K_a K_{m2} f F X_0}{V_{m2}} \left[\frac{1}{(K_{el} + K_{m1} + K_{m2} - K_a)(K_{mel1} - K_a)} e^{-K_a t} \right.$$

$$+ \frac{1}{(K_a - K_{el} - K_{m1} - K_{m2})(K_{mel1} - K_{el} - K_{m1} - K_{m2})} e^{-(K_{el} + K_{m1} + K_{m2})t}$$

$$\left. + \frac{1}{(K_{el} + K_{m1} + K_{m2} - K_{mel2})(K_a - K_{mel2})} e^{-K_{mel2} t} \right] \tag{2.34}$$

The equations describing the model in stage 4 are

$$C = \frac{K_a f F X_0}{V_c} \left[\frac{K_{21} - K_a}{(\lambda_1 - K_a)(\lambda_2 - K_a)} e^{-K_a t} + \frac{K_{21} - \lambda_1}{(K_a - \lambda_1)(\lambda_2 - \lambda_1)} e^{-\lambda_1 t} \right.$$

$$\left. + \frac{K_{21} - \lambda_2}{(K_a - \lambda_2)(\lambda_1 - \lambda_2)} e^{-\lambda_2 t} \right] \tag{2.35}$$

$$M_1 = \frac{K_a K_{m1} f F X_0}{V_{m1}} \left[\frac{K_{21} - K_a}{(\lambda_1 - K_a)(\lambda_2 - K_a)(K_{mel1} - K_a)} e^{-K_a t} \right.$$

$$+ \frac{K_{21} - \lambda_1}{(K_a - \lambda_1)(\lambda_2 - \lambda_1)(K_{mel1} - \lambda_1)} e^{-\lambda_1 t}$$

$$+ \frac{K_{21} - \lambda_2}{(K_a - \lambda_2)(\lambda_1 - \lambda_2)(K_{mel1} - \lambda_2)} e^{-\lambda_2 t}$$

$$\left. + \frac{K_{21} - K_{mel1}}{(\lambda_1 - K_{mel1})(\lambda_2 - K_{mel1})(K_a - K_{mel1})} e^{-K_{mel1} t} \right] \tag{2.36}$$

$$M_2 = \frac{K_a K_{m2} f F X_0}{V_{m2}} \left[\frac{K_{21} - K_a}{(\lambda_1 - K_a)(\lambda_2 - K_a)(K_{mel2} - K_a)} e^{-K_a t} \right.$$

$$+ \frac{K_{21} - \lambda_1}{(K_a - \lambda_1)(\lambda_2 - \lambda_1)(K_{mel2} - \lambda_1)}e^{-\lambda_1 t}$$

$$+ \frac{K_{21} - \lambda_2}{(K_a - \lambda_2)(\lambda_1 - \lambda_2)(K_{mel2} - \lambda_2)}e^{-\lambda_2 t}$$

$$+ \left. \frac{K_{21} - K_{mel2}}{(\lambda_1 - K_{mel2})(\lambda_2 - K_{mel2})(K_a - K_{mel2})}e^{-K_{mel2}t} \right] \qquad (2.37)$$

where

$$\lambda_1 = \frac{1}{2}\sqrt{(K_{el} + K_{m1} + K_{m2} + K_{12} + K_{21})^2 - 4(K_{el} + K_{m1} + K_{m2})K_{21}}$$
$$(2.38)$$

$$\lambda_2 = \frac{1}{2}\sqrt{(K_{el} + K_{m1} + K_{m2} + K_{12} + K_{21})^2 + 4(K_{el} + K_{m1} + K_{m2})K_{21}}$$
$$(2.39)$$

As one can see, the equations become discouragingly complicated as the models are developed into stage 4. These models in stages 2, 3, and 4 are fitted to the concentration profiles using PCNONLIN® with different weighting schemes, and the estimated rate constants are listed in Table 2.3. It seems that the model in stage 4 with a weight of −1 gives the best estimation of the rate constants among all other models. However, the percent deviation associated with the compartmental modeling (Table 2.3) is significantly higher than that with the Time Constant Approach (Table 2.2). Inconsistent results from different models are another drawback in the compartmental modeling. The estimated rate constants using the model in stage 4 cannot be reasonably reproduced as the weighting scheme changes. The simulated concentration profiles in this example are rather smooth. When the real-life data are more variable, the difference in the estimated rate constants by different weighting schemes or from different initial guess values could be tremendous. This produces an uncertainty regarding the reproducibility and robustness of the compartmental modeling. Another drawback of the compartmental modeling is that the simpler models in the earlier stages do not provide the correct estimation of the rate constants. Since, frequently, one cannot be sure that tissue distribution may be important or other metabolites may be discovered later in time, there is always an uncertainty associated with the results from compartmental modeling.

TABLE 2.3. The Estimated Rate Constants (percent deviation from the theoretical value) by Compartmental Modeling, Compared with the Theoretical Values.

Parameter	Stage 2 (wt = −1)	Stage 3 (wt = −1)	Stage 4 (wt = −1)	Stage 4 (wt = 0)	Stage 4 (wt = 1)	Theoretical Value
K_{m1}	0.092 (−69.3%)	0.423 (41.0%)	0.246 (−18.0%)	0.180 (−40.0%)	0.143 (−52.3%)	0.3
K_{m2}		0.225 (125.0%)	0.129 (29.0%)	0.104 (4.0%)	0.103 (3.0%)	0.1
K_{c1}	0.268 (78.6%)	0.725 (383.3%)	0.188 (25.3%)	0.132 (−12.0%)	0.125 (−16.7%)	0.15
K_{mel1}	0.100 (16.7%)	0.099 (−17.5%)	0.142 (18.3%)	0.157 (30.8%)	0.177 (47.5%)	0.12
K_{mel2}		0.206 (−17.6%)	0.308 (23.2%)	0.328 (31.2%)	0.346 (38.4%)	0.25

We have seen that, as the complexity of the model increases, the equations for the Time Constant Approach become considerable (Table 2.1). We have seen in the present section that, for the same level of complexity, the equations for the compartmental approach are much more complex than those of the Time Constant Approach. The reason is simple: the computations of the two approaches are similar; both are best handled by transforming from the time domain to the frequency domain (with the Laplace transform), but the compartmental approach requires a return to the time domain (via the inverse Laplace transform) whereas the Time Constant Approach requires only evaluations (and a differentiation) in the frequency domain (steps 5 and 6 described in Appendix 2). The inverse transformation is much more difficult than differentiation. The simulations in this section suggest that the compartmental approach, which requires extra effort, does not always produce consistent results like the simple Time Constant Approach does.

An alternative to going in the direction of more complexity, from the Time Constant Approach to the compartmental approach, is to go in the direction of less complexity, to the noncompartmental approach. The noncompartmental approach, with its simple calculations of descriptive parameters such as C_{max} and AUC, is currently the method of choice in most of the literature. (Of more than 400 references cited in this text, only less than ten apply compartmental modeling, and the rest use the noncompartmental approach.) Clearly, the noncompartmental approach takes on the role of describing the concentration profiles without examining the pharmacokinetic processes. This eliminates the possibility of prediction and reduces the role of the clinical trial to demonstrating the relationship between clinical factor and pharmacokinetic outcome. The Time Constant Approach offers an alternative that may strike an optimal medium between the noncompartmental and compartmental approaches.

DRUG-DEFINED MODELS

Throughout Chapters 5–19, the simplest model is selected for each drug in individual cases and examples. We establish these pharmacokinetic models based on a concept called "drug-defined model." A drug-defined model is the simplest possible model consisting of only the physicochemical compartments of parent drug and metabolites or physiological compartments where drug concentrations can be measured. In the model, compartments are connected by pharmacokinetic processes based on the knowledge of the metabolic pathways, urine, and/or bile recovery. If biexponential decay is observed from a concentration profile or tissue concentrations are measured, a reversible distribution compartment can be added to the model. In essence, the drug defines the pharmacokinetic model, and there will be little confusion about which model should be used.

The models shown in Table 2.1 are good examples of a drug-defined model. In stage 1, only the parent drug can be assayed, and the model consists of only one compartment. Surrounding the compartment, two processes are involved: the absorption and the renal elimination. In stage 2, one metabolite is discovered, and the revised model consists of two compartments—one for the parent drug and one for the metabolite. A process is added, which is responsible for converting the parent drug to the metabolite, and another process accounts for the renal elimination of the metabolite. In stage 3, a second metabolite is discovered, of which the pathway is parallel to the first metabolite. Therefore, one additional compartment is added to the model, and new processes are defined based on the metabolic pathways. As the knowledge of the drug accumulates, the drug-defined model can be modified accordingly. However, very importantly, the time constants estimated from the different models in various stages of a drug development process are consistent, as discussed earlier in this chapter.

Each pharmacokinetic process in a drug-defined model can contain multiple subprocesses in parallel and/or series. For example, an absorption process can consist of paracellular, intracellular, and active absorptions, which are parallel to each other, and a metabolic pathway converting a parent drug to a metabolite may go through several intermediates in series. Therefore, in a drug-defined model, the time constant characterizing a process is a lumped value accounting for all the subprocesses involved. When a series of subprocesses are lumped together, it is important that none of the intermediate processes is a rate limiting step, except for the first one. Take the following model as an example:

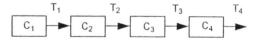

In order to combine the three processes corresponding to time constants T_1, T_2 and T_3 and to estimate T_4 based on the concentration profiles in compartments C_1 and C_4, it is necessary that T_2 and T_3 are not rate limiting (i.e., T_2 and T_3 must be much less than T_4). Therefore, when we estimate T_4 from the equation $T_4 = \bar{t}_4 - \bar{t}_1$, it will not be grossly overestimated since, in fact, $T_2 + T_3 + T_4 = \bar{t}_4 - \bar{t}_1$.

From a micro-model point of view, each local model describing a process connecting two compartments is valid as long as the direction of the process is defined correctly. Take the stage 3 model in Table 2.1 as an example. The local process connecting C and M2, characterized by T_{m2}, is valid as long as it is true that the parent drug is converted to metabolite M2. This is because it is certain a pharmacokinetic process is responsible for converting C to M2 and the local model defines just that. The next question is whether the time constant estimated for a process is affected by the other processes in the model. We can have confidence in the estimated time constant of a process when (1) the local model is valid and (2) the estimated value is not affected by the complexity and linearity of the other processes. Fortunately, the estimation of time constants is based on the local model and independent of the global model. The model-independent nature in estimation of time constants will be discussed next.

MODEL-INDEPENDENT ESTIMATION OF TIME CONSTANTS

As discussed in the previous section, we can have confidence about the estimated values of time constants if the estimation is not affected by complexity of the other processes involved in the model. In all the models examined in this text, the estimations of time constants are based on local models and independent of global models. Most of the models used in this text can be summarized by the following three basic cases.

Case 1

When two compartments are connected by a lumped process and no other process enters the second compartment, as shown in the diagram below, the estimation of T_1 and T_2 is independent of our knowledge of the rest of the model (shown by the dashed lines):

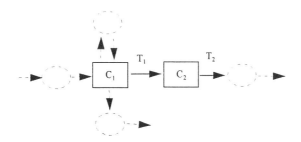

The values of T_1 and T_2 can be correctly estimated as long as the concentration profiles of C_1 and C_2 are measured. The following is the mathematical proof. Assuming the processes corresponding to T_1 and T_2 have first-order linear kinetics, then the following equations can be written based on material balance over compartment C_2:

$$\frac{dC_2}{dt}V_2 = \frac{1}{T_1}C_1V_1 - \frac{1}{T_2}C_2V_2 \qquad (2.40)$$

and multiplying the above equation by t on both sides yields

$$\frac{dC_2}{dt}V_2t = \frac{1}{T_1}C_1V_1t - \frac{1}{T_2}C_2V_2t \qquad (2.41)$$

Integrating Equations (2.40) and (2.41) from time 0 to infinity gives

$$C_2V_2\big|_\infty - C_2V_2\big|_0 = 0 - 0 = \frac{1}{T_1}\int_0^\infty C_1V_1 dt$$

$$- \frac{1}{T_2}\int_0^\infty C_2V_2 dt = \frac{AUC_1}{T_1}V_1 - \frac{AUC_2}{T_2}V_2 \qquad (2.42)$$

and

$$C_2V_2t\big|_\infty - C_2V_2t\big|_0 - \int_0^\infty C_2V_2 dt = 0 - 0 - AUC_2V_2 = \frac{1}{T_1}\int_0^\infty C_1V_1 t dt$$

$$- \frac{1}{T_2}\int_0^\infty C_2V_2 t dt = \frac{AUMC_1}{T_1}V_1 - \frac{AUMC_2}{T_2}V_2$$

$$(2.43)$$

by assuming the decay of concentration C_2 is faster than a linear decay (e.g., exponential and Michaelis-Menten). Rearranging Equations (2.42) and (2.43) and dividing Equation (2.43) by Equation (2.42) produces

$$T_2 = \frac{AUCM_2}{AUC_2} - \frac{AUCM_1}{AUC_1} \qquad (2.44)$$

and

$$\frac{T_1}{V_1}V_2 = \frac{AUC_1}{AUC_2}T_2 \qquad (2.45)$$

Based on this derivation, the values of T_2 and $T_1 V_2 / V_1$ can be correctly estimated, as long as we know (1) C_1 is converted to C_2 and (2) the concentration profiles of C_1 and C_2. The knowledge of the rest of the model is not required for the estimation of the two indicated time constants. The kinetics of the other processes (linear, nonlinear, or Michaelis-Menten) do not affect the calculation either, since no assumption regarding these processes is made during the calculation.

Case 2

When the urine and/or bile concentrations of all final metabolic products derived from an intermediate are known, as shown in the model below, the elimination time T_{el} of the intermediate can be estimated without the knowledge of the rest of the model (shown by the dashed lines). This estimation is most feasible in the practical situations when all the final metabolites are excreted renally.

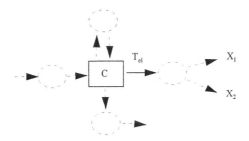

Assuming the elimination process corresponding to T_{el} follows first-order kinetics, it is straightforward to prove the following:

$$\frac{T_{el}}{V} = \frac{X_1 + X_2}{\text{AUC}} \tag{2.46}$$

Therefore, the estimated value of T_{el}/V is valid and meaningful as long as (1) the pathways are correct and (2) C, X_1, and X_2 are measured. Again, the estimation of T_{el}/V is independent of the knowledge of other processes in the model. The time constant can be correctly estimated from Equation (2.46), regardless of the kinetics of other processes.

Case 3

In the cases when reversible kinetics are involved, such as when tissue concentrations are measured or reversible metabolic pathways are identified, the estimation of time constants is also dependent only on the local model. An example is shown below:

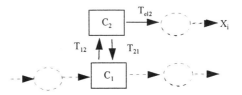

Assuming linear kinetics for the processes corresponding to T_{12}, T_{21}, and T_{el2}, the following equations can be written:

$$\frac{dC_2}{dt}V_2 = \frac{1}{T_{12}}C_1V_1 - \left(\frac{1}{T_{21}} + \frac{1}{T_{el2}}\right)C_2V_2 \tag{2.47}$$

and multiplying the above equation by t on both sides yields

$$\frac{dC_2}{dt}V_2t = \frac{1}{T_{12}}C_1V_1t - \left(\frac{1}{T_{21}} + \frac{1}{T_{el2}}\right)C_2V_2t \tag{2.48}$$

Similar to the derivation in Cases 1 and 2, we can obtain the following:

$$T_{el2,t} = \frac{1}{1/T_{21} + 1/T_{el2}} = \frac{AUCM_2}{AUC_2} - \frac{AUCM_1}{AUC_1} \tag{2.49}$$

$$\frac{T_{12}}{V_1}V_2 = \frac{AUC_1}{AUC_2}T_{el2,t} \tag{2.50}$$

$$\frac{T_{el2}}{V_2} = \frac{\Sigma X_i}{AUC_2} \tag{2.51}$$

Therefore, the local time constants $T_{el2,t}$, $T_{12}V_2/V_1$ and T_{el2}/V_2 can be correctly estimated as long as (1) the pathways are known, and (2) C_1 and C_2 concentration profiles are measured. The estimated values of these time constants are independent of the knowledge of the global model.

With the demonstrations of these three cases, we can be confident that, in most cases, the time constants estimated for individual processes are valid and independent of the global model. The next question is whether we can ever obtain the true global model describing a drug. The answer is "not likely." Frequently, we cannot be certain that there may be another metabolite existing, tissue distribution may be important, protein binding may play a role in pharmacokinetics, or gastric emptying and dissolution processes may be important in some clinical conditions. But one thing we can be certain of is that the estimation of individual time constants is always accurate, regardless of how well we know the global model.

REFERENCES

1. Aarons L., "Mean residence time for drugs subject to reversible metabolism," *J. Pharm. Pharmacol.*, 1987; 39:565–567.

2. Benet L. Z., "Mean residence time in the body versus mean residence time in the central compartment," *Journal of Pharmacokinetics and Biopharmaceutics*, 1985; 13(5):555–558.

3. Brockmeier D. and Ostrowski J., "Mean time and first-pass metabolism," *Eur. J. Clin. Pharmacol.*, 1985; 29:45–48.

4. Chan K. K., "A simple integrated method for drug and derived metabolite kinetics. An application of the statistical moment theory," *Drug Metabolism and Disposition*, 1982; 10(5):474–479.

5. Chan K. K. and Bolger M. B., "Statistical moment theory in chemical kinetics," *Anal. Chem.*, 1985; 57:2145–2151.

6. Chan K. K. H. and Gibaldi M., "Estimation of statistical moments and steady-state volume of distribution for a drug given by intravenous infusion," *Journal of Pharmacokinetics and Biopharmaceutics*, 1982; 10(5):551–558.

7. Chan K. K. H. and Gibaldi M., "Effects of first-pass metabolism on metabolite mean residence time determination after oral administration of parent drug," *Pharmaceutical Research*, 1990; 7(1):59–63.

8. Chanter D. O., "The determination of mean residence time using statistical moments: Is it correct?" *Journal of Pharmacokinetics and Biopharmaceutics*, 1985; 13(1):93–100.

9. Cheng H., "A method for calculating the mean transit times and distribution rate parameters of interconversion metabolites," *Biopharmaceutics & Drug Disposition*, 1993; 14:635–641.

10. Cheng H., Jusko W. J., and Gillespie W. R., "Relationships between the area under the first moment curve after single bolus injection and the integral of blood concentrations after constant-rate intravenous infusion," *Journal of Pharmaceutical Sciences*, 1991; 80(5):507–510.

11. Cheng H., Staubus A. E., and Shum L., "An area function method for estimating the apparent absorption rate constant," *Pharmaceutical Research*, 1988; 5(1):57–60.

12. Cheng H., "A general method for calculating the mean transit times and distribution rate parameters of catenary metabolites," *Biopharmaceutics & Drug Disposition*," 1992; 13:179–186.

13. Cheng H., "A method for calculating the mean transit times and distribution rate parameters of metabolites without separate intravenous administration of metabolite," *Journal of Pharmaceutical Sciences*, 1992; 81(5):488–490.

14. Cheng H., "A method for calculating the mean residence times of catenary metabolites," *Biopharmaceutics & Drug Disposition*, 1991; 12:335–342.

15. Cheng H. and Jusko W., "Mean residence time concepts for pharmacokinetic systems

with nonlinear drug elimination described by the Michaelis-Menten Equation," *Pharmaceutical Research*, 1988; 5(3):156–164.

16. Cheng H. and Jusko W. J., "An area function method for calculating the apparent elimination rate constant of a metabolite," *Journal of Pharmacokinetics and Biopharmaceutics*, 1989; 17(1):125–130.

17. Cheng H. and Jusko W. J., "Mean residence times and distribution volumes for drugs undergoing linear reversible metabolism and tissue distribution and linear or nonlinear elimination from the central compartments," *Pharmaceutical Research*, 1991; 8(4):508–511.

18. Cheng H. and Jusko W. J., "Mean interconversion times and distribution rate parameters for drugs undergoing reversible metabolism," *Pharmaceutical Research*, 1990; 7(10):1003–1010.

19. Cheng H. and Jusko W. J., "Constant-rate intravenous infusion methods for estimating steady-state volumes of distribution and mean residence times in the body for drugs undergoing reversible metabolism," *Pharmaceutical Research*, 1990; 7(6):628–632.

20. Cheng H. and Jusko W. J., "Mean residence time of oral drugs undergoing first-pass and linear reversible metabolism," *Pharmaceutical Research*, 1993; 10(1):8–13.

21. Cheng H. and Justko W. J., "Mean residence times of multicompartmental drugs undergoing reversible metabolism," *Pharmaceutical Research*, 1990; 7(1):103–107.

22. Cheng H. and Shum L., "A method for calculating the mean absorption time of drugs undergoing reversible and first pass metabolism," *Biopharmaceutics & Drug Disposition*, 1993; 14:71–79.

23. Chow A. T. and Jusko W. J., "Application of moment analysis to nonlinear drug disposition described by the Michaelis-Menten Equation," *Pharmaceutical Research*, 1987; 4(1):59–61.

24. Chung M., "Computation of model-independent pharmacokinetic parameters during multiple dosing," *Journal of Pharmaceutical Sciences*, 1984; 73(4):570–571.

25. Cobelli C. and Toffolo G., "Compartmental vs. noncompartmental modeling for two accessible pools," *Am. J. Physiol.*, 1984; 247:R488–R496.

26. Collier P. S., "Some considerations on the estimation of steady state apparent volume of distribution and the relationships between volume terms," *Journal of Pharmacokinetics and Biopharmaceutics*, 1983: 11(1):93–105.

27. Covel D. G., Berman M., and Delisi C., "Mean residence time-theoretical development, experimental determination, and practical use in tracer analysis," *Mathematical Biosciences*, 1984; 72:213–244.

28. Cutler D. J., "Theory of the mean absorption time, an adjunct to conventional bioavailability studies," *J. Pharm. Pharmac.*, 1978; 30:476–478.

29. Cutler D. J., "Definition of mean residence times in pharmacokinetics," *Biopharmaceutics & Drug Disposition*, 1987; 8:87–97.

30. Ebling W. F. and Jusko W. J., "The determination of essential clearance, volume, and residence time parameters of recirculating metabolic systems: The reversible metabolism of methylprednisolone and methylprednisone in rabbits," *Journal of Pharmacokinetics and Biopharmaceutics*, 1986; 14(6):557–599.

31. Eisenfeld J., "On mean residence time in compartments," *Mathematical Biosciences*, 1981; 57:265–278.

32. Gillespie W. R. and Veng-Pedersen P., "The determination of mean residence time using statistical moments: Is it correct?" *Journal of Pharmacokinetics and Biopharmaceutics*, 1985; 13(5):549–554.

33. Jackson A. J. and Chen M., "Application of moment analysis in assessing rates of absorption for bioequivalency studies," *Journal of Pharmaceutical Sciences*, 1987; 76(1):6–9.

34. Kakutani T., Atsumi R., Sumimoto E., and Hashida M., "Deconvolution of the regeneration process of mitomycin from prodrug in a muscle perfusion system based on statistical moment theory," *Chem. Pharm. Bull.*, 1987; 35(12):4907–4914.

35. Kakutani T., Nara E., and Hashida M., "Statistical moments and disposition parameters in a local perfusion system under mammillary nonequilibrium condition," *Journal of Pharmacokinetics and Biopharmaceutics*, 1990; 18(5):449–458.

36. Kakutani T., Yamaoka K., Hashida M., and Sezaki H., "A new method for assessment of drug disposition in muscle: Application of statistical moment theory to local perfusion systems," *Journal of Pharmacokinetics and Biopharmaceutics*, 1985; 13(6):609–631.

37. Kasuya Y., Hirayama H., Kubota N., and Pang K. S., "Interpretation and estimates of mean residence time with statistical moment theory," *Biopharmaceutics & Drug Disposition*, 1987; 8:223–234.

38. Kong A. and Jusko W. J., "Definitions and applications of mean transit and residence times in reference to the two-compartment mammillary plasma clearance model," *Journal of Pharmaceutical Sciences*, 1988; 77(2):157–165.

39. Landaw E. M. and Katz D., "Comments on mean residence time determination," *Journal of Pharmacokinetics and Biopharmaceutics*, 1985; 13(5):543–547.

40. Matis J. H., Wehrly T. E., and Metzler C. M., "On some stochastic formulations and related statistical moments of pharmacokinetic models," *Journal of Pharmacokinetics and Biopharmaceutics*, 1983; 11(1):77–92.

41. Mayer P. R. and Brazzell R. K., "Application of statistical moment theory to pharmacokinetics," *J. Clin. Pharmacol.*, 1988; 28:481–483.

42. Midha K. K., Roscoe R. M. H., Wilson T. W., Cooper J. K., Loo J. C. K., Ho-Ngoc A., and McGilveray I. J., "Pharmacokinetics of glucuronidation of propanolol following oral administration in humans," *Biopharmaceutics & Drug Disposition*, 1983; 4:331–338.

43. Nakashima E. and Benet L. Z., "General treatment of mean residence time, clearance, and volume parameters in linear mammillary models with elimination from any compartment," *Journal of Pharmacokinetics and Biopharmaceutics*, 1988; 16(5):475–492.

44. Perrier D. and Mayersohn M., "Noncompartmental determination of the steady-state volume of distribution for any mode of administration," *Journal of Pharmaceutical Sciences*, 1982; 71(3):372–373.

45. Pfeffer M., "Estimation of mean residence time from data obtained when multiple-dosing steady state has been reached," *Journal of Pharmaceutical Sciences*, 1984; 73(6):854–856.

46. Rescigno A., "On transfer times in tracer experiments," *J. Theo. Biol.*, 1973; 39:9–27.

47. Riegelman S. and Collier P., "The application of statistical moment theory to the evaluation of in vivo dissolution time and absorption time," *Journal of Pharmacokinetics and Biopharmaceutics*, 1980; 8(5):509–534.

48. Roberts G. W., Larson K. B., and Spaeth E. E., "The interpretation of mean transit time measurements for multiphase tissue system," *J. Theo. Biol.*, 1973; 39:447–475.

49. Smith I. L. and Schentag J. J., "Noncompartmental determination of the steady-state volume of distribution during multiple dosing," *Journal of Pharmaceutical Sciences*, 1984; 73(2):281–282.

50. Tanigawara Y., Yamaoka K., Nakagawa T., and Uno T., "New method for the evaluation of in vitro dissolution time and disintegration time," *Chem. Pharm. Bull.*, 1982; 30(3):1088–1090.

51. Veng-Pedersen P., "A simple method for obtaining the mean residence time of metabolites in the body," *Journal of Pharmaceutical Sciences*, 1986; 75(8):818–819.

52. Veng-Pedersen P., Cheng H., and Jusko W. J., "Regarding dose-independent pharmacokinetic parameters in nonlinear pharmacokinetics," *Journal of Pharmaceutical Sciences*, 1991; 80(6):608–612.

53. Veng-Pedersen P. and Gillespie W., "The mean residence time of drugs in the systemic circulation," *Journal of Pharmaceutical Sciences*, 1985; 74(7):791–792.

54. Veng-Pedersen P. and Gillespie W., "Single pass mean residence time in peripheral tissues: a distribution parameter intrinsic to the tissue affinity of a drug," *Journal of Pharmaceutical Sciences*, 1986; 75(12):1119–1126.

55. Veng-Pedersen P. and Gillespie W., "Mean residence time in peripheral tissue: A linear disposition parameter useful for evaluating a drug's tissue distribution," *Journal of Pharmacokinetics and Biopharmaceutics*, 1984; 12(5):535–543.

56. Veng-Pedersen P. and Gillespie W. R., "A method for evaluating the mean residence time of metabolites in the body, systemic circulation, and the peripheral tissue not requiring separate i.v. administration of metabolite," *Biopharmaceutics & Drug Disposition*, 1987; 8:395–401.

57. Wagner J. G., "Types of mean residence times," *Biopharmaceutics & Drug Disposition*, 1988; 9:41–57.

58. Weiss M., "Hemodynamic influences upon the variance of disposition residence time distribution of drugs," *Journal of Pharmacokinetics and Biopharmaceutics*, 1983; 11(1):63–75.

59. Weiss M., "Residence time and accumulation of drugs in the body," *International Journal of Clinical Pharmacology*, 1981; 19(2):82–85.

60. Weiss M., "A general model of metabolite kinetics following intravenous and oral administration of the parent drug," *Biopharmaceutics & Drug Disposition*, 1988; 9:159–176.

61. Weiss M., "Drug metabolite kinetics: Noncompartmental analysis," *Br. J. Clin. Pharmac.*, 1985; 19:855–856.

62. Weiss M. and Forster W., "Pharmacokinetic model based on circulatory transport," *Eur. J. Clin. Pharmacol.*, 1979; 16:287–293.

63. Yamaoka K., Nakagawa T., and Uno T., "Statistical moments in pharmacokinetics," *Journal of Pharmacokinetics and Biopharmaceutics*, 1978; 6(6):547–558.

64. Yamaoka K., Nakagawa T., and Tanaka H., "Recirculatory moment analysis of drugs in mean: Estimation of extraction ratio and mean cycle time for single systemic and pulmonary circulation," *Chem. Pharm. Bull.*, 1985; 33:784–794.

CHAPTER 3

Evaluation of Time Constants by Visual Inspection of Concentration-Time Profiles

In Chapter 2, the time constants were defined as the concentration-average time required to move a drug from one compartment to another, and the advantages in the application of the Time Constant Approach to pharmacokinetic analysis was demonstrated. In this chapter, an intuitive way to visually observe time constants from concentration-time profiles will be discussed. Many time constants can be observed from the slope of the semi-log plot of the concentration-time profile. There are certain principles, based on the structure of models, governing which time constants will appear on the concentration-time profile. Based on these principles, one can visually identify the observable time constants from a model structure with ease. These principles are discussed in the following sections.

NOT ALL THE TIME CONSTANTS CAN BE OBSERVED

First, let's determine from the structure of models which time constants can be visually observed from concentration profiles and which cannot. There are always multiple time constants involved in any model, but not all of the constants will be observed from the concentration-time profiles. Only some of the time constants are observable, and these time constants can be called the "characteristic time constant" to distinguish them from those that are not observable. Here, a "characteristic time constant" means that the time constant is able to be observed from concentration profiles, except for some special cases. Sometimes the "characteristic time constants" cannot be identified from the concentration profiles due to reasons such as "interference" among the time constants. Later in this chapter the special cases where these "characteristic time constants" cannot be observed from the

61

concentration-time profiles will be discussed. But now, let us examine the three principles of identifying the characteristic time constants based on the structure of a model.

(1) The first principle for identifying the characteristic time constants from the structure of a model is that all the characteristic time constants in a compartment will also be the characteristic time constants in the compartments positioned later in the model. Take the model in Figure 3.1 as an example. All the characteristic time constants in compartment C will also be the characteristic time constants in compartment M1.

(2) The characteristic time constants can be easily identified from a model involving only irreversible processes, while the identification is more complicated when reversible processes are involved. In the case where only irreversible processes are involved, the characteristic time constants include the absorption time and the total elimination time of each compartment. Take the model in Figure 3.1 as an example. There are three compartments as well as three concentration profiles involved in the model. For the concentration profile in compartment C, the characteristic time constants are the absorption time (T_a) and the total elimination time $[T_{el,t} = 1/(1/T_{el} + 1/T_{m1} + 1/T_{m2})]$. According to the first principle, for the concentration profile in compartment M1, the characteristic time constants include those of compartment C, and according to the second principle the characteristic time constants in compartment M1 also include the elimination time T_{mel1}. Similarly, in compartment M2, the characteristic time constants are T_a, $T_{el,t}$, and T_{mel2}.

(3) In the case where reversible processes are involved, the characteristic time constants must be derived from the equations describing the model. For example, the model in Figure 3.2 involves one reversible process. The concentration profile of C can be described by Equation (2.35) in Chapter

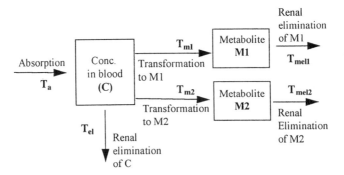

FIGURE 3.1. A multi-compartment model as an example for identifying "characteristic time constants" based on the structure of a model.

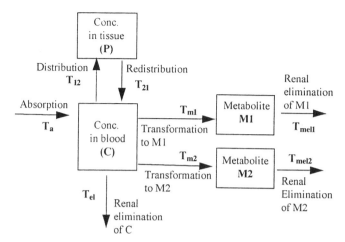

FIGURE 3.2. A multi-compartment model with reversible tissue distribution. The equations describing the concentration-time profile are listed in Equation (2.35) in Chapter 2.

2. Clearly, there are three characteristic exponents involved in this equation, which correspond to three characteristic time constants: T_a, T_1 ($= 1/\lambda_1$), and T_2 ($= 1/\lambda_2$). According to the first principle, for a metabolite concentration profile, the characteristic time constants consist of those for the parent drug, and according to the second principle, the characteristic time constants of a metabolite also include the elimination time of the metabolite. Therefore, in compartment M1, the characteristic time constants include those of compartment C and the elimination time T_{mel1}, while in compartment M2, the characteristic time constants are those of compartment C and the elimination time T_{mel2}.

TIME CONSTANTS APPEAR ON THE CONCENTRATION-TIME PROFILE ACCORDING TO THE ORDER OF MAGNITUDE

Now we know how to identify, based on the model structure, the "characteristic time constants" that may potentially be observed from the concentration-time profiles. The next question is in what order the time constants will appear on the concentration profiles. The principle here is that the time constants appear according to their order of magnitude. In general, there is a period of time for a time constant to be observed in the concentration-time profile, ranging approximately from two to three times the time constant. As a result, a "time window" specifies the segment (time period) of the concentration-time profile where a time constant can be

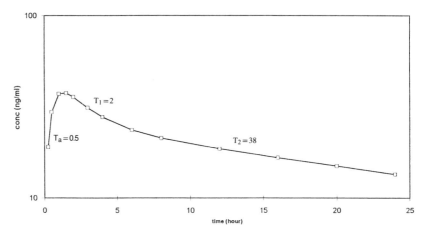

FIGURE 3.3. The simulated concentration profile based on the model in Figure 3.2. The order of appearance of time constant along the concentration profile is according to their order of magnitude.

observed. At any specific time point t, only one time constant will be observed. Take the model in Figure 3.2 as an example. The three characteristic time constants in compartment C can be identified from Equation (2.35), which are T_a, T_1 $(= 1/\lambda_1)$, and T_2 $(= 1/\lambda_2)$. The graph in Figure 3.3 gives an example of the concentration profile of C based on this model, where $T_a = 0.5$ hr, $T_1 = 2$ hr, and $T_2 = 38$ hr.

As shown in Figure 3.3, the time constants appear according to the order of magnitude. The smaller time constants appear earlier in the concentration-time profile. Each time constant is observed on the concentration profile within a certain "time window," ranging approximately from 0 to 2 hr for T_a, 2 to 6 hr for T_1, and 6 hr and later for T_2. This divides the observation time (24-hour total) into three time windows. In the situation where the total observation time is shorter than the lower limit of the time window of T_2, the longest time constant (T_2) will not be observed. The quantitative values of these time constants can be obtained by a stripping method.

FLIP-FLOP AND DOMINANT TIME CONSTANT OF TERMINAL PHASE

It is usually assumed that the absorption time should be observed earlier than the elimination time in a concentration-time profile, since the absorption process itself starts earlier than the elimination process in the human body; however, this is not always the case. The order of appearance of time constants along the concentration profile is strictly dependent on the order of magnitude as stated above. When the absorption time is longer than the elimination time, the absorption process starts earlier but also lasts longer so that the absorption time is observed in the distal portion of the concentration profile; in contrast, the elimination process starts later but immediately catches up and exceeds the absorption process, such that the elimination time is observed in the proximal portion of the concentration profile. When this occurs ($T_a > T_{el}$), it is called a flip-flop. Figure 3.4 is a graph that shows an example of concentration profile based on a simple one-compartment model (Model 1 of Table 2.1 in Chapter 2).

By just visually examining Figure 3.4, one cannot determine whether $T_a < T_{el}$ or $T_a > T_{el}$. In fact, the only way to definitely determine T_a and T_{el} is to conduct a study administering both an oral and an intravenous dose (discussed in Chapter 5). Another parameter (characterizing absorption) that can be unambiguously determined from the oral administration alone is $T_a*V/f/F$ (discussed in Chapter 6). In either case, with or without flip-flop, the dominant time constant in the terminal phase of the concentration profile is the longest time constant. This rule for determining the dominant time constant also applies to all other models with multiple characteristic times. But one has to remember that the longest time constant is not always the elimination time!

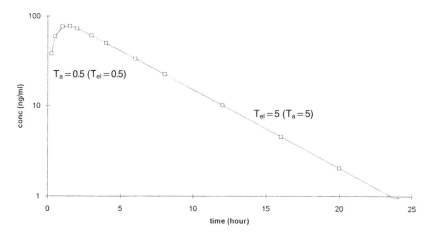

FIGURE 3.4. Simulated concentration profiles based on a one-compartment model with two cases (1) $T_a > T_{el}$ or (2) $T_a < T_{el}$. The other parameters in the model (i.e., *F*, *D*, and *V*) are adjusted so that the two concentration profiles overlap each other.

INDISTINGUISHABLE TIME CONSTANTS WITH OVERLAPPING TIME WINDOWS

The characteristic time constants are not always visually identifiable in concentration-time profiles. As stated earlier, the characteristic time constants are time constants possible to be observed from the concentration profiles. We will discuss several situations where some of the characteristic time constants cannot be actually observed. The first situation is that the time windows of several time constants are overlapped. This means the time constants are too close to be distinguished from each other on the concentration profile. Figure 3.5 shows an example of the concentration profile of C based on the model in Figure 3.2, where absorption time (T_a) = 1 hr, first decay time (T_{z1}) = 4.5 hr, and second decay time (T_{z2}) = 5.3 hr.

In Figure 3.5, the time constants appear on the concentration profile according to the order of magnitude. However, two of the constants, T_1 and T_2, are relatively close to each other so that their time windows for observation are overlapped. As a result, only two time constants are clearly observed in the concentration-time profile. To be precise, the larger one of T_1 and T_2 is observed at the terminal phase of the profile. When this situation occurs, the two-compartment model collapses to a one-compartment model. The details of many cases where this type of collapse happens will be discussed in Chapter 6.

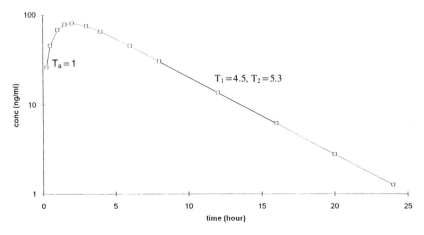

FIGURE 3.5. Simulated concentration profile based on the model in Figure 3.2. Two of the time constants $(T_1$ and $T_2)$ in this case are close and cannot be distinguished from each other on the concentration-time profile.

TIME CONSTANT WINDOWS INTERRUPTED BY PEAK CONCENTRATION

Another situation where a characteristic time constant cannot actually be observed is when the time window of the time constant is interrupted by a peak concentration. The interruption makes the visual observation of the time constant difficult from real-life data, especially when the data involve some variabilities. This type of overlapping between the time window of time constant and the peak concentration frequently occurs for metabolites of drugs. As discussed above, the characteristic time constants of a metabolite concentration profile include those of the parent drug and the elimination time of the metabolite. Take the model in Figure 3.2 again as an example. There are four characteristic time constants on the concentration profile of metabolite M1: T_a, T_1, T_2, and T_{mel}. Presumably, if the time windows of the four characteristic time constants are well separated, all four of them should be identifiable in the M1 concentration profile; however, this is usually not the case, depending on the location of the peak concentration of M1. First, the principle based on which the peak concentration of M1 locates is discussed. The lag time between the peak concentrations of metabolite and parent drug can be approximated by the lag between the two mean residence times. The lag between the mean residence times of metabolite M1 and parent drug C is equal to the elimination time of the metabolite, T_{mel}. Therefore, the peak concentration of M1 is approximately delayed by T_{mel} relative to the peak concentration of C. The smaller the values of T_{mel}, the earlier the peak concentration of M1 occurs, and the earlier T_{mel} appears in the M1 concentration profile. As a result, when T_{mel} is small, the distal portion of the M1 profile is parallel to that of C since the time window of T_{mel} and the peak concentration occur much earlier. On the other hand, if T_{mel} is large, the peak concentration of M1 occurs late and overlaps with most of the other time constant windows and only T_{mel} is likely to be observed in the M1 concentration profile. Figures 3.6 and 3.7 show examples of concentration profiles of M1 and C based on the model in Figure 3.2, with small and large T_{mel} values.

As shown in Figure 3.6, the peak concentration of M1 occurs much earlier when the elimination time of the metabolite is smaller. In this case, the elimination time of the metabolite is small, and the terminal portions of the two concentration profiles are parallel to each other. This is because the peak concentration of M1, as well as the time window of T_{mel}, occurs relatively early. As a result, two time constants of the parent drug, T_1 and T_2, are observed again on the metabolite concentration profile, while T_{mel} cannot be observed since its time window is interrupted by the peak concen-

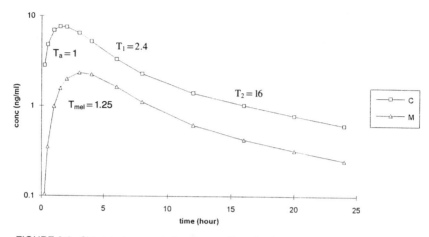

FIGURE 3.6. Simulated concentration-time profiles of a drug and its metabolite based on the model in Figure 3.2. The metabolite has a short elimination time (T_{mel}).

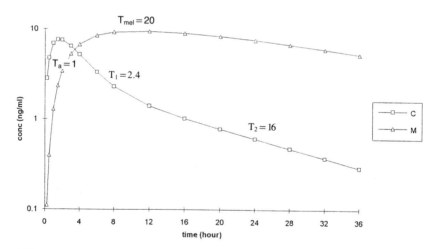

FIGURE 3.7. Simulated concentration-time profiles of a drug and its metabolite based on the model in Figure 3.2. The metabolite has a long elimination time (T_{mel}).

tration. In Figure 3.7, T_{mel} is relatively long. As a result, the peak of M1 is delayed and broadened and interrupts the time windows of time constants T_a, T_1, and T_2. In this case, only the elimination time T_{mel} is observed from the metabolite concentration profile.

OBSERVATION TIME SCALE AND IDENTIFICATION OF TIME CONSTANT

As discussed above, each time constant has a time window to be observed along the concentration profile. This time window is a specific range of time within which the time constant can be clearly determined from the semi-log plot of concentration-time profile. In the situation where the observation time scale, i.e., the interval between every two observation time points, is longer than the range of time window of a time constant, the time constant cannot be visually identified. In other words, the observation may not be detailed enough to pick up the time constants that are with narrow time windows. This situation frequently occurs in intravenous administrations, where the initial distribution time is usually very short. An example is shown in Figure 3.8, based on the model in Figure 3.2 with $T_1 = 0.6$ and $T_2 = 29$ (intravenous dose).

In Figure 3.8, the first observation is much more detailed than the second one. In the first observation, the observation time points in the first 2 hours are 0, 0.25, 0.5, 1, 1.5, and 2 hours. In the second observation, time points are separated by 2 hours. One of the time constants, $T_1 = 0.6$ hr, is relatively short and cannot be picked up by the second observation. Therefore, the two-compartment model collapses to a one-compartment model when the observation time scale is much greater than T_1. The collapsed model can only give a rough prediction of the concentration-time profile but fails to describe the initial distribution phase immediately following the intravenous administration. The concept of observation time scale is also important in multiple dose study, where a dose is repeatedly given for many days. If the observation time scale is short (say 1–4 hours), then one will observe that the concentration profile rises and falls. If the observation time scale is one time point per every 24 hours, then one will observe that the concentration increases and reaches a "steady-state concentration."

SUPERPOSITION PRINCIPLE AND TIME SHIFTING

When the pharmacokinetics of all processes involved in the disposition of a drug are linear, the superposition principle can be applied to predict, from

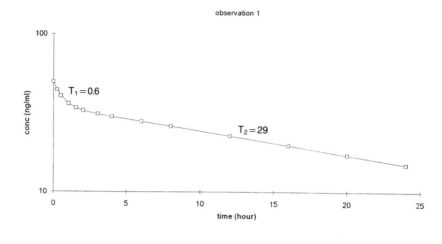

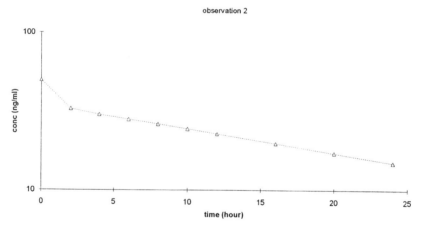

FIGURE 3.8. Simulated concentration-time profile based on the model in Figure 3.2 following an intravenous bolus dose. The observation in the upper plot is more detailed than that in the lower plot.

70

the single-dose profile, the concentration profile following a multiple dose. The superposition principle assumes that the early doses of drug do not affect the pharmacokinetics of subsequent doses. Therefore, the concentration after the second and later doses will overlay or superimpose the concentration attained after the first dose. Figure 3.9 shows an example of superposition principle applied to two doses of a drug following the model in Figure 3.2.

The concentration produced by the second dose is assumed to be the same as that by the first dose; therefore, the concentration profile contributed by the second dose can be predicted by shifting the concentration profile after a single dose forward by 24 hours. The summation of the two concentration profiles contributed by the first and the second doses gives the profiles for the multiple doses.

Similarly, the superposition principle can be applied to predict the concentration profile following an intravenous infusion administration. An intravenous infusion for a finite time can be viewed as a summation of a continuous infusion and a bolus infusion. This means that the drug is continuously infused for a period of time T and the infusion stops. When the infusion stops, there is still a certain amount of drug left in the body. This residual amount of drug will continue to be eliminated as if it is given as a bolus dose at time T.

Figure 3.10 shows an example of superposition principle applied to an intravenous infusion for 2 hours, based on Model 1 in Table 2.1 of Chapter 2.

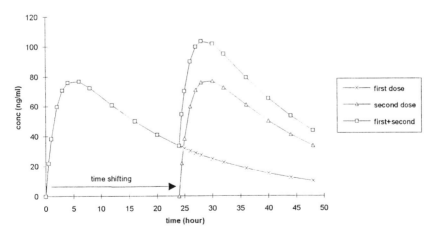

FIGURE 3.9. Simulated concentration profiles following multiple doses based on superposition principle using the model in Figure 3.2. The concentration profile after the multiple doses is a summation of those of two single doses.

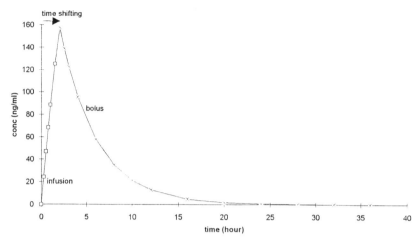

FIGURE 3.10. Simulated concentration-time profile following a short-term intravenous infusion based on the superposition principle using Model 1 in Table 2.1 of Chapter 2.

In this example, the drug is intravenously infused for 2 hours. Therefore, the concentration profile (Figure 3.10) in the first 2 hours can be predicted by the equation describing a continuous infusion:

$$C = \frac{R}{VK_{el}} (1 - e^{-K_{el} \cdot t}) \tag{3.1}$$

where R is the infusion rate. After 2 hours, the concentration decays according to an intravenous bolus model but with the time shifted forward by 2 hours ($T = 2$).

$$C = C_0 e^{-K_{el}(t - T)} \tag{3.2}$$

where C_0 is the concentration at time T, which is equal to $[R/(VK_{el})]$ $(1 - e^{-K_{el} \cdot T})$ according to Equation (3.1). To summarize, the concentration profile following an intravenous infusion (short time length) can be predicted from the concentration profiles following a continuous infusion (long time length) and a bolus dose, applying the superposition principle.

The superposition principle is very useful in predicting concentration profiles following complicated dosing regimens, such as variable dosing intervals or dose amount or combined dosing routes; however, one must bear in mind that this principle only applies to linear kinetics. The determination of linearity of pharmacokinetics is presented in Chapter 7.

PHARMACOKINETIC AND PHARMACODYNAMIC LINKS— ISOLATED MULTI-COMPARTMENT MODEL

The ultimate goal of pharmacokinetic/pharmacodynamic analysis in a clinical trial is to provide a prediction of the temporal profiles of pharmacological effects after a single or multiple dose under clinical settings. One of the most complicated, but not necessarily the most accurate, ways to predict pharmacodynamic effects of a drug is to calculate the effects from the dose amount based on a full pharmacokinetic model, which may include all possible disposition processes: dissolution, gastric emptying, absorption, distribution, metabolism, eliminations, and so on. Due to the tremendous variability accumulated from each time constant and the complexity of the mathematical equations involved, it is not always feasible to estimate pharmacological effects based on the full pharmacokinetic/pharmacodynamic model.

Alternatively, the pharmacological effects can be correlated with the plasma drug concentration using a simplified model, where the central and effect compartments are isolated from other compartments in the full pharmacokinetic model. An example of the isolated multi-compartment model is shown below:

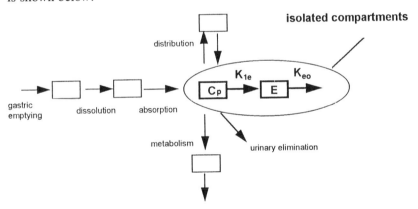

The pharmacological effects can be predicted from the plasma drug concentration with a simple relationship

$$E = C_p * T \tag{3.3}$$

where $T = K_{1e} e^{-k_{eo} \cdot t}$ and the symbol "*" represents convolution, which can be easily accomplished in a spreadsheet software such as EXCEL® or LOTUS®. The formula for convolution is

$$E = \int_0^t C_p(u) \cdot T(t - u)du \qquad (3.4)$$

The pictorial representation of the convolution calculation is shown in Figure 3.11. It illustrates the convolution of C_p with T at $t = 8$ hr. The upper part of the figure shows a typical serum concentration profile $C_p(u)$, and the lower part shows the exponential function $T(t - u)$, which decays retrogressively from the time point $t = 8$ hr. The curve in the middle represents the product of $C_p(u)$ and $T(8 - u)$, and the area under this curve is equal to the effect according to Equation (3.4). Because $T(t - u)$ decays retrogressively, the serum drug concentration at a time point closer to 8 hours contributes more to the pharmacological effects at $t = 8$ hr.

The relative contribution of drug concentrations at earlier time points to the pharmacological effects can be determined by the value of $T(t - u)$ as shown in Table 3.1. According to the table, the contribution to $E(t)$ from the drug serum concentration at time $t - (2/K_{eo})$ is less than 15% of the contribution from a same amount of drug at time t. When the value of K_{eo} is relatively large, the lag time between C_p and E (which is equal to $1/K_{eo}$) becomes small, and the pharmacological effect is directly correlated with the drug concentration at t, not affected by the concentrations at the earlier time points.

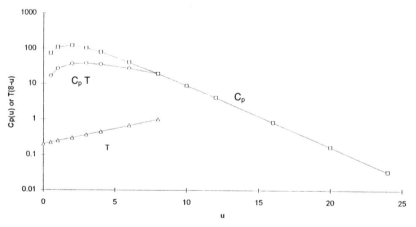

FIGURE 3.11. The calculation of convolution based on Equation (3.4). Function $T(t)$ decays retrogressively and exponentially. The area under the C_p*T curve determines the contribution of plasma concentration (C_p) to the effect (E).

*TABLE 3.1. Relative Contribution of
Drug Concentration at Different Time Point to
Pharmacological Effect.*

Early Time Point (u)	Value of $T(t - u)$ $= e^{-K_{eo}(t - u)}$
t	100%
$t - \dfrac{1}{K_{eo}}$	37%
$t - \dfrac{1}{K_{eo}}$	15%
$t - \dfrac{3}{K_{eo}}$	5%
$t - \dfrac{4}{K_{eo}}$	2%

Equation (3.3) can be applied to any formulation, administration route, or dose regimen, assuming the relationship between central compartment concentration and effect remains the same with time (linear and no tolerance developed). The detail of the Time Constant Approach in pharmacokinetics/pharmacodynamics will be discussed in Chapter 12.

CHAPTER 4

Scaling of Time Constants among Different Animal Species

One of the fundamental problems in drug development process is to extrapolate human pharmacokinetic parameters from animal data. The extrapolated human parameters can be used to predict the concentration and toxicity of the drug in humans before the first dose of the drug in any man. This prediction provides a quantitative safety consideration for the first clinical experiment of the drug. Traditionally, pharmacokinetic parameters are scaled among animal species, assuming a linear relationship between the logarithm of the parameters and the logarithm of the body weight. This relationship is empirical and without any physiological basis. In this chapter, we attempt to provide a rationale for scaling time constants among animal species by establishing relationships between time constants and physiological time scales.

PHARMACOKINETIC TIME CONSTANTS AND PHYSIOLOGICAL TIME SCALES

Since pharmacokinetic processes, such as hepatic elimination, renal elimination, and tissue distribution, occur in specific organs in the body, the pharmacokinetic time constants associated with the pharmacokinetic processes can be correlated to the physiological time scales in these organs. The most useful physiological time scale in an organ is the time required for the total volume of the central compartment (V_c) to pass through the organ. For example, the times required for the central compartment volume to pass through liver and glomeruli are

$$\text{Hepatic perfusion time } (T_{\text{hepatic}}) = \frac{V_c}{\text{HBF}} \qquad (4.1)$$

77

$$\text{Glomerular perfusion time } (T_{\text{glomerular}}) = \frac{V_c}{\text{GFR}} \qquad (4.2)$$

where HBF is the hepatic blood flow and GFR is the glomerular filtration rate as shown below:

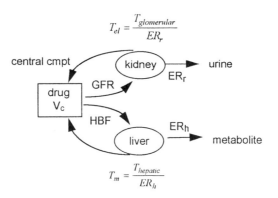

The hepatic elimination time (T_m) and renal elimination time (T_{el}) can be correlated with T_{hepatic} and $T_{\text{glomerular}}$ as follows:

$$\text{Hepatic elimination time } (T_m) = \frac{V_c}{\text{ER}_h \text{HBF}} = \frac{T_{\text{hepatic}}}{\text{ER}_h} \qquad (4.3)$$

$$\text{Renal elimination time } (T_{el}) = \frac{V_c}{\text{ER}_r \text{HBF}} = \frac{T_{\text{glomerular}}}{\text{ER}_r} \qquad (4.4)$$

where ER_h and ER_r are the hepatic extraction ratio and renal extraction ratio, respectively. Therefore, for drugs with a large central compartment volume, it requires a long time for the drug in the central compartment to pass through the liver (T_{hepatic}) and glomerular $(T_{\text{glomerular}})$, and the resulting hepatic elimination time (T_m) and renal elimination time (T_{el}) are relatively long. In addition, drugs with a low extraction ratio have a long elimination time.

Similarly, the absorption time can be correlated to the physiological time, $T_{\text{intestine}}$, as shown in the following diagram:

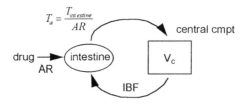

The time required for the central compartment volume to pass through the intestine is

$$\text{Intestinal perfusion time } (T_{\text{intestine}}) = \frac{V_c}{\text{IBF}} \qquad (4.5)$$

where IBF is the intestinal blood flow. The absorption time T_a can be correlated to $T_{\text{intestine}}$ as follows:

$$\text{Absorption time } (T_a) = \frac{V_c}{\text{AR} \cdot \text{IBF}} = \frac{T_{\text{intestine}}}{\text{AR}} \qquad (4.6)$$

where the absorption ratio AR is defined as the fraction of the drug absorbed per each unit volume of blood passing through the intestine.

For drugs that follow a one-compartmental model, the mean residence time of the plasma concentration curve is the sum of absorption time and elimination time:

$$\text{Mean residence time of one-compartment model } (\bar{t}) = T_a + T_{\text{el},t} \qquad (4.7)$$

where the total elimination time can be determined from the hepatic elimination time and the renal elimination time

$$\frac{1}{T_{\text{el},t}} = \frac{1}{T_m} + \frac{1}{T_{\text{el}}} \qquad (4.8)$$

For drugs that follow the two-compartmental model shown below, the distribution of the drugs into and out of the peripheral compartment prolongs the mean residence time of the drug in the body.

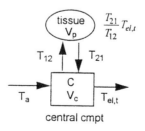

As a result, the distribution process contributes one additional term to the mean residence time, compared with the one-compartmental model:

Mean residence time of two-compartment model $(\bar{t}) = T_a + T_{el,t} + T_{el,t} \dfrac{T_{21}}{T_{12}}$

$$(4.9)$$

where T_{12} is the distribution time and T_{21} is the redistribution time. For drugs with strong tissue binding, the apparent volume of distribution will be large, the redistribution time (T_{21}) of the drug from the tissue to the central compartment will be long, and consequently, the mean residence time of the drug will be long. Therefore, drugs with a large apparent volume of distribution usually exhibit a long mean residence time in the plasma.

INTERSPECIES SCALING OF TIME CONSTANTS

Since the pharmacokinetic time constants are proportional to the organ perfusion time, if the organ blood perfusion rates can be scaled among species, it is likely that the pharmacokinetic time constants can also be scaled. Examples of organ blood perfusion rates in different animals are shown in Table 4.1. The organ blood perfusion rates, in general, increase with the body size, as does the organ perfusion time, Therefore, organ perfusion time can be scaled up from animal to human based on the body weight.

It has also been demonstrated that pharmacokinetic parameters can be extrapolated from animal data to man [1,4,8,9,13,32,38], based on body weight or body surface area. The basic equation for allometric scaling is

$$Y = a \cdot \mathrm{BW}^{b} \qquad (4.10)$$

where Y is a pharmacokinetic parameter, BW is body weight, a is a constant, and b is the exponent of the scaling equation. Examples of parameters that may be extrapolated from animal to man include Cl_r [5,11,12], Cl_{tot} [12,21,31,40], $t_{1/2}$ [12,22], V_d [12,15,21,31,40], V_{max} [38], k_m [38], and organ weight [1]. The allometric scaling formula has also been used when Y is a pharmacodynamic variable [7,39].

Volume of Distribution

Volume of distribution of drugs is likely to correlate with the body weight of different species since the blood volume and organ size are proportional to the body weight. Examples of the scaling exponent of several drugs are shown in Table 4.2. In general, the exponent for scaling volume of distribution is approximately one [38]. An existing relationship between the

TABLE 4.1. Blood Perfusion Rates (ml/min) through Organs and Organ Perfusion Time (min) (in parentheses) in Various Species. (Reproduced from Reference [44] with permission.)

Organ or Tissue	Mouse (0.02 kg)	Rat (0.25 kg)	Rabbit (2.5 kg)	Monkey (5 kg)	Dog (10 kg)	Human (70 kg)
Brain	—	1.3 (6.00)	—	72 (3.11)	45 (11.44)	700 (4.28)
Liver	1.8 (0.56)	13.8 (0.57)	177 (0.62)	218 (1.03)	309 (1.67)	1450 (2.07)
Kidneys	1.3 (0.77)	9.2 (0.85)	80 (1.38)	138 (1.62)	216 (2.38)	1240 (2.42)
Heart	0.28 (3.57)	3.9 (2.00)	16 (6.88)	60 (3.73)	54 (9.53)	240 (12.5)
Spleen	0.09 (11.11)	0.63 (12.38)	9 (12.22)	21 (10.67)	25 (20.60)	77 (38.96)
Gut	1.5 (0.67)	7.5 (1.04)	111 (0.99)	125 (1.79)	216 (2.38)	1100 (2.72)
Muscle	0.91 (1.10)	7.5 (1.04)	155 (0.71)	90 (2.48)	250 (2.06)	750 (4.00)
Adipose	—	0.4 (19.5)	32 (3.43)	20 (11.2)	35 (14.7)	260 (11.53)
Skin	0.41 (2.44)	5.8 (1.34)	—	54 (4.15)	100 (5.15)	300 (10.0)
Hepatic artery	0.35 (2.85)	2.0 (3.9)	37 (2.97)	51 (4.39)	79 (6.52)	300 (10.0)
Portal vein	1.45 (0.69)	9.8 (0.80)	140 (0.79)	167 (1.34)	230 (2.24)	1150 (2.61)
Cardiac output	8.0	74.0	530	1086	1200	5600

TABLE 4.2. The Exponent in the Scaling Equation (4.10) for the Volume of
Distribution of Several Drugs.

Drug	Exponent	Reference
Blood volume	0.99	[1]
Organ volume	1.0	[1]
Caffeine	1.005	[32]
FCE22101	1.19	[33]
Pentachlorophenol	0.941	[31]
Enprofylline	1.048	[40]
Panipenem	0.956	[21]
Betamipron	1.008	[21]
Sematilide	0.89	[16]

volume of distribution and body weight is a necessary criterion for a possible relationship between the hepatic/renal elimination times and the body weight, since the elimination times depend on the volume of distribution [Equations (4.3) and (4.4)].

Renal Elimination Time

The renal elimination time is expressed as a function of volume of distribution, renal extraction ratio, and glomerular filtration rate in Equation (4.4). Assuming the scaling exponent of volume of distribution is one and the renal extraction ratio is the same between species, then the scaling exponent of the renal elimination time is equal to one minus the scaling exponent of glomerular filtration rate. Since the glomerular filtration rate is estimated from inulin clearance, the scaling exponent of the glomerular filtration rate is 0.72 to 0.77 (Table 4.3). The renal elimination time can be estimated from the renal clearance as follows:

$$\text{Renal elimination time } (T_{el}) = \frac{V_c}{Cl_r} \qquad (4.11)$$

The exponents for the scaling equation of renal elimination time (T_{el}) of several drugs are shown in Table 4.3. A general scaling law with an exponent of 0.25 ($= 1 - 0.75$) is proposed for the renal elimination time (exponent $= 0.75$ for renal clearance) [38].

Hepatic Elimination Time

The hepatic elimination time is difficult to scale up from small animals to man, since metabolite profiles between species are usually very different [3,19,26–28]. Examples of the ratio of hepatic elimination time to renal elimination time of several drugs are shown in Table 4.4. In general, the ratio is higher with greater body weight.

The hepatic elimination time can be estimated from the following equation:

$$\text{Hepatic elimination time } (T_m) = \frac{V_c}{\text{ER}_h \cdot \text{HBF}} \qquad (4.12)$$

The volume of distribution can be accurately scaled up from animals to man with an exponent of one, as discussed earlier in this chapter. The hepatic blood flow is known in many species [4,9]: 1.8 ml/min for mouse, 11.8 ml/min for rat, 153 ml/min for monkey, 270 ml/min for dog, 1450 ml/min for man. The hepatic extraction ratio can be estimated from the following equation [30]:

$$\text{Hepatic extraction ratio } (\text{ER}_h) = \frac{f_B \text{Cl}'_{\text{intrinsic}}}{\text{HBF} + f_B \text{Cl}'_{\text{intrinsic}}} \qquad (4.13)$$

where f_B is the fraction of the drug bound to plasma proteins and $\text{Cl}'_{\text{intrinsic}}$ is the hepatic intrinsic clearance and can be estimated as follows. First, the Michaelis-Menten kinetics is assumed for the metabolic rate:

TABLE 4.3. The Exponent in the Scaling Equation (4.10) for the Renal Elimination Time of Several Drugs, Estimated from the Scaling Law of Renal Clearance Assuming the Exponent for Scaling Volume of Distribution is One.

Drug	Exponent	Reference
Urea	0.28	[1]
Inulin	0.23	[1]
Inulin	0.28	[11]
Creatinine	0.31	[1]
Creatinine	0.32	[11]
Diodrast	0.11	[1]
Hippurate	0.20	[1]
Uracil arabinoside	0.20	[9]
para-Aminohippuric acid	0.23	[11]
FCE22101	0.26	[12]
Sematilide	0.31	[16]

TABLE 4.4. Intrinsic Clearance V_{max}/k_m and Ratio of Hepatic Elimination Time to Renal Elimination Time of Several Drugs.

Drug	Parameters	Mouse	Rat	Hamster	Guinea Pig	Rabbit	Dog	Monkey	Man	Reference
Butadiene Monoxide	V_{max}/k_m (nmol·L/min/mg/nmol)	15	11						8	[20]
Flunarizine	V_{max}/k_m (pmol·L/μmol/min)						28.0		5.7	[23]
Remoxipride	T_m/T_{el}	0.068	0.175	0.0077			0.67		0.55	[41]
Imidapril	T_m/T_{el}						0.125	0.075		[43]
Dofetilide	T_m/T_{el}	0.89	0.69				2.08		9.33	[35]
Enciprazine	T_m/T_{el}	0					0.072		0.284	[34]
Mianserin	T_m/T_{el}	0.017	0.011		0.027				0.023	[10]
Fenfluramine	T_m/T_{el}	0.032	0			0			0	[25]
Venlafaxine	T_m/T_{el}	0.149	0.019				0.092	0.0035	0.051	[17]

The ratio T_m/T_{el} is estimated from the ratio of urine recovery of the parent drug to the total urine recovery of all metabolites.

$$\text{Metabolic rate } (v) \; = \; \frac{V_{max} \cdot C}{k_m + C} \tag{4.14}$$

The maximum rate of metabolism V_{max} and the Michaelis-Menten constant k_m can be measured in vitro from microsomes and cytosol of liver fractions. Assuming a first-order metabolic kinetics when $C \ll k_m$, the intrinsic clearance is equal to the ratio of V_{max} to k_m:

$$\text{Intrinsic clearance } (\text{Cl}'_{intrinsic}) \; = \; \frac{V_{max}}{k_m} \tag{4.15}$$

It has been proposed that the maximum metabolic rate can be scaled between species with an exponent of 0.75 [38]. Unfortunately, information on interspecies scaling of metabolic rate is inadequate to validate this scaling exponent. However, hepatic extraction ratios of several drugs in the rat have been accurately estimated [Equation (4.15)] from in vitro measurement of intrinsic clearance [30].

To summarize, the hepatic elimination time in man can be estimated from Equation (4.12), with the volume of distribution scaled up from animals using Equation (4.10) and the extraction ratio estimated from Equation (4.13) with in vitro measurement of intrinsic clearance.

Absorption

The rate and extent of absorption of drugs depend on a number of physiological factors, which may be different between species. These physiological factors include permeability, pH, transit time, intestinal metabolism, bile secretion, and gastric emptying. The transport characteristics of rat and human intestinal brush-border membranes of cephalosporins are comparable, while that of rabbits is an inadequate animal model for investigating absorption of β-lactam antibiotics [36]. The gastric emptying of tablets and granules in humans, dogs, pigs, and rabbits were compared under the fasting condition [2]. It appeared that the dog is a better animal model for bioavailability studies under fasting conditions than the pig and the rabbit. There may be interspecies differences in the extent of intestinal metabolism; for example, the extent of intestinal hydrolysis of certain glucuronide conjugates is different between mouse, rat, and rabbit [18]. The difference in metabolism may be due to a difference in intestinal pH or bacterial-derived enzyme activity. The intestinal transit time may affect the extent of drug absorption. The effect of interspecies difference in intestinal transit time on drug absorption has been estimated using a compartmental model [6]. The bioavailability and urine recovery of several drugs after oral

TABLE 4.5. The Interspecies Difference in Bioavailability and Urine Recovery of Several Drugs after Oral Administration.

Drug	Parameters	Mouse	Rat	Hamster	Guinea Pig	Rabbit	Dog	Monkey	Man	Reference
Remoxipride	fF (%)	8	<1	4			94		93	[41]
Verapamil	fF (%)		13.0						22.0	[24]
Dofetilide	fF (%)	66	35				72		83	[35]
Oxiracetam	$X_{u.tot}/D$ (%)		39.7				80.7		56.4	[14]
Imidapril	$X_{u.tot}/D$ (%)		46.3				37.1	29.0		[43]
Bepridil	$X_{u.tot}/D$ (%)	48.1	28.2			53.0		40.3	66.6	[42]
H-FCE22178	$X_{u.tot}/D$ (%)		64.6						91.0	[37]
Enciprazine	$X_{u.tot}/D$ (%)	32.2					44.7		59.3	[34]
Mianserin	$X_{u.tot}/D$ (%)	29.5	44		41.5	72.0			41.5	[10]
Fenfluramine	$X_{u.tot}/D$ (%)	96	97				92		92	[25]
Venlafaxine	$X_{u.tot}/D$ (%)	92.6	97.0				86.0	85.3	92.1	[17]

administration are shown in Table 4.5. In general, the dog is a better animal model for investigating the extent of absorption than the rat and mouse.

REFERENCES

1. Adolph E. F., "Quantitative relations in the physiological constitutions of mammals," *Science,* 1949; 109:579–585.
2. Aoyagi N., Ogata H., Kaniwa N., Uchiyama M., Yasuda Y., and Tanioka Y., "Gastric emptying of tablets and granules in humans, dogs, pigs, and stomach-emptying-controlled rabbits," *Journal of Pharmaceutical Sciences,* 1992; 81(12):1170–1174.
3. Benschop H. P. and De Jong L. P. A., "Toxicokinetics of soman: Species variation and stereospecificity in elimination pathways," *Neuroscience & Biobehavioral Reviews,* 1991; 15:73–77.
4. Bernareggi A. and Rowland M., "Physiologic modeling of cyclosporin kinetics in rat and man," *Journal of Pharmacokinetics and Biopharmaceutics,* 1991; 19(1):21–50.
5. Bischoff K. B., Dedrich R. L., Zaharko D. S., and Longstreth J. A., "Methotrexate pharmacokinetics," *Journal of Pharmaceutical Sciences,* 1971; 60(8):1128–1133.
6. Bischoff K. B., Dedrich R. L., and Zaharko D. S., "Preliminary model for methotrexate pharmacokinetics," *Journal of Pharmaceutical Sciences,* 1970; 59(2):149–154.
7. Davis C. D., Schut H. A. J., Adamson R. H., Thorgeirsson U. P., Thorgeirsson S. S., and Snyderwine E. G., "Mutagenic activation of IQ, PhIP and MeIQx by hepatic microsomes from rat, monkey and man: Low mutagenic activation of MeIQx in cynomolgus monkey in vitro reflects low DNA adduct levels in vivo," *Carcinogenesis,* 1993; 14(1):61–65.
8. Dedrick R. L., Bischoff K. B., and Zaharko D. S. "Interspecies correlation of plasma concentration history of methotrexate (NSC-740)," *Cancer Chemotherapy Reports,* 1970; part 1, 54(2):95–101.
9. Dedrick R. L. and Bischoff K. B. "Species similarities in pharmacokinetics," *Federation Proceedings,* 1980; 39(1):54–59.
10. Delbressine L. P. C., Moonen N. E. M., Kasperson F. M., Jacobs P. L., and Wagenaars G. L., "Biotransformation of mianserin in laboratory animals and man," *Xenobiotica,* 1992; 22(2):227–236.
11. Edwards N. A. "Scaling of renal functions in mammals," *Comp. Biochem. Physiol.,* 1975; 52A:63–66.
12. Efthymiopoulos C., Battaglia R., and Benedetti M. S. "Animal pharmacokinetics and interspecies scaling of FCE 22101, a penem antibiotic," *Journal of Antimicrobial Chemotherapy,* 1991; 27:517–526.
13. Gillette, J. R., "Application of pharmacokinetic principals in the extrapolation of animal data to humans," *Clinical Toxicology,* 1976; 9(5):709–722.
14. Gschwind H. P., Schutz H., Wigger N., and Bentley P., "Absorption and disposition of ¹⁴C-labelled oxiracetam in rat, dog and man," *European Journal of Drug Metabolism and Pharmacokinetics,* 1992; 17(1):67–82.
15. Gunnarsson P. O., Andersson S., Sandberg A. A., and Ellman M., "Accumulation of estramustine and estromustine in adipose tissue of rates and humans," *Cancer Chemother. Pharmacol.* 1991; 28:361–364.

16. Hinderling P. H., Dilea C., Koziol T., and Millington G., "Comparative kinetics of sematilide in four species," *Drug Metabolism and Disposition*, 1993; 21(4):662–669.

17. Howell S. R., Husbands G. E. M., Scatina J. A., and Sisenwine S. F., "Metabolic disposition of ¹⁴C-enlafaxine in mouse, rat, dog, rhesus monkey and man," *Xenobiotica*, 1993; 23(4):349–359.

18. Kenyon E. M. and Calabrese E. J. "Extent and implications of interspecies differences in the intestinal hydrolysis of certain glucuronide conjugates," *Xenobiotica*, 1993; 23(4):373–381.

19. Krause W., Kuhne G., Jakobs U., and Hoyer G. A., "Biotransformation of the antidepressant DL-rolipram I. Isolation and identification of metabolites from rat, monkey, and human urine," *Drug Metabolism and Disposition*, 1993; 21(4):682–689.

20. Kreuzer P. E., Kessler W., Welter H. F., Baur C., and Filser J. G., "Enzyme specific kinetics of 1,2-epoxybutene-3 in microsomes and cytosol from livers of mouse, rat, and man," *Arch. Toxicol.*, 1991; 65:59–67.

21. Kurihara A., Naganuma H., Hisaoka M., Tokiwa H., and Kawahara Y., "Prediction of human pharmacokinetics of panipenem-betamipron, a new carbapenem, from animal data," *Antimicrobial Agents and Chemotherapy*, 1992; 36(9):1810–1816.

22. Lashev L. D. and Pashov D. V., "Interspecies variations in plasma half-life of ampicillin, amoxycillin, sulphadimidine and sulphacetamide related to variations in body mass," *Research in Veterinary Science*, 1992; 53:160–164.

23. Lavrijsen K., Van Houdt J., Van Dyck D., Hendrickx J., Bockx M., Hurkmans R., Meuldermans W., Le Jeune L., Lauwers W., and Heykants J., "Comparative metabolism of flunarizine in rats, dogs and man: An in vitro study with subcellular liver fractions and isolated hepatocytes," *Xenobiotica*, 1992; 22(7):815–836.

24. Manitpisitkul P. and Chiou W. L., "Intravenous verapamil kinetics in rats: Marked arteriovenous concentration difference and comparison with humans," *Biopharmaceutics & Drug Disposition*, 1993; 14:555–566.

25. Marchant N. C., Btreen M. A., Wallace D., Bass S., Taylor A. R., Ings R. M. J., Campbell D. B., and Williams J., "Comparative biodisposition and metabolism of ¹⁴C-(±)-fenfluramine in mouse, rat, dog and man," *Xenobiotica*, 1992; 22(11):1251–1266.

26. Matsuda M., Sakashita M., Mizuki Y., Yamaguchi T., Fujii T., and Sekine Y., "Comparative pharmacokinetics of the histimine H1-receptor antagonist ebastine and its active metabolite carebastine in rats, guinea pigs, dogs and monkeys," *Arzneim.*, 1994; 44(I)1:55–59.

27. Midgley I., Hood A. J., Proctor P., Chasseaud L. F., Irons S. R., Cheng K. N., Brindley C. J., and Bonn R., "Metabolic fate of ¹⁴C-camostat mesylate in man, rat and dog after intravenous administration," *Xenobiotica*, 1994; 24(1):79–92.

28. Ohmori S., Taniguchi T., Rikihisa T., Kanakubo Y., and Kitada M., "Species differences of testosterone 16-hydroxylases in liver microsomes of guinea pig, rat and dog," *Xenobiotica*, 1993; 23(4):419–426.

29. Paxton J. W., Young D., and Robertson G. G., "Pharmacokinetics of acridine-4-carboxamide in the rat, with extrapolation to humans," *Cancer Chemother. Pharmacol.*, 1993; 32:323–325.

30. Rane A., Wilkinson G. R. and Shand D. G., "Prediction of hepatic extraction ratio from in vitro measurement of intrinsic clearance," *The Journal of Pharmacology and Experimental Therapeutics*, 1977; 200(2):420–424.

31. Reigner B. G., Bois F. Y., and Tozer T. N., "Pentachlorophenol carcinogenicity: Ex-

trapolation of risk from mice to humans," *Human & Experimental Toxicology,* 1993; 12:215–225.

32. Ritschel W. A., Vachharajani N. N., Johnson R. D., and Hussain A. S., "The allometric approach for interspecies scaling of pharmacokinetic parameters," *Comp. Biochem. Physiol.,* 1992; 103C(2):249–253.

33. Ritschel W. A., Johnson R. D., Vachharajani N. N., and Hussain A. S., "Prediction of the volume of distribution of 7-hydroxycoumarin in man from in vitro and ex vivo data obtained in rate," *Biopharmaceutics & Drug Disposition,* 13:389–402.

34. Scatina J. A., Lockhead S. R., Cayen M. N., and Sisenwine S. F., "Metabolic disposition of enciprazine, a non-benzodiazepine anxiolytic drug, in rat, dog and man," *Xenobiotica,* 1991; 21(12):1591–1604.

35. Smith D. A., Rasmussen H. S., Stopher D. A. and Walker D. K., "Pharmacokinetics and metabolism of dofetilide in mouse, rat, dog and man," *Xenobiotica,* 1992; 22(6):709–719.

36. Sugawara M., Toda T., Iseki K., Miyazaki K., Shiroto H., Kondo Y., and Uchino J., "Transport characteristics of cephalosporin antibiotics across intestinal brush-border membrane in man, rat and rabbit," *J. Pharm. Pharmacol.,* 1992; 44:968–972.

37. Thomassin J., Battablia R., Allievi C., Castelli M. G., and Benedetti M. S., "In vivo glucuronidation in rat and humans of 5,6-dihydro-7-(1H-imidazol-1-YL)-naphthalene-2-carboxylic acid, a selective inhibitor of thromboxane synthase," *Drug Metabolism and Disposition,* 1993; 21(1):151–155.

38. Travis C. C., White R. K. and Ward R. C., "Interspecies extrapolation of pharmacokinetics," *J. Theor. Biol.,* 1990; 142:285–304.

39. Travis C. C. and Bowers J. C., "Interspecies scaling of anesthetic potency," *Toxicology and Industrial Health,* 1991; 7(4):249–260.

40. Tsunekawa Y., Hasegawa T., Nadai M., Takagi K., and Nabeshima T., "Interspecies differences and scaling for the pharmacokinetics of xanthine derivatives," *J. Pharm. Pharmacol.,* 1992; 44:594–599.

41. Widman M., Nilsson L. B., Bryske B., and Lundstrom J., "Disposition of remoxipride in different species," *Arzneim.,* 1993; 43(I)3:287–297.

42. Wu W. N., Fritchard J. F., Ng K. T., Hills J. F., Uetz J. A., Yorgey K. A., McKown L. A., and O'Neill P. J., "Disposition of bepridil in laboratory animals and man," *Xenobiotica,* 1992; 22(2):153–169.

43. Yamada Y., Endo M., Otsuka M., and Takaiti O., "Metabolic fate of the new angiotensin-converting enzyme inhibitor imidapril in animal," *Arzneim.,* 1992; 42(I)4:499–506.

44. Davis B. and Morris T., "Physiological parameters in laboratory animals and humans," *Pharm. Research,* 1993; 10(7):1093–1095.

FORMULATION FACTORS

CHAPTER 5

Influence of Administration Route on Pharmacokinetics—Bioavailability

INTRODUCTION

The relative availability of a drug and its metabolites may change as the drug is administered by different routes to the systemic circulation. A bioavailability study is designed to detect such differences in availability of drugs. A difference in bioavailability between two administration routes may be caused by the difference in permeability of the drug through the barriers between the blood vessels and absorption sites; in the available surface area for absorption; in secretion at the sites, which may help or hinder the absorption; or in transit time limit at the sites. Typical administration routes include intravenous, oral [1,4,5], intramuscular [12,13], intracolonic [3], intranasal [14,15], topical [2], and subcutaneous [16,17] administration. The most common bioavailability study is a comparison between oral and intravenous administrations, where the intravenous administration can be given as a bolus or infusion [6–8]. A relative bioavailability is also frequently conducted between oral and intramuscular, intranasal and oral, or intracolonic and oral administrations.

The key pharmacokinetic parameters in a bioavailability study are defined to capture the difference in pharmacokinetics between administration routes: the rate and extent of absorption. The rate at which a drug is presented to the systemic circulation can be instantaneous (intravenous bolus), zero-order (intravenous infusion), or first-order (most of oral, intranasal, intracolonic), depending on the route and the method of administration and the absorption kinetics. Therefore, in order to characterize the absorption, the key time constants and pharmacokinetic parameters in a bioavailability study are the absorption time constant (defining the rate of absorption) and the bioavailability (defining the extent of absorption).

When a drug is given orally, the bioavailability is a function of two parameters: the fraction absorbed (f) and the extent of first pass effects ($1 - F$), where f is the fraction of the drug absorbed in the intestine and $1 - F$ is the first pass loss of the drug.

Some common themes in time constant view may be observed in bioavailability as well as other studies. For example, the first pass effect may be observed in many pharmacokinetic studies. If the first pass metabolism is confirmed in a bioavailability study, then the appearance of metabolites in the blood will be faster following oral administration than intravenous administration. This will result in a shorter mean residence time of metabolites following oral administration than intravenous administration since the metabolites will be formed earlier after the oral dose [18]. Rapid appearance of metabolites in the blood will also be observed in other studies. The first pass effect may also be detected in a food study, where the drug is administered under fed and fasting conditions. It is likely that food will reduce the first pass metabolism and increase the bioavailability of the drug (Chapter 13); therefore, food will prolong the mean residence time of metabolites. If the first pass effect is extensive, it can be expected that hepatic elimination time may be shorter than the renal elimination time. In this case, hepatic diseases will have great impact on the total elimination time (Chapter 18), while renal impairment will have less influence on the total elimination time (Chapter 17). When the total elimination time becomes shorter than the absorption time, a flip-flop of the plasma concentration profile occurs after the oral administration, where the terminal decay time represents the absorption time instead of the elimination time. If a flip-flop is identified in the bioavailability study, the decay time in other studies must be interpreted with caution. For example, the hepatic elimination time may be different between young and elderly subjects in an age study (Chapter 15), while the decay time may be similar between the two subject groups due to the flip-flop.

In this chapter, four models are used to describe the absorption through different routes: (1) one-compartment model with intravenous bolus, intravenous infusion, and first-order absorption; (2) two-compartment model with intravenous bolus and first-order absorption; (3) first pass model with intravenous bolus and first-order absorption; and (4) bioavailability model with intravenous bolus and first-order absorption. Four simulated case studies and three literature examples are discussed in this chapter to illustrate the utilities of these models in bioavailability studies. Additional examples of bioavailability studies can be found in References [1–11]. The derivation of the relationship between the area under the curve and the area under the first moment curve with time constants for each model is listed in Appendix 3.

PHARMACOKINETIC MODELS

This section presents four models that are useful in describing absorption through different administration routes. The goal is to establish simple relationships between time constants and measurable parameters such as (1) mean residence time, which is the sum of input and output times, and (2) area under the curves. The derivations of these relationships are straightforward and are discussed in Chapter 2.

Model 1: One-Compartment Model with Intravenous Bolus, Intravenous Infusion, or First-Order Absorption

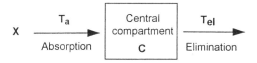

This is the classic one-compartmental model, which can be applied to drugs with a concentration profile exhibiting monoexponential elimination phase. In this model, the absorption and elimination rates are assumed to be of first-order linear kinetics, with time constants being T_a and T_{el}, respectively. The volume of distribution is represented by V. The bioavailability of the drug following an oral dose is equal to the product of the fraction absorbed from the intestine (f) and the fraction not metabolized by the first pass effect (F).

In the analysis of a bioavailability study, the goal is to obtain estimates of the key parameters T_a and fF. These estimates can be obtained simply by measuring AUCs and AUMCs. The mean residence time of the plasma concentration profile is the ratio of AUMC to AUC.

ORAL ADMINISTRATION

Following an oral administration, the mean residence time is simply the sum of input and output times

$$\text{Mean residence time following oral administration } (\bar{t}_{po}) = \frac{\text{AUMC}_{po}}{\text{AUC}_{po}}$$

$$(5.1)$$

$$= \text{Input time } (T_{po,in}) + \text{Output time } (T_{po,out}) = T_a + T_{el}$$

Therefore, the mean residence time is the sum of the absorption time (T_a) and the elimination time (T_{el}).

The decay time constant of the terminal phase is calculated from the inverse of the terminal slope of the logarithm concentration-time curve. The slope is typically calculated by a curve-fitting technique. An alternative to curve-fitting is the following formula:

$$\frac{1}{\text{Decay time } (T_z)} = \lambda_z = 2\frac{(t_{\text{last}} - t_{\text{ref}}) \ln C_{\text{ref}} - \text{AU} \ln C_{t_{\text{ref}} - t_{\text{last}}}}{(t_{\text{last}} - t_{\text{ref}})^2}$$

(5.2)

where t_{last} is the time point of the last measurable concentration, t_{ref} is a time point that exceeds three times the half-life of either absorption or elimination (see Appendix 2) and $\text{AU} \ln C_{t_{\text{ref}} - t_{\text{last}}} = \int_{t_{\text{ref}}}^{t_{\text{last}}} \ln (C)dt$. The estimate for T_z after an oral dose gives an estimate to T_{el} or T_a, whichever one is larger.

$$T_{z,\text{po}} = \text{Max } \{T_a, T_{\text{el}}\}$$

(5.3)

If it turns out that T_a is larger than T_{el}, we have an estimate for this key time constant, T_a, from T_z. However, one can never be sure which of the T_a and T_{el} is greater, unless the intravenous data are available for a direct estimate of T_{el}.

INTRAVENOUS ADMINISTRATION

The mean residence time of the concentration profile after an intravenous dose is equal to the output time:

Mean residence time following

$$\text{intravenous administration } (\bar{t}_{\text{iv}}) = \frac{\text{AUMC}_{\text{iv}}}{\text{AUC}_{\text{iv}}}$$

(5.4)

$$= \text{Output time } (T_{\text{iv,out}}) = T_{\text{el}}$$

Thus, $\bar{t}_{\text{iv}}$ provides an estimate of T_{el}. This estimation of T_{el} should be accurate as long as AUMC and AUC, especially AUMC, can be accurately estimated. There are two additional methods for estimating T_{el}. One of the alternatives is that the estimate for T_z after an intravenous dose gives an estimate to T_{el}.

$$\text{Elimination time } (T_{\text{el}}) = T_{z,\text{iv}}$$

(5.5)

T_z can be estimated by either curve stripping or Equation (5.2). Apparently, the accuracy of this estimation of T_{el} depends on the accuracy of the estimated $T_{z,iv}$. Another alternative of estimating T_{el} is

$$\text{Elimination time } (T_{el}) = \text{AUC}_{iv}/C_0 \qquad (5.6)$$

where C_0 is the initial concentration obtained by extrapolation to time 0. The advantage of this estimation of T_{el} is that Equation (5.6) holds even when a peripheral compartment is added to Model 1 (as the two-compartmental model in Model 2), while Equations (5.4) and (5.5) do not apply in the case of a two-compartmental model. However, the error involved in the extrapolated value of C_0 may be great, especially when the first few time points of concentration data are not close enough to time 0.

The mean residence time following the intravenous administration is shorter than that after an oral administration, and the difference between the two, from Equations (5.1) and (5.4), is the mean absorption time:

$$\text{Absorption time } (T_a) = \bar{t}_{po} - \bar{t}_{iv} \qquad (5.7)$$

The bioavailability of the oral dose is equal to the ratio AUC of the oral dose to that of the intravenous dose (see Appendix 3).

$$\text{Bioavailability } (fF) = \frac{\text{AUC}_{po}}{\text{AUC}_{iv}} \qquad (5.8)$$

This completes the estimations of T_a, T_{el}, and fF without the use of extrapolations or curve-fitting techniques.

Further dissection of the bioavailability factor (fF) can be done with urine data. Assuming renal excretion is the predominant elimination route, then the fraction absorbed is the ratio of urine recovery to the dose.

$$\text{Fraction absorbed } (f) = \frac{X_u}{X_0} \qquad (5.9)$$

From Equations (5.8) and (5.9), the first pass effect $(1 - F)$ can be estimated.

The volume of distribution of the central compartment can be estimated only with an intravenous dose, not with an oral dose. To estimate the volume of the central compartment, the initial concentration at time 0 is first obtained by extrapolation. Then the volume of distribution is equal to the ratio of the dose to the initial concentration.

$$\text{Volume of distribution of central compartment } (V) = \frac{X_0}{C_0} \quad (5.10)$$

When the error in the extrapolated value of C_0 is great, Equation (5.10) would not provide a good estimate of V. The following equation should then be used to estimate V_c from T_{el}.

$$\text{Volume of distribution of central compartment } (V) = \frac{T_{el}X_0}{AUC_{iv}} \quad (5.11)$$

where T_{el} could be estimated from Equation (5.4) or Equation (5.5) [in the latter case, T_{ziv} could be estimated by Equation (5.2) or curve-stripping technique].

INTRAVENOUS INFUSION

The mean residence time of the plasma concentration profile after an intravenous infusion is longer than that after a bolus intravenous dose because of the prolonged infusion time (T). The mean residence time of plasma concentration curves is simply the sum of input and output times:

$$\text{Mean residence time following iv infusion } (\bar{t}_{infu}) = \frac{AUMC_{infu}}{AUC_{infu}}$$

$$= \text{Input time } (T_{infu,in}) + \text{Output time } (T_{infu,out}) = T_{el} + \frac{T}{2} \quad (5.12)$$

This equation provides a way to estimate T_{el}. From the mean residence time of plasma concentration curves after oral administration and intravenous infusion, the absorption time constant can be estimated as follows:

$$\text{Absorption time } (T_a) = \bar{t}_{po} - \bar{t}_{infu} + \frac{T}{2} \quad (5.13)$$

The absolute bioavailability of the oral dose compared with the intravenous infusion is the ratio of the area under the concentration curve between the two dosing routes:

$$\text{Bioavailability } (fF) = \frac{AUC_{po}}{AUC_{infu}} \quad (5.14)$$

In this way, the parameters T_{el}, T_a, and fF can be estimated from intravenous infusion and oral administration data.

The volume of the central compartment can be estimated by first calculating T_{el} from Equation (5.2) and then using the following equation:

$$\text{Volume of distribution } (V) = \frac{X_0 T_{el}}{\text{AUC}} \qquad (5.15)$$

Model 2: Two-Compartment Model with Intravenous Bolus and First-Order Absorption

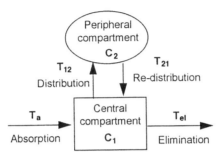

Plasma drug concentration profiles after intravenous bolus doses frequently show biexponential elimination phases [6], especially when the first few sampling points are taken within a short time following the dose. The biexponential phase is a result of distinctly different distribution and elimination rates. Model 2 is a classic two-compartmental model, accounting for distribution as well as elimination. The mean residence time can be calculated as the ratio of area under the first moment of the concentration curve to the area under the concentration curve. Following an oral administration, the mean residence time is the sum of input and output times (see Chapter 2).

$$\text{Mean residence time following oral administration } (\bar{t}_{po}) = \frac{\text{AUMC}_{po}}{\text{AUC}_{po}}$$

$$= \text{Input time } (T_{po,in}) + \text{Output time } (T_{po,out}) = T_a + T_{el} + T_{el}\frac{T_{21}}{T_{12}}$$

$$(5.16)$$

The third term , $T_{el}(T_{21}/T_{12})$, of the above equation does not appear in the mean residence time of the one-compartmental model [Equation (5.1)]. The third term in the above equation represents the contribution of the distribution to the mean residence time. If a drug can easily penetrate into the tissue compartment but slowly release back to the blood, indicated by a small T_{12} value and a large T_{21}, the mean residence will be prolonged.

Following an intravenous dose, the mean residence time is equal to the output time:

$$\text{Mean residence time following iv administration } (\bar{t}_{iv}) = \frac{\text{AUMC}_{iv}}{\text{AUC}_{iv}}$$

$$= \text{Output time } (T_{iv,out}) = T_{el} + T_{el}\frac{T_{21}}{T_{12}} \tag{5.17}$$

The absorption time constant can then be estimated from the difference in mean residence time between the oral and intravenous doses:

$$\text{Absorption time } (T_a) = \bar{t}_{po} - \bar{t}_{iv} \tag{5.18}$$

The absolute bioavailability of the oral dose is equal to the ratio of the area under the curve after the oral dose to that after the intravenous dose.

$$\text{Bioavailability } (fF) = \frac{\text{AUC}_{po}}{\text{AUC}_{iv}} \tag{5.19}$$

The formulars for estimation of absorption time T_a and the bioavailability fF in the two-compartmental model [Equations (5.18) and (5.19)] are the same as those for the one-compartmental model [Equations (5.7) and (5.8)]. The volume of the central compartment can be estimated from the extrapolated initial concentration in the blood:

$$\text{Volume of central compartment } (V_1) = \frac{X_0}{C_0} \tag{5.20}$$

The elimination time constant can then be calculated from the volume of the central compartment, dose, and the area under the concentration curve after the intravenous dose:

$$\text{Elimination time } (T_{el}) = \frac{\text{AUC}_{iv}V_1}{X_0} \tag{5.21}$$

Model 3: First Pass Model with Intravenous Bolus and First-Order Absorption

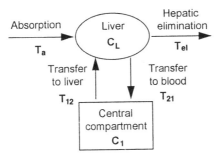

Drugs with extensive metabolism may be subjected to the first pass effect. After a drug is absorbed, it is immediately metabolized by the liver enzymes before it enters the systemic circulation. Model 3 is a classic first pass model, in which the drug is absorbed and passes through the liver immediately, where it may be metabolized or distribute to the central compartment. The difference between Models 2 and 3 is that the drug is absorbed into the central compartment in the former, but into the liver compartment in the latter. Notice that, in most of the cases, only the concentration in the central compartment is available.

In Model 3, after the first pass effect, the drug may recirculate between the central compartment and the liver, and further metabolism will occur in the liver. As a result of the distribution between the liver and the central compartment, there may be a biexponential elimination phase according to this model. The mean residence time of the concentration curve after an oral dose is the sum of input and output times (see Chapter 2):

$$\text{Mean residence time following oral administration } (\bar{t}_{po}) = \frac{\text{AUMC}_{po}}{\text{AUC}_{po}}$$

$$= \text{Input time } (T_{po,in}) + \text{Output time } (T_{po,out}) = T_a + T_{el} + T_{12} + T_{el}\frac{T_{12}}{T_{21}}$$

$$(5.22)$$

where the mean residence time can be estimated from the ratio of the area under the first moment of the concentration curve to the area under the curve. Following an intravenous administration, the mean residence time of the concentration curve is equal to the output time:

Mean residence time following iv administration $(\bar{t}_{iv}) = \dfrac{\text{AUMC}_{iv}}{\text{AUC}_{iv}}$

$$= \text{Output time } (T_{iv,out}) = -\dfrac{1}{1/T_{21} + 1/T_{el}} + \dfrac{1}{\lambda_1} + \dfrac{1}{\lambda_2} = T_{el} + T_{el}\dfrac{T_{21}}{T_{12}}$$

$$(5.23)$$

where the definitions of λ_1 and λ_2 can be found in Appendix 3. The absorption can be estimated as follows:

$$\text{Absorption time } (T_a) = \bar{t}_{po} - \bar{t}_{iv} \qquad (5.24)$$

The bioavailability of the oral dose is the ratio of the elimination time constant to the sum of elimination and distribution time constants from the liver.

$$\text{Bioavailability } (F) = \dfrac{\text{AUC}_{po}}{\text{AUC}_{iv}} = \dfrac{T_{el}}{T_{21} + T_{el}} \qquad (5.25)$$

Model 4: Bioavailability Model with Intravenous Bolus and First-Order Absorption

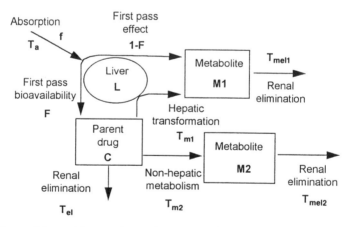

This model provides an alternative way to describe the first pass effect in addition to Model 3. The drug is absorbed with an absorption time constant T_a. Immediately after the absorption, a fraction $(1 - F)$ of the drug is metabolized in the liver and converted to metabolite M1, and the rest of the drug (F) enters the systemic circulation; therefore, the bioavailability is equal to the fraction absorbed f times F. The first pass effect is assumed to occur immediately after the absorption and is not a rate limited step. The drug in the blood can further be metabolized to M1 through the hepatic enzymes or to M2 through other enzymes. The parent drug and metabolites can be excreted renally with first-order elimination rates. The bioavailabilities of the parent drug and the metabolites can be obtained from the area under the concentration curves:

$$\frac{AUC_{C,po}}{AUC_{C,iv}} = fF \tag{5.26}$$

$$\frac{AUC_{M1,po}}{AUC_{M1,iv}} = fF + \frac{f(1 - F)(T_{m2}T_{el} + T_{m1}T_{m2} + T_{m1}T_{el})}{T_{m2}T_{el}} \tag{5.27}$$

$$\frac{AUC_{M2,po}}{AUC_{M2,iv}} = fF \tag{5.28}$$

Notice that the first pass effect contributes a second term to the bioavailability of metabolite M1 [Equation (5.27)]. Therefore, if the oral bioavailability of the parent drug is smaller than the oral bioavailability of a metabolite, the drug is subjected to the first pass effect. The volume of the central compartment can be obtained by first estimating the initial plasma concentration after the intravenous dose.

$$\text{Volume of central compartment } (V_c) = \frac{X_0}{C_0} \tag{5.29}$$

Then the elimination time constant is calculated as follows:

$$\text{Elimination time } (T_{el}) = \frac{AUC_{iv}V_c}{X_0} \tag{5.30}$$

The renal clearance time of a metabolite (T_{mel}/V_m) is equal to the ratio of the area under the plasma concentration curve to the cumulative amount of the metabolite in the urine:

$$\text{Renal clearance time of metabolite } \left(\frac{T_{mel}}{V_m}\right) = \frac{AUC_M}{X_{um}} \tag{5.31}$$

The elimination time of a metabolite can be estimated from the decay time constant of the metabolite concentration profile by Equation (5.2), if the elimination of metabolite is slower than the elimination of the parent drug.

However, the elimination time of the parent drug may dominate the decay time of the metabolite, if the elimination time of the parent drug is longer than that of the metabolite. A more reliable method for estimating the elimination time constant is based on the following equation:

$$\text{Elimination time of metabolite } (T_{\text{mel}}) = \bar{t}_{\text{M}} - \bar{t}_{\text{C}} \qquad (5.32)$$

Then the volume of distribution of the metabolite in the central compartment can be estimated by

$$\text{Volume of distribution of metabolite } (V_{\text{m}}) = \frac{T_{\text{mel}} X_{\text{um}}}{\text{AUC}_{\text{M}}} \qquad (5.33)$$

The hepatic elimination time constant can be estimated from the intravenous data:

$$\text{Hepatic elimination time } (T_{\text{m}}) = \frac{\text{AUC}_{\text{Civ}} V_{\text{c}}}{X_{\text{umiv}}} \qquad (5.34)$$

where AUC_{Civ} is the area under the curve of the parent drug after it is given intravenously. The absorption time constant can be estimated from the difference in the mean residence time between oral and intravenous doses.

$$\text{Absorption time } (T_{\text{a}}) = \bar{t}_{\text{po}} - \bar{t}_{\text{iv}} \qquad (5.35)$$

The fraction absorbed f can be estimated from the urine recovery data, assuming renal excretion is the predominant elimination route of the drug and metabolite.

$$\text{Fraction absorbed } (f) = \frac{X_{\text{uc}} + X_{\text{um}}}{X_{0}} \qquad (5.36)$$

CASE STUDIES

Case 1: Intravenous Bolus, Infusion, and Oral Administrations

In this example, a drug is administered to a subject orally and intravenously (bolus and 30-minute infusion) to assess the bioavailability of the oral formulation. There is no metabolite for this drug, and the drug is eliminated renally. The objective is to determine the extent (f) and the absorption time (T_a) after the drug is given orally. The plasma drug concentrations after the administration of the drug through three different routes, oral, intravenous bolus, and intravenous infusion, are simulated using Model 1 and shown in Figure 5.1. In this example, the intravenous infusion is given in a 30-minute interval at a constant rate.

Theoretically, the estimated oral bioavailability relative to intravenous bolus or intravenous infusion should be the same. In practice, the use of intravenous infusion can avoid a high initial serum concentration and reduce the possibility of adverse events associated with the high concentration. However, an intravenous bolus dose will give a direct estimate for the volume of the central compartment from the initial plasma concentration at time 0. The estimated pharmacokinetic parameters applying the time constant analysis are shown in Table 5.1, and the estimated time constants are presented in Figure 5.2. The assumption made when estimating oral bioavailability by comparing the area under the curve after oral and intravenous administrations is that the elimination time is the same in the two treatments. In order to estimate the elimination time constant, a portion of terminal phase must be selected where the absorption no longer occurs. One reasonable choice of the terminal phase for the calculation of elimination time is the portion after two times the mean residence time $(2T_a + 2T_{el})$, which is longer than three times the absorption half-life $(3 \cdot 0.693*T_a)$, and after which time most of the absorption has been completed. Therefore, the elimination time constant can be estimated 14 hours $(= 2 \cdot \bar{t}_{po})$ after the oral dose by assuming a single exponential phase.

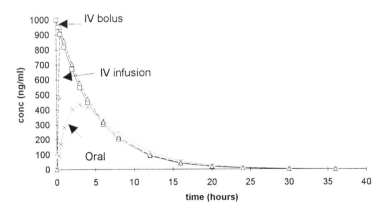

FIGURE 5.1. Simulated plasma drug concentration profiles with monoexponential decay, following intravenous bolus, infusion, and oral administration using Model 1. The time constant plot comparing the three administrations is shown in Figure 5.2. The parameters used in this simulation are $X_0 = 10,000$ μg (oral or intravenous dose), $f = 0.8$, $F = 1$, $V = 10$ L, $K_a = 0.5$ hr^{-1}, $K_{el} = 0.2$ hr^{-1}, $T = 0.5$ hr, and $R = 20,000$ $\mu g/hr$.

TABLE 5.1. The Estimated and Model Values of the Pharmacokinetic
Parameters for the Example Shown in Figure 5.1.

Parameter	Time Constant Analysis	Model Value	Equation
$\bar{t}_{iv}$ (hr)	4.91	5.0	(5.4)
$\bar{t}_{inf}$ (hr)	5.16	5.25	(5.12)
t_{po} (hr)	6.91	7.0	(5.1)
T_{el} (hr)	5.0	5.0	(5.4)
T_{a} (hr)	2.0	2.0	(5.7)
$fF = AUC_{po}/AUC_{iv}$	0.79	0.8	(5.8)
$fF = AUC_{po}/AUC_{infu}$	0.79	0.8	(5.14)

Now let us examine the time constant plot (Figure 5.2). The estimated
elimination time is equal to the mean residence time following the intravenous bolus dose and is longer than the absorption time. The bioavailabilities for the oral administration relative to either the intravenous bolus
or the infusion are the same. Compared to the two intravenous doses, the
oral bioavailability is about 79%. The mean residence time after the oral
administration is 6.9 hours, which is a sum of absorption time and elimination time. The mean residence time after the intravenous infusion is slightly
longer than that after the intravenous bolus dose, because of the prolonged
infusion time. A bioavailability study is a good opportunity to estimate the
absorption time since both oral and intravenous data are available. The ab-

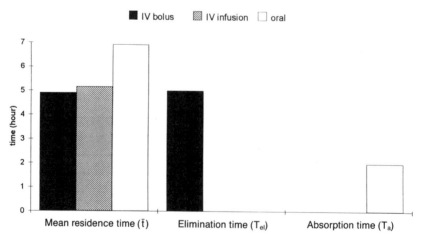

FIGURE 5.2. The time constant plot comparing intravenous bolus, infusion, and oral administrations in the example shown in Figure 5.1. The mean residence time ($\bar{t}$) after the oral
administration is 6.9 hours, which is a sum of absorption time (T_a) and elimination time (T_{el}).

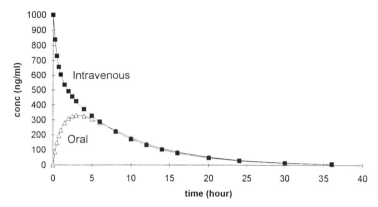

FIGURE 5.3. Simulated plasma drug concentration profiles with biexponential terminal phase, following oral and intravenous administrations using Model 2. The time constant plot comparing the two treatments is shown in Figure 5.4. The parameters used in this simulation are $X_0 = 10,000$ μg, $f = 0.8$, $F = 1$, $V_1 = 10$ L, $V_2 = 20$ L, $K_a = 0.5$ hr^{-1}, $K_{el} = 0.2$ hr^{-1}, $K_{12} = 0.6$ hr^{-1}, and $K_{21} = 1.25$ hr^{-1}.

sorption time is relatively short (2 hours) in this example. In this case, the absorption of the drug can be characterized as rapid and almost complete by the last measurement.

Case 2: Biexponential Terminal Phase

If the plasma concentration profile of a drug exhibits biexponential phase, a two-compartment model should be used for the time constant analysis. The plasma concentration profiles of a drug with biexponential terminal phase after intravenous and oral doses are simulated using Model 2 and shown in Figure 5.3. In this example the distribution rate (K_{12}) is three times faster than the elimination rate (K_{el}), resulting in a distinct biexponential terminal phase.

The estimation of oral bioavailability of drugs with a biexponential terminal phase is also based on the area under the curve like drugs with a monoexponential terminal phase. The sampling time for drugs with a biexponential terminal phase should be sufficiently long enough for the estimation of the second decay time. The estimated pharmacokinetic parameters applying the time constant analysis are listed in Table 5.2, and the estimated time constants are presented in Figure 5.4. The analysis shows that 80% of the drug is absorbed orally compared to the intravenous dose. The plasma drug concentration profile after the intravenous bolus dose shows multiple phases, and the elimination time constant (T_{el}) cannot be estimated from

TABLE 5.2.   *The Estimated and Model Values of the Pharmacokinetic Parameters for the Example Shown in Figure 5.3.*

Parameter	Time Constant Analysis	Model Value	Equation
$\bar{t}_{iv}$ (hr)	7.35	7.4	(5.17)
t_{po} (hr)	9.36	9.4	(5.16)
T_a (hr)	2.0	2.0	(5.18)
T_z (hr)	7.4	7.69	(5.2)
V_1 (L)	10	10	(5.20)
T_{el} (hr)	5.0	5.0	(5.21)
$fF = AUC_{po}/AUC_{iv}$	0.80	0.8	(5.19)

the terminal slope in the semi-log plot of the concentration profile but can be determined from Equation (5.20) using the intravenous data. Now let us examine the time constant plot (Figure 5.4). The elimination time is shorter than the decay time, indicating a significant tissue distribution. The absorption time is relatively short, reflecting a rapid absorption and resulting in a short time to reach the maximum concentration.

Case 3: First Pass Model

When a drug is extensively metabolized by the liver, the first pass elimination may significantly reduce the bioavailability [6,18]. Model 3 can be

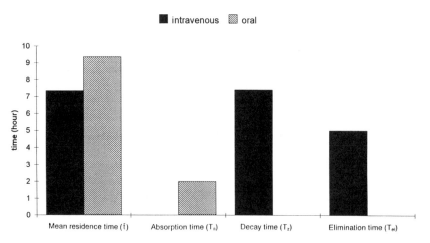

FIGURE 5.4.   The time constant plot comparing intravenous and oral administrations in the example in Figure 5.3. The absorption time (T_a) is relatively short, reflecting a rapid absorption and resulting in a short time to reach the maximum concentration.

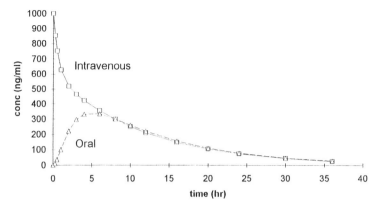

FIGURE 5.5. Simulated plasma drug concentration profiles with first pass effect, following intravenous and oral administrations using Model 3. The parameters used in this simulation are $X_0 = 10,000\ \mu g$, $f = 1$, $F = 0.8$, $V = 10\ L$, $K_a = 0.5\ hr^{-1}$, $K_{el} = 0.2\ hr^{-1}$, $K_{12} = 0.7\ hr^{-1}$, and $K_{21} = 0.8\ hr^{-1}$.

used to explain the first pass metabolism. The model assumes that the drug is subjected to the first pass metabolism in the liver immediately after it is absorbed but before it enters the systemic circulation. The plasma drug concentration profiles after an oral and an intravenous administration are simulated by the model and shown in Figure 5.5. In this example, an extraction ratio of 0.2 is assumed (i.e., 20% of the absorbed drug is subjected to the first pass effect).

The plasma concentration profiles, simulated by the first pass model, for the intravenous dose show a biphasic exponential decay in Model 2. The parameters estimated from the time constant analysis are shown in Table 5.3. The analysis results show an 80% bioavailability through the oral administration compared to the intravenous dose. Intuitively, the bioavailability is the ratio of T_{el} to $(T_{21} + T_{el})$, which gives the fraction of the drug entering the central compartment after it is absorbed. However, there are several

TABLE 5.3. The Estimated and Model Values of the Pharmacokinetic Parameters for the Example Shown in Figure 5.5.

Parameter	Time Constant Analysis	Model Value	Equation
$\bar{t}_{iv}$ (hr)	10.99	11.14	(5.23)
$\bar{t}_{po}$ (hr)	14.03	14.14	(5.22)
T_λ (hr)	11.24	11.49	(5.2)
$F = AUC_{po}/AUC_{iv}$	0.80	0.8	(5.25)

limitations of this model; first, the hepatic elimination time constant (represented by T_{el} in this model) cannot be estimated from the terminal phase since a multiple compartment model is used, nor can it be determined from the mean residence time of the intravenous dose, where T_{12} cannot be solved independently from T_{21} [(Equations (5.a24) and (5.a25) in Appendix 3], and second, the bioavailability of the metabolites cannot be estimated from the model.

Case 4: First Pass Effects

A more complicated case is presented in this example. A drug is extensively metabolized into two metabolites M1 and M2. The ratios of AUC_{M1} to AUC_C are different after the oral and the intravenous administrations, indicating a classic first pass effect. On the other hand, the ratios of AUC_{M2} to AUC_C are the same after the oral and the intravenous doses. The oral bioavailability for C and M2 is the same, while the bioavailability of M1 is higher than C. Based on these results, metabolite M1 is affected by the first pass elimination, but metabolite M2 is not affected by the first pass effect. The pharmacokinetics of drug C and its metabolites M1 and M2 can be described by Model 4, and the simulated plasma drug concentration profiles are shown in Figure 5.6. In this example, 30% of the drug is converted to metabolite M1 by a first pass effect, while metabolite M2 is not produced by the first pass effect.

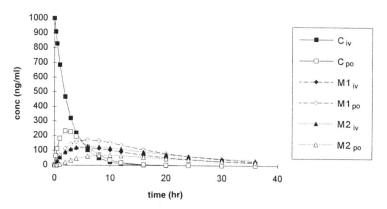

FIGURE 5.6. Simulated plasma concentration profiles of a drug and its metabolite with first pass effect, following oral and intravenous administrations using Model 4. The time constant plot comparing the two treatments is shown in Figure 5.7. The parameters used in this simulation are $X_0 = 10,000$ μg, $f = 0.8$, $F = 0.7$, $V_c = 10$ L, $V_{m1} = 15$ L, $V_{m2} = 12$ L, $K_a = 0.5$ hr^{-1}, $K_{el} = 0.2$ hr^{-1}, $K_{m1} = 0.1$ hr^{-1}, $K_{m2} = 0.08$ hr^{-1}, $K_{mel1} = 0.7$ hr^{-1}, $K_{mel2} = 0.05$ hr^{-1}.

TABLE 5.4. *The Estimated and Model Values of the Pharmacokinetic Parameters for the Example Shown in Figure 5.6.*

Parameter	Time Constant Analysis	Model Value	Equation
$\bar{t}_{iv}$ (hr)	2.59	2.63	
$\bar{t}_{po}$ (hr)	4.63	4.63	
$T_{el,t} = 1/(1/T_{el} + 1/T_{m1}$ $+ 1/T_{m2})$ (hr)	2.44	2.63	(5.2)
T_{mel1} (hr)	14.5	14.3	(5.32)
T_{mel2} (hr)	20.4	20.0	(5.32)
T_a (hr)	2.04	2.0	(5.35)
$X_{u,c}$ (μg)	5358	5263	
$X_{u,m1}$ (μg)	2635	2631	
$X_{u,m2}$ (μg)	2113	2105	
V_c (L)	10	10	(5.29)
V_{m1} (L)	15.2	15	(5.33)
V_{m2} (L)	12.3	12	(5.33)
T_{m1} (L)	10.0	10.0	(5.34)
f	0.77	0.8	(5.36)
F	0.71	0.7	(5.26)
$AUC_{C,po}/AUC_{C,iv}$	0.55	0.56	(5.26)
$AUC_{M1,po}/AUC_{M1,iv}$	1.47	1.47	(5.27)
$AUC_{M2,po}/AUC_{M2,iv}$	0.57	0.56	(5.28)
$AUC_{M1,po}/AUC_{C,po}$	2.50	2.5	
$AUC_{M2,po}/AUC_{C,po}$	1.35	1.33	
$AUC_{M1,iv}/AUC_{C,iv}$	0.94	0.95	
$AUC_{M2,iv}/AUC_{C,iv}$	1.31	1.33	

It is shown in the model that metabolite M1 is produced by the liver, and a nonhepatic metabolism is responsible for M2. After the absorption, a portion of the drug is converted to M1 before it reaches the systemic circulation. Once in the central compartment, the drug is then further eliminated to the two metabolites or excreted into urine. The key pharmacokinetic parameters in this example are absorption time constant (T_a), first pass effect $(1 - F)$, and the bioavailability of all three compounds (C, MI, and M2). The pharmacokinetic parameters determined from the time constant analysis are listed in Table 5.4, and the estimated time constants are presented in Figure 5.7. The drug is 77% (f) absorbed, of which 29% $(1 - F)$ is eliminated by the first pass metabolism. The resulting oral bioavailability of C is 55% compared to the intravenous administration. The first pass metabolism converts a portion of the drug into metabolite M1; therefore, the AUC_{M1}/AUC_C ratio is higher after the oral dose than the intravenous dose, and the oral bioavailability of M1 is higher than C. On the other hand, metabolite M2 is produced through a nonhepatic route; thus, the

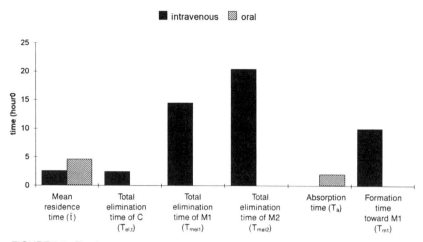

FIGURE 5.7. The time constant plot of the drug and its metabolite for the example in Figure 5.6, comparing intravenous and oral administrations. The absorption (T_a) and elimination time ($T_{el,t}$) constants are relatively short, reflected by the sharp concentration profile of the parent drug following the oral administration.

AUC_{M2}/AUC_C ratio is the same after both oral and intravenous administrations, and M2 has the same oral bioavailability as C.

Now let us examine the time constant plot (Figure 5.7). The elimination times of both metabolites (T_{mel1} and T_{mel2}) are much longer than the elimination time of the parent drug ($T_{mel,t}$), resulting in long decay times for the metabolites. The absorption and elimination time constants are relatively short, reflected by the sharp concentration profile of the parent drug following the oral administrations. On the other hand, the concentration profiles of the metabolites are broad because of their long mean residence time and elimination time.

So far we have discussed three simulated case studies that demonstrate the accuracy of the Time Constant Approach by comparing the estimated time constants with the theoretical values. To further illustrate the utility of the Time Constant Approach, we will examine three examples from the literature next.

EXAMPLES

Example 1: Monoexponential Terminal Phase

Benzydamine was given to six healthy adult males as a 5-mg intravenous dose and a 50-mg oral dose [2]. The mean plasma concentration profiles of benzydamine following the two treatments are shown in Figure 5.8. Based

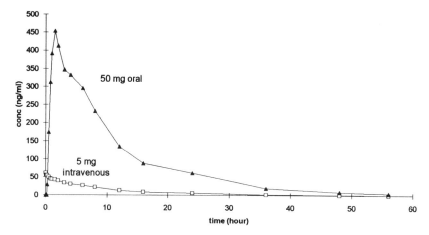

FIGURE 5.8. Mean concentration profiles of benzydamine after administration of a 5-mg intravenous dose and a 50-mg oral dose to six healthy male subjects. (Reproduced from Reference [2] with permission.) The time constant plot comparing the two treatments is shown in Figure 5.9.

on the concentration profiles, benzydamine can be characterized as a drug with a relatively long decay time and a relatively large volume of distribution. The concentration profiles follow a one-compartmental model, and there is no metabolism involved. Therefore, the pharmacokinetic parameters are estimated using Model 1. The estimated pharmacokinetic parameters are listed in Table 5.5, and the estimated time constants are presented in Figure 5.9. The bioavailability of the oral dose is 100%. As shown in the time constant plot (Figure 5.9), the absorption time is very short, indicating a relatively fast absorption. The elimination time constant is much longer than the absorption time constant, resulting in a sharp absorption phase and a long elimination decay time following the oral administration.

TABLE 5.5. Estimated Pharmacokinetic
Parameters of Benzydamine Using the Time
Constant Analysis for the Example in Figure 5.8.

Parameter	Value*	Equation
$\bar{t}_{iv}$ (hr)	10.8	(5.4)
$\bar{t}_{po}$ (hr)	11.4	(5.1)
T_{el} (hr)	11.1	(5.4)
T_a (hr)	0.61	(5.7)
$fF = AUC_{po}/AUC_{iv}$	1.0	(5.8)

*Estimated from the mean concentration profiles and the reported mean values.

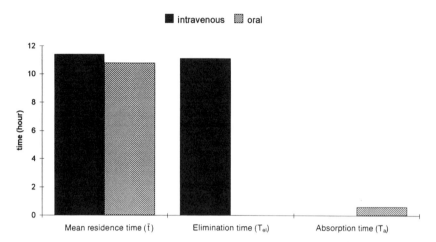

FIGURE 5.9. The time constant plot of benzydamine using Model 1, comparing intravenous and oral administrations. The elimination time constant (T_{el}) is much longer than the absorption time constant (T_a), resulting in a sharp absorption phase and a long elimination decay time following the oral administration.

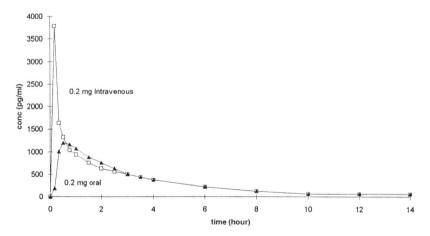

FIGURE 5.10. Mean concentration profiles of moxonidine after administration of a 0.2-mg intravenous dose and a 0.2-mg oral dose to eighteen healthy male subjects. (Reproduced with permission from the *European Journal of Drug Metabolism and Pharmacokinetics* [9].) The time constant plot comparing the two treatments is shown in Figure 5.11.

Example 2: Biexponential Terminal Phase

Moxonidine was given to eighteen healthy subjects with two formulations (0.2-mg tablet and 0.2-mg solution) to investigate the absolute bioavailability of the oral formulation [9]. The mean concentration profiles of moxonidine following the two treatments are shown in Figure 5.10. The concentration profiles follow a two-compartmental model; therefore, the pharmacokinetic parameters of moxonidine are estimated using Model 2. The estimated pharmacokinetic parameters are listed in Table 5.6, and the estimated time constants are presented in Figure 5.11. The bioavailability of the oral dose is 88% relative to the intravenous dose. The amount of moxonidine excreted unchanged in the urine (58% after oral dose 61% after intravenous dose) also shows a relatively complete absorption after the oral administration. The urine recovery data show a similar amount of the parent drug after both treatments, indicating a minimum first pass effect.

Now let us examine the time constant plot (Figure 5.11). The absorption time is shorter than the decay time, reflected by the sharp absorption phase and prolonged terminal phase of the concentration profile. The decay time is much longer than the elimination time, indicating a significant tissue distribution. To summarize, moxonidine can be characterized as a drug with rapid and complete absorption.

Example 3: First Pass Effects

Levoprotiline was given to twelve healthy subjects (eleven women, one man) as a 15-mg intravenous dose and a 75-mg oral dose to investigate the

TABLE 5.6. Estimated Pharmacokinetic
Parameters of Moxonidine Using the Time Constant
Analysis for the Example in Figure 5.10.

Parameter	Value*	Equation
$\bar{t}_{iv}$ (hr)	3.08	(5.17)
$\bar{t}_{po}$ (hr)	3.49	(5.16)
T_a (hr)	0.41	(5.18)
T_λ (hr)	3.15	(5.2)
V_1 (L)	34.5	(5.20)
T_{el} (hr)	0.64	(5.21)
fF	0.88	(5.19)
$X_{u,po}/X_0$ (%)	58.0	
$X_{u,iv}/X_0$ (%)	61.0	

*Estimated from the mean concentration profiles and the reported mean values.

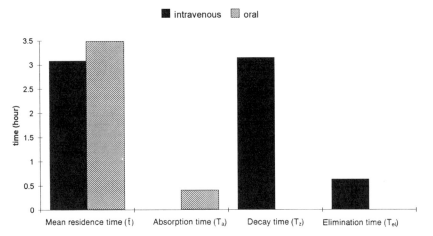

FIGURE 5.11. The time constant plot of moxonidine using Model 2, comparing intravenous and oral administrations. The absorption time (T_a) is shorter than the decay time (T_z), reflected by the sharp absorption phase and prolonged terminal phase of the concentration profile. The decay time (T_z) is much longer than the elimination time (T_{el}), indicating a significant tissue distribution.

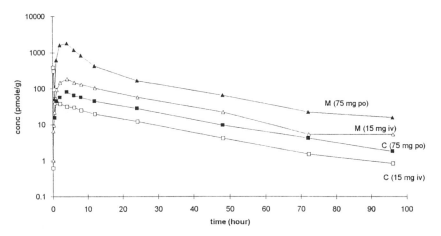

FIGURE 5.12. Mean concentration profiles of levoprotiline and its metabolite after administration of a 15-mg intravenous dose and a 75-mg oral dose to twelve healthy subjects. (Reproduced from Reference [6] with permission.) The time constant plot comparing the two treatments is shown in Figure 5.13.

116

TABLE 5.7. Estimated Pharmacokinetic
Parameters of Levoprotiline Using the Time
Constant Analysis for the Example in Figure 5.12.

Parameter	Value*	Equation
$\bar{t}_{iv}$ (hr)	18.2	
$\bar{t}_{po}$ (hr)	22.0	
T_{el} (hr)	103.1	(5.30)
T_{mel}/V_m (hr/L)	1.33	(5.31)
T_a (hr)	3.85	(5.35)
V_c (L)	99	(5.29)
T_m (hr)	250.0	(5.34)
f	0.57	(5.36)
F	0.7	(5.26)
$AUC_{C,po}/AUC_{C,iv}$	0.4	(5.26)
$AUC_{M,po}/AUC_{M,iv}$	0.99	(5.27)
$AUC_{M,po}/AUC_{C,po}$	10.1	
$AUC_{M,iv}/AUC_{C,iv}$	4.0	

*Estimated from the mean concentration profiles and the reported
mean values.

pharmacokinetics of the drug and assess the absolute bioavailability [6].
The mean concentration profiles of levoprotiline following the two treatments are shown in Figure 5.12. The ratio of metabolite concentration to
levoprotiline is higher after the oral administration than the intravenous administration, indicating a significant first pass effect. Therefore, Model 4 is

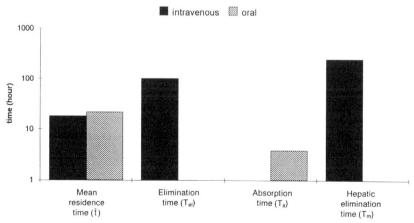

FIGURE 5.13. The time constant plot of levoprotiline using Model 4, comparing intravenous and oral administrations. The long renal (T_{el}) and hepatic (T_m) elimination time
constants may result in a long decay time of the concentration time profiles.

used to estimate the pharmacokinetic parameters. The estimated pharmacokinetic parameters of levoprotiline are listed in Table 5.7, and the estimated time constants are presented in Figure 15.13. The ratio of the area under the metabolite concentration curve to the area under the parent drug concentration curve is higher after the oral dose than the intravenous dose, indicating a first pass effect. The large volume of distribution of the central compartment indicates an extensive tissue binding or tissue distribution. The long renal and hepatic elimination time constants and extensive tissue distribution may result in a long decay time (Figure 5.13). The fraction absorbed f is equal to the total urine recovery of the drug (57%), assuming that elimination from nonrenal routes is insignificant. The bioavailability fF of the parent drug is 40%, and the first pass effect $(1 - F)$ is then 30%.

REFERENCES

1. Aweeka F. T., Tomlanovich S. J., Prueksaritanont T., Gupta S. K., and Benet L. Z., "Pharmacokinetics of orally and intravenously administered cyclosporine in pre-kidney transplant patients,"*J. Clin. Pharmacol.*, 1994; 34:60–67.
2. Baldock G. A., Brodie R. R., Chasseaud L. F., Taylor T., and Walmsley L. M. "Pharmacokinetics of benzydamine after intravenous, oral, and topical doses to human subjects," *Biopharmaceutics & Drug Disposition*, 1991; 12:481–492.
3. Beglinger C., Born W., Muff R., Drewe J., Dreyfuss J. L., Bock A., Mackray M., and Fischer J. A., "Intracolonic bioavailability of human calcitonin in man," *Eur. J. Clin. Pharmacol.*, 1992; 43:527–531.
4. Flor S. C., Rogge M. C., and Chow A. T. "Bioequivalence of oral and intravenous ofloxacin after multiple-dose administration to healthy male volunteers," *Antimicrobial Agents and Chemotheraphy*, July 1993; 37(7):1468–1472.
5. Hutt V., Theodor R., Pabst G., Bonn R., Fritschi E., and Jaeger H. "Evaluation of bioavailability and pharmacokinetics of two isosorbide-5-mononitrate preparations in healthy volunteers," *J. Clin. Pharmacol.*, 1992; 553–557.
6. Kaiser G., Ackermann R., and Dieterle W., "Pharmacokinetics of the antidepressant levoprotiline after intravenous and peroral administration in healthy volunteers," *Biopharmaceutics & Drug Disposition*, 1992; 13:83–93.
7. Obach R., Torrent J., Colom H., Prunonosa J., Peraire C, and Domenech J., "Pharmacokinetics and oral bioavailability of carbimide in man," *Biopharmaceutics & Drug Disposition*, 1991; 12:425–434.
8. Ryde M., Huitfeldt B., and Pettersson R., "Relative bioavailability of olsalazine from tablets and capsules: A drug targeted for local effect in the colon," *Biopharmaceutics & Drug Disposition*, 1991; 12:233–246.
9. Theodor R., Weimann H. J., Weber W., and Michaelis K., "Absolute bioavailability of moxonidine," *European Journal of Drug Metabolism and Pharmacokinetics*, 1991; 16(2):153–159.
10. Woodworth J. R., Delong A. F., Fasola A. F., and Oldham S., "Isomazole disposition in man as a function of dose and route of administration," *Biopharmaceutics & Drug Disposition*, 1991; 12:673–686.

11. Wyss P. A., Rosenthaler J., Nuesch E., and Aellig W. H., "Pharmacokinetic investigation of oral and IV dihydroergotamine in healthy subjects," *Eur. J. Clin. Pharmacol.*, 1991; 41:597–602.

12. Heykants J., Van-Peer A., Woestenborghs R., Gould S., and Mills J., "Pharmacokinetics of ketanserin and its metabolite ketanserin-ol in man after intravenous, intramuscular and oral administration," *Eur. J. Clin. Pharmacol.*, 1986; 31(3):343–350.

13. Puigdellivol E., Carral M. E., Moreno J., Pla-Delfina J. M., and Jane F., "Pharmacokinetics and absolute bioavailability of intramuscular tranexamic acid in man," *Int. J. Clin. Pharmacol. Ther. Toxicol.*, 1985; 23(6):298–301.

14. Laursen T., Ovesen P., Grandjean B., Jensen S., Jorgensen J.O., Illum P., and Cristiansen J. S., "Nasal absorption of growth hormone in normal subjects: Studies with four different formulations," *Ann. Pharmacother.*, 1994; 28(78):845–848.

15. Bioavailability of leuprolide acetate following nasal and inhalation delivery to rats and healthy humans," *Pharm. Res.*, 1992; 9(2):244–249.

16. Gustavson L. E., Nadeau R. W., and Oldfield N. F., "Pharmacokinetics of teceleukin (recombinant human interleukin-2) after intravenous or subcutaneous administration to patients with cancer," *J. Biol. Response Mod.*, 1989; 8(4):440–449.

17. Bratt G., Thornebohm E., Windlund L., and Lockner D., "Low molecular weight heparin (KABI 2165, Fragmin): Pharmacokinetics after intravenous and subcutaneous administration in human volunteers," *Thromb. Res.*, 1986; 42(5):613–620.

18. Midha K. K., Roscoe R. M. H. Wilson T. W., Cooper J. K., Loo J. C. K., Ho-Ngoc A., and McGilveray I. J., "Pharmacokinetics of glucuronidation of propranolol following oral administration in humans," *Biopharmaceutics & Drug Disposition*, 1983; 4:331–338.

CHAPTER 6

Influence of Formulation on Pharmacokinetics—Bioequivalence

INTRODUCTION

The influence of formulation on the pharmacokinetics of a drug is determined in a bioequivalence study. The difference in pharmacokinetics between formulations can be caused by a difference in disintegration or the dissolution rate of the formulations or by excipients (i.e., pH buffers or surfactants) that may affect the dissolution or absorption rate. Since a change in formulation affects only the dissolution and permeability, the key time constants and pharmacokinetic parameters of concern in a bioequivalence trial are dissolution time constant, absorption time constant, and extent of absorption. The two processes, dissolution and absorption, can be lumped together in a pharmacokinetic model and can be characterized by a single time constant.

The guidance of statistical procedures for bioequivalence studies has been provided by the FDA [17]. For a single-dose bioequivalence study, the guideline requires, at a minimum, the following pharmacokinetic parameters to be tested: AUC_{0-t}, $AUC_{0-\infty}$ (denoted by AUC in this text), and C_{max}. It is recommended that the logarithmic transformation of $AUC_{0-\infty}$ and C_{max} be performed and that the transformed parameters be used for the statistical test. The Division of Bioequivalence has employed the one-sided procedure to determine whether average values for pharmacokinetic parameters measured after administration of the test and reference products are comparable. The statistical procedure involves the calculation of a confidence interval for the ratio (or difference) between the test and reference product pharmacokinetic variable averages. The observed confidence interval should fall into a predefined range for the ratio (or difference). If μ_T and μ_R

denote the expected medians for the test and reference, respectively, the test problem can be described as follows

$$H_0: \theta \leq \theta_1 \text{ or } \theta \geq \theta_2 \text{ (bioinequivalence)}$$

$$H_1: \theta_1 \leq \theta \leq \theta_2 \text{ (bioequivalence)}$$

where $\theta = \mu_T/\mu_R$ (or $= \mu_T - \mu_R$) and θ_1 and θ_2 are the predefined range of the ratio (or difference) for bioequivalence. The FDA guidance has stated the criterion for bioequivalence. The Division of Bioequivalence has decided to use an equivalence of criterion of 80 to 125% for the ratio (μ_T/μ_R) of the averages.

A number of pharmacokinetic parameters have been identified for the assessment of rate and extent of absorption in bioequivalence studies, including the area under the concentration curve from time 0 to infinity ($AUC_{0-\infty}$) [1,2], the maximum concentration (C_{max}) [4,8], the time to reach the maximum concentration (T_{max}) [10,11], the terminal slope (λ_z), mean residence time (MRT) [13], mean absorption time (MAT) [13], partial AUCs (such as AUC_{0-1} and $AUC_{0-T_{max}}$) [3], and $C_{max}/AUC_{0-\infty}$ [5]. Recently, the intestinal permeabilities of several drugs have been successfully measured in humans [7], which is the most direct estimation of the absorption rate constant. In this chapter, we will discuss the application of the time constant analysis to bioequivalence studies. The major considerations in selecting appropriate parameters for the assessment of absorption are (1) that the parameter measures absorption and (2) that the variability in the estimation of the parameter is low. The key time constant discussed in this chapter is $T_a V_c$, which fits these two criteria.

Some common themes in the time constant view are shared by bioequivalence studies and other types of studies. For example, in bioequivalence studies, the variability of hepatic elimination time is usually large for drugs with extensive metabolism, while the variability of absorption time is usually large for drugs with low dissolution rates. Similar effects on the variability of time constants can be observed in other studies. If a long absorption time is observed in the bioequivalence study, the absorption time may be shortened under the fed condition in food study, since food may improve the dissolution (Chapter 13). Lipophilicity of drugs is a common factor affecting time constants in many pharmacokinetics studies, including the bioequivalence study. Lipophilic drugs may show a long dissolution time in the bioequivalence study due to their low water solubility. Some of the basic lipophilic drugs are susceptible to a first pass effect, which can be identified in a bioavailability or food study. Lipophilic drugs also tend to have large apparent volumes of distribution because of easy tissue penetration, and this will be reflected by long mean residence times in all pharmacokinetic studies. The mean residence time of lipophilic drugs will be a key time constant in age (Chapter 15) and gender (Chapter 16) studies, since the body mass content of fat is different between populations of different age or gender. The pK values (pK = $-\log K$, where K is dissociation constant) of a drug are another common factor affecting time constants in bioequivalence as well as other studies. The dissolution time and the absorption time are also dependent on whether a drug is basic or acidic, since the pH in the gastrointestinal tract varies. In addition, the pK values of a drug can be used to predict the characteristics of its protein binding. In general, acidic drugs bind to albumin and basic drugs bind to α_1-acid glycoprotein. Change in protein binding affects the distribution time and redistribution time, especially in renal impairment (Chapter 17), inflammatory diseases (Chapter 19), age (Chapter 15), and drug interaction (Chapter 14) studies.

Two models are used for the estimation of the parameter T_aV_c: (1) the first model describes pharmacokinetics of drugs with monoexponential terminal phase; (2) the second model describes pharmacokinetics of drugs with biexponential terminal phase. Three simulated case studies and two literature examples are discussed in this chapter to illustrate the utility of these models in bioequivalence studies. Additional literature examples of bioequivalence studies can be found in References [1–16].

PHARMACOKINETIC MODELS

This section presents two models that are useful in the estimation of T_a*V. The goal is to establish simple relationships between time constants and measurable parameters such as (1) mean residence time, which is the sum of input and output times, and (2) area under the curves. The derivations of these relationships are straightforward and are discussed in Chapter 2.

Model 1: Monoexponential Terminal Phase

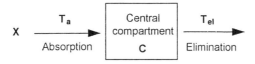

The objective of the pharmacokinetic analysis in a bioequivalence is to determine the absorption characteristics of different formulations of a drug. The absorption rate may be affected by the disintegration, dissolution, release rate, particle size, surface area of the drug powder, and other factors associated with formulations [18]. Model 1 describes the pharmacokinetics of drugs with first-order absorption and elimination rates. The elimination may be via a combination of renal, hepatic, biliary, and other routes.

The mean residence time of the concentration curve is simply the sum of input and output times

$$\text{Mean residence time } (\bar{t}) = \frac{\text{AUMC}}{\text{AUC}}$$

$$= \text{Input time } (T_{\text{in}}) + \text{Output time } (T_{\text{out}}) = T_{\text{a}} + T_{\text{el}} \quad (6.1)$$

where the mean residence time can be estimated from the ratio of the area under the first moment curve to the area under the curve. The mean residence time of different formulations in a bioequivalence study may be different due to a difference in the absorption time between formulations. When the predominant route of elimination is through the kidney, the bioavailability can be estimated as the ratio of the urine recovery to the dose.

$$\text{Bioavailability } (f) = \frac{X_{\text{u}}}{X_0} \quad (6.2)$$

The decay time constant T_z of the concentration curve can be estimated from the following equation, by selecting $t_{\text{ref}} > 2\bar{t}$ (see Appendix 2):

$$\frac{1}{\text{Decay time } (T_z)} = \lambda_z = 2 \frac{(t_{\text{ref}} - t_{\text{last}}) \ln (C_{t_{\text{ref}}}) - \text{AU} \ln C_{t_{\text{ref}} - t_{\text{last}}}}{(t_{\text{ref}} - t_{\text{last}})^2} \quad (6.3)$$

The estimated decay time T_z is equal to the absorption time T_{a} or the elimination time T_{el}, whichever is longer, and the initial time constant T_0 ($= 1/\lambda_0$) of the concentration curve can be calculated from the mean residence time [Equation (6.1)]. However, there is an uncertainty about whether T_z or T_0 represents the absorption time constant. A less ambiguous parameter than T_0 to characterize the absorption rate is $T_{\text{a}} \cdot V$, which is estimated as follows. First, the terminal portion of the concentration curve is fitted to a monoexponential function, and the intercept of this monoexponential function with the y-axis is

$$A = \frac{fFX_0}{V} \frac{K_{\text{a}}}{\lambda_0 - \lambda_z} \quad (6.4)$$

The ratio of area under the curve [Equation (6.a3) in Appendix 3] to the intercept [Equation (6.4)] gives an expression containing only the initial time constant and the decay time constant on the right-hand side of the equation:

$$\frac{\text{AUC}}{A} = \frac{1}{\lambda_z} - \frac{1}{\lambda_0} = T_z - T_0 \tag{6.5}$$

Then the initial time constant can be calculated from the values of mean residence time $\bar{t}$, area under the curve AUC and the intercept A.

$$\frac{1}{T_0} = 2 \bigg/ \left(\bar{t} - \frac{\text{AUC}}{A} \right) \tag{6.6}$$

The estimation of $\bar{t}$, AUC, and A is likely more robust than the estimation of λ_0 directly by a curve-stripping technique, especially when few time points are located in the absorption phase. The accuracy of the stripping method may be improved with a large number of data points along the rising phase of the concentration curve. In that case, the curve-stripping method can be an alternative for the estimation of λ_0. With known λs and fF, the value of $T_a \cdot V$ can be expressed as follows:

$$\frac{1}{\text{Absorption time} \times \text{Volume} (T_a V)} = \frac{A(\lambda_0 - \lambda_z)}{fFX_0} \tag{6.7}$$

From this equation, the value of $T_a \cdot V$ can be estimated whether a flip-flop occurs or not. Therefore, $T_a \cdot V$ is a more direct and less ambiguous parameter for characterizing the absorption rate than T_0.

Model 2: Biexponential Terminal Phase

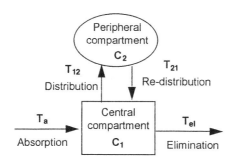

When the drug concentration profile shows a biexponential terminal phase, the possible scenarios of flip-flops become more complicated, since the absorption, distribution, and elimination phases (or time constants) may be arranged in any order. Care must be taken to identify which exponential phase represents absorption in a bioequivalence study. In this case, the pharmacokinetics can be described by a two-compartmental model.

The mean residence time of the concentration curve is the sum of input and output times (see Chapter 2):

$$\text{Mean residence time of } C_1 \ (\bar{t}_{C1}) \ = \ \frac{\text{AUMC}_{C1}}{\text{AUC}_{C1}}$$

$$= \text{ Input time } (T_{c1,in}) \ + \ \text{Output time } (T_{c1,out}) \ = \ T_a \ + \ T_{el} \ + \ T_{el} \frac{T_{21}}{T_{12}} \quad (6.8)$$

When the distribution time to the peripheral compartment (T_{12}) is short or the redistribution time back to the central compartment (T_{21}) is long, the third term of the above equation will contribute a large portion of the mean residence time. As a result, the mean residence time does not correlate well with the absorption time in the case of significant peripheral distribution.

The renal clearance time is the ratio of the area under the curve to the cumulative urine recovery.

$$\text{Renal clearance time } \left(\frac{T_{el}}{V_1}\right) \ = \ \frac{\text{AUC}_C}{X_{uc}} \quad (6.9)$$

The absorbed fraction of the drug can be calculated from the cumulative urine recovery, if (1) the renal excretion dominates the elimination of the drug or (2) all the metabolites, as well as the parent drug, are recovered in the urine.

$$\text{Fraction absorbed } (f) \ = \ \frac{X_{uc}}{X_0} \quad \text{or Fraction absorbed } (f) \ = \ \frac{\Sigma X_{ui}}{X_0}$$

$$(6.10)$$

The slopes of the three exponential phases can be estimated from the curve-stripping technique. Let λ_{z0}, λ_{z1} and λ_{z2} represent the three exponents, where $\lambda_{z0} > \lambda_{z1} > \lambda_{z2}$. Thus, $1/\lambda_{z1}$ and $1/\lambda_{z2}$ represent the first and second decay time constants of the terminal portion of the concentration curve, and $1/\lambda_{z0}$ represents the initial time constant of the concentration curve. The first and second phases of the terminal portion of the concentration curve can be fitted to two exponential terms:

$$C = Ae^{-\lambda_{z1}} + Be^{-\lambda_{z2}} \tag{6.11}$$

where A and B are the intercepts of the first and second terminal phases.

The sequence of appearance of T_a (resulting from absorption) and time constants $1/\lambda_1$ and $1/\lambda_2$ [resulting from distribution and elimination, Equations (6.a11) and (6.a12), Appendix 3] along the concentration profile cannot be clearly determined. Therefore, it is difficult to identify which one of the time constants, T_0, T_{z1}, and T_{z2}, represents the absorption time T_a. A less ambiguous parameter than λs for characterizing the absorption rate is $T_a \cdot V_1$. The value of $T_a \cdot V_1$ can be obtained from the following expression:

$$\frac{1}{\text{Absorption time} \times \text{Volume } (T_a V_1)} = \frac{A + B}{fFX_0} \frac{(\lambda_{z1} - \lambda_{z0})(\lambda_{z2} - \lambda_{z0})}{\lambda_{z0} - K_{21}} \tag{6.12}$$

The three exponents obtained from the curve-stripping method, λ_0, λ_{z1}, and λ_{z2}, represent the following three constants: K_a, λ_1, and λ_2, but not necessarily in this particular order. The relationships between λ_1 and λ_2 and rate constants are defined in Appendix 3. It is worth mentioning that the relationship between K_{21}, λ_1, and λ_2 is $\lambda_1 > K_{21} > \lambda_2$. Under condition (1), only two of the three exponential phases can be identified using the curve-stripping method because the first decay phase lasts for a very short period of time. Therefore, in this case, the two-compartmental model collapses to a one-compartmental model. Under condition (2), the second decay phase lasts very long, and the variability involved in estimating λ_{z2} can be large. Two special cases of condition (2) are discussed below [conditions (3) and (5)]:

(1)   if $K_{21} \rightarrow \lambda_1$ and $\lambda_1 = \lambda_{z1}$ then $A \rightarrow 0$ (6.13)

(2)   if $K_{21} \rightarrow \lambda_2$ and $\lambda_2 = \lambda_{z2}$ then $B \rightarrow 0$ (6.14)

In conditions (3) to (5), the concentration profiles typically show long tails, and the error involved in the estimation of λ_{z2} ($\lambda_{z2} = \lambda_2$ unless $K_a < \lambda_2$) can be large. Fortunately, under conditions (3) and (5), the denominator in Equation (6.12) cancels out with one term in the numerator (when $\lambda_{z2} = \lambda_2$). In addition, under conditions (3) to (5), exponent λ_{z2} in the numerator of Equation (6.12) is very small and can be ignored compared with λ_0. Thus, the estimation of $T_a \cdot V_1$ is not affected by the large variability of λ_{z2} under conditions (3) to (5).

(3)   if K_{el}, $K_{21} \gg K_{12}$ then $\lambda_1 \rightarrow K_{el}$, $\lambda_2 \rightarrow K_{21}$ (6.15)

(4)   if K_{12}, $K_{21} \gg K_{el}$ then $\lambda_1 \rightarrow K_{12} + K_{21}$, $\lambda_2 \rightarrow K_{el}$ (6.16)

(5)   if K_{el}, $K_{12} \gg K_{21}$ then $\lambda_1 \rightarrow K_{el} + K_{12}$, $\lambda_2 \rightarrow K_{21}$ (6.17)

Therefore, under the above five conditions, Equation (6.12) collapses and contains only one of the two decay exponents. In other conditions (e.g., $\lambda_{z2} = K_a$), when the second decay time is much longer than the first decay time, λ_{z2} in the numerator of Equation (6.12) is very small and can be ignored compared with λ_0.

Another equation for estimating T_a*V_1 is shown below (see Appendix 3 for derivation):

$$\frac{\text{Absorption time} \times \text{Volume } (T_aV_1)}{\text{Bioavailability } (fF)} = \frac{X_0}{A(\lambda_0 - \lambda_{z1}) + B(\lambda_0 - \lambda_{z2})}$$

(6.18)

When the second decay is much longer than the first decay time, the value of B becomes very small and can be dropped out of Equation (6.18). As a result, Equation (6.18) collapses to Equation (6.7) when the second decay time is long. Therefore, the large variability (or error) involved in estimating λ_{z2} does not affect the accuracy of $T_a*V_1/f/F$.

CASE STUDIES

Case 1: Large Intrasubject Variability in Elimination

The intrasubject variability of the plasma concentration of a drug depends on the variability of the elimination rate, as well as the variability of the absorption. When an extensive metabolism is involved, the variability associated with the elimination can be relatively large compared with the variability of the absorption. An example of large intrasubject variability in elimination is illustrated by Model 1, and the simulated plasma concentration profiles of two different formulations are shown in Figure 6.1. In this example, the intrasubject variability of the elimination rate constant is 40%, resulting in a significant difference in the maximum concentration between the two formulations.

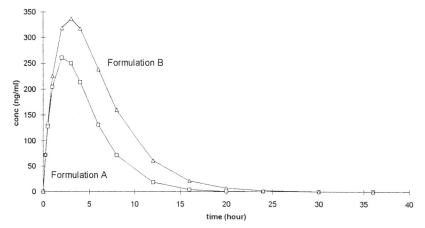

FIGURE 6.1. Simulated (Model 1) plasma concentration profiles after dosing two formulations of a drug to a same subject with large variability in elimination. The time constant plot comparing the two formulations is shown in Figure 6.2. The parameters used in this simulation are as follows: formulation A: $X_0 = 10$ mg, $fF = 0.8$, $V = 10$ L, $K_a = 0.4$ hr^{-1}, $K_{el} = 0.5$ hr^{-1}; formulation B: $X_0 = 10$ mg, $fF = 0.8$, $V = 10$ L, $K_a = 0.4$ hr^{-1}, $K_{el} = 0.3$ hr^{-1}.

Because of the large variability in elimination time, time constants and parameters associated with the elimination time, including area under the curve, decay time, maximum concentration, and mean residence time, are expected to vary significantly between formulations. The estimated pharmacokinetic parameters of the above example using the time constant analysis are listed in Table 6.1, and the estimated time constants are presented in Figure 6.2. The extent of absorption is given by the total urine recovery (X_u), which is the combined amount of the drug and its metabolite in the urine. The intrasubject variability of the elimination rate affects the area under the concentration curve (66.4%) the most and affects $T_a \cdot V$ (1.2%) the least.

Now let us examine the time constant plot (Figure 6.2). The difference in the absorption time between the two formulations determined by $T_a \cdot V$ is small, but the difference in the initial time constant T_0 is relatively large. This is because T_0 of formulation B represents the absorption time, while T_0 of formulation A represents the elimination time due to a flip-flop. To summarize, the area under the curve and the maximum concentration are not equivalent between the two formulations; however, the rate and the extent of absorption are equivalent between the formulations. If T_0 were to be indiscriminately adopted to indicate the rate of absorption, the result would be the erroneous conclusion that the rate of absorption varies with formulation. Use of $T_a \cdot V$ leads to the correct conclusion.

TABLE 6.1. Estimated Time Constants of Model for the Example Shown in Figure 6.1.

Parameter	Formulation A		Formulation B			Equation
	Time Constant Analysis	Model Value	Time Constant Analysis	Model Value	Percent Difference	
$\bar{t}$ (hr)	4.5	4.5	5.8	5.8	28.9%	(6.1)
T_0 (hr)	1.85	2.0 (T_{el})	2.33	2.5 (T_a)	25.6%	(6.3)
T_z (hr)	2.63	2.5 (T_a)	3.45	3.3 (T_{el})	31.0%	(6.3)
$T_a \cdot V$ (hr·L)	24.4	25.0	24.2	25.0	1.2%	(6.7)
X_u (μg)	8108	8000	8089	8000		
fF	0.81	0.8	0.81	0.8		
C_{max} (ng/ml)	260		337		29.6%	(6.2)
AUC (ng·hr/ml)	1621	1600	2696	2666	66.4%	

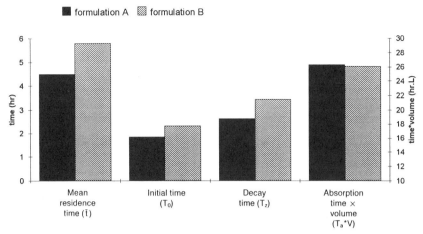

FIGURE 6.2. The time constant plot comparing the two formulations of the example in Figure 6.1. The difference in the absorption time between the two formulations determined by $T_a \cdot V$ is small, but the difference in the initial time constant T_0 is relatively large.

Case 2: Large Variability in Elimination and Distribution

If the concentration curve of a drug involves a biexponential terminal phase, a two-compartmental model, Model 2, is required for the estimation of absorption time constant. Simulated plasma concentration profiles using the model for two different formulations of a drug are shown in Figure 6.3. In this simple example, the intrasubject variability associated with K_{el} is 28.6%, with K_{12} 16.7%, and with K_{21} 28.6%. The difference in plasma concentration between the two formulations is more significant in the terminal phase than at the earlier time points, due to a greater variability in elimination and distribution than in absorption.

For drugs with an extensive metabolism, the intrasubject variability of the elimination rate is frequently high. For drugs with outstanding tissue distribution and tissue binding, the second decay time can be relatively long, and the serum concentrations in the second decay phase are usually low. A large variability in the second decay time may be introduced by a low assay sensitivity or a short sampling period. The significant intrasubject variability in elimination and distribution rates may result in large differences in the area under the curve and the mean residence time between formulations. The estimated pharmacokinetic parameters of the above example using the time constant analysis are listed in Table 6.2, and the estimated time constants are presented in Figure 6.4. As a result of the intrasubject variability, the difference in the area under the concentration

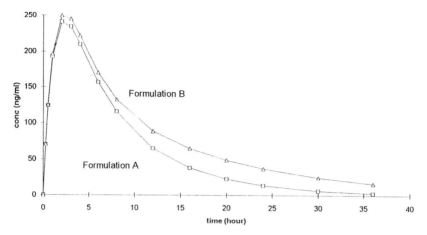

FIGURE 6.3. Simulated plasma concentration profiles of two different formulations of a drug with large variability in elimination and distribution using Model 2. The time constant plot comparing the two formulations is shown in Figure 6.4. The parameters used in this simulation are as follows: formulation A: $X_0 = 10$ mg, $fF = 0.8$, $V_1 = 10$ L, $V_2 = 20$ L, $K_a = 0.4$ hr^{-1}, $K_{12} = 0.3$ hr^{-1} $K_{21} = 0.3$ hr^{-1}, $K_{el} = 0.35$ hr^{-1}; formulation B: $X_0 = 10$ mg, $fF = 0.8$, $V_1 = 10$ L, $V_2 = 20$ L, $K_a = 0.4$ hr^{-1}, $K_{12} = 0.35$ hr^{-1}, $K_{21} = 0.2$ hr^{-1}, $K_{el} = 0.25$ hr^{-1}.

curve and mean residence time between formulations is significant, while the maximum concentration is not much different between the formulations. From the time constant plot (Figure 6.4), the intrasubject variability only results in a 1.5% difference in the estimated $T_a \cdot V$ of the two formulations. Among the three time constants, T_0, T_{z1}, and T_{z2}, only the first decay time constant T_{z1} is not affected by the intrasubject variability. This is because, as a result of flip-flops, T_{z1} represents the absorption time constant, which does not vary between the formulations. To summarize, the area under the curve and the mean residence time are not equivalent between the two formulations, while the bioavailability and rate of absorption are equivalent between the two. Once again, the use of $T_a \cdot V$ leads to the correct conclusion about the rate of absorption. By comparison, we would not know whether to use T_0, T_{z1}, and T_{z2} to draw conclusions about absorption unless we knew the relative order of T_a, $1/\lambda_1$, and $1/\lambda_2$.

Case 3: Relatively Long Second Decay Time

If the pharmacokinetics of a drug involves biexponential elimination with a long decay time, the variabilities of the estimated mean residence time and mean absorption time are often significant due to the large variability

TABLE 6.2. *Estimated Time Constants of Model 2 for the Example Shown in Figure 6.3.*

	Formulation A		Formulation B			
Parameter	Time Constant Analysis	Model Value	Time Constant Analysis	Model Value	Percent Difference	Equation
$\bar{t}$ (hr)	8.1	8.2	13.3	13.5	64.2%	(6.8)
T_0 (hr)	1.19	1.22	1.37	1.32	15.1%	(6.3)
T_{z1} (hr)	2.22	2.5	2.27	2.5	2.2%	(6.3)
T_{z2} (hr)	7.81	7.87	14.71	14.71	88.2%	(6.3)
$T_a \cdot V$ (hr·L)	24.8	25.0	24.4	25.0	1.5%	(6.12)
X_u (μg)	8048	8000	8015	8000		
fF	0.8	0.8	0.8	0.8		
C_{max} (ng/ml)	240		249		3.7%	(6.10)
AUC (ng·hr/ml)	2299	2285	3206	3200	39.5%	

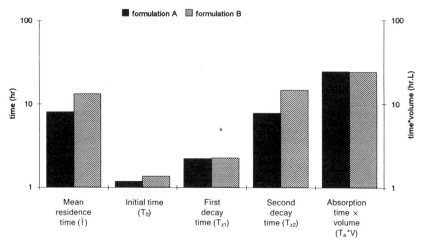

FIGURE 6.4. The time constant plot comparing the two formulations of the example in Figure 6.3. The intrasubject variability only results in a 1.5% difference in the estimated $T_a \cdot V$ of the two formulations. Among the three time constants T_0, T_{z1}, and T_{z2}, only the first decay time constant T_{z1} is not affected by the intrasubject variability.

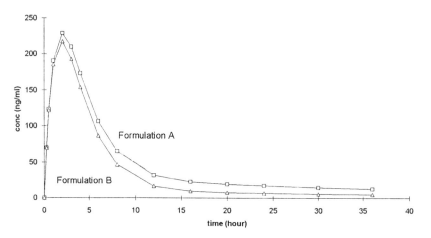

FIGURE 6.5. Simulated plasma concentration profiles of two different formulations of a drug with long second decay time using Model 2. The time constant plot comparing the two formulations is shown in Figure 6.6. The parameters used in this simulation are as follows: formulation A: $X_0 = 10$ mg, $fF = 0.8$, $V_1 = 10$ L, $V_2 = 20$ L, $K_a = 0.4$ hr^{-1}, $K_{12} = 0.3$ hr^{-1}, $K_{21} = 0.05$ hr^{-1}, $K_{el} = 0.35$ hr^{-1}; formulation B: $X_0 = 10$ mg, $fF = 0.8$, $V_1 = 10$ L, $V_2 = 20$ L, $K_a = 0.4$ hr^{-1}, $K_{12} = 0.2$ hr^{-1}, $K_{21} = 0.03$ hr^{-1}, $K_{el} = 0.5$ hr^{-1}.

134

TABLE 6.3. Estimated Time Constants of Model 3 for the Example Shown in Figure 6.5.

Parameter	Formulation A		Formulation B			Equation
	Time Constant Analysis	Model Value	Time Constant Analysis	Model Value	Percent Difference	
$\bar{t}$ (hr)	21.5	22.5	15.7	17.8	30%	(6.8)
T_0 (hr)	1.39	1.49	1.35	1.41	2.7%	(6.3)
T_{z1} (hr)	2.26	2.5	2.27	2.5	0.7%	(6.3)
T_{z2} (hr)	35.7	38.5	37.0	37.0	3.7%	(6.3)
$T_a \cdot V$ (hr·L)	25.0	25.0	24.2	25.0	3.4%	(6.12)
X_u (μg)	7969	8000	7923	8000		
fF	0.8	0.8	0.79	0.8		
C_{max} (ng/ml)	229		217		5.2%	
AUC (ng·hr/ml)	2276	2285	1584	1600	30.4%	(6.10)

and inaccuracy usually associated with the estimation of the second decay exponent λ_{z2}. However, in the process of estimating $T_a \cdot V$ from a concentration profile with long decay time using Equation (6.12), the value of λ_{z2} can be ignored (see discussion in Model 2), and the variability of the estimated $T_a \cdot V$ is reduced to a minimum. Such an example is described by Model 2 and shown in Figure 6.5. In this example, the variability associated with K_{el} is 43%, with K_{12} 33%, and with K_{21} 40%. The drug has a long decay time because of its small K_{21}.

As a result of the large intrasubject variability in the second decay time, a large difference in the area under the curve and mean residence time can be expected between the two formulations. The estimated pharmacokinetic parameters for the above example using the time constant analysis are listed in Table 6.3, and the estimated time constants are presented in Figure 6.6. The intrasubject variability results in a large difference in the area under the concentration curve and the mean residence between the two formulations.

Now let us examine the time constant plot (Figure 6.6). Interestingly, there is not much difference in time constants T_0, T_{z1}, and T_{z2} of the two formulations, despite the large variability in K_{el} (43%), K_{12} (33%), and K_{21} (40%). The resulting variability in the estimated $T_a \cdot V$ is also small. However, the variability in the rate constants is reflected in the mean residence time, which shows a 30% difference between the two formulations.

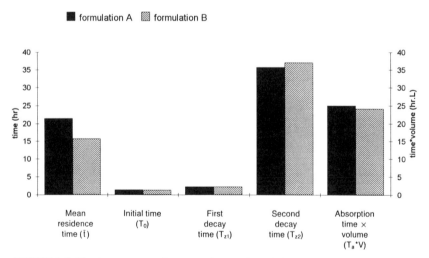

FIGURE 6.6. The time constant plot comparing two formulations of the examples in Figure 6.5. There is not much difference in time constants T_0, T_{z1}, and T_{z2} of the two formulations, despite the large variability in K_{el} (43%), K_{12} (33%), and K_{21} (40%).

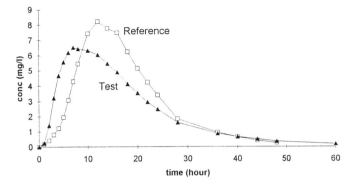

FIGURE 6.7. Mean plasma concentration profiles of theophylline following a single dose of two different formulations of 600 mg theophylline to eighteen subjects. (Reproduced with permission from Reference [11].) The time constant plot comparing the two formulations is shown in Figure 6.8.

EXAMPLES

Example 1: Monoexponential Terminal Phase

Theophylline was given to eighteen healthy subjects to assess the bioequivalence of two 600-mg oral sustained release formulations [11]. The mean plasma concentration profiles of the two formulations are shown in Figure 6.7. The concentration curves show a clear difference in the maximum concentration and the time to reach the maximum concentration. Since the formulations are sustained release, the extent and rate of absorption may be significantly affected by the performance of the formulations,

TABLE 6.4. Pharmacokinetic Parameters of Theophylline for the Example in Figure 6.7 Estimated by the Time Constant Analysis.

Parameter	Reference*	Test*	Percent Difference	Equation
$\bar{t}$ (hr)	18.0	17.7	1.7%	(6.1)
T_0 (hr)	5.56	4.17	25.0%	(6.3)
T_z (hr)	9.52	12.35	29.6%	(6.3)
$T_a \cdot V/fF$ (hr·L)	207.9	210.1	1.1%	(6.7)
C_{max} (mg/L)	8.22	6.51	20.8%	
AUC (mg·hr/L)	146.9	137.1	6.6%	

*Estimated from the mean concentration profiles.

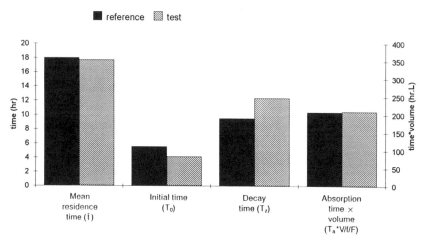

FIGURE 6.8. The time constant plot for theophylline using Model 1, comparing two different formulations. The between-formulation variabilities of T_0 and T_z are much higher than the variability of $T_a \cdot Vl(fF)$.

as well as the intrasubject variability. Both concentration profiles exhibit monoexponential elimination phases. Therefore, Model 1 was used for the estimation of pharmacokinetic parameters. The estimated parameters are listed in Table 6.4, and the estimated time constants are presented in Figure 6.8. The intrasubject variability of C_{max} is much higher than the variability of AUC and $T_a \cdot Vl(fF)$. Similarly, from the time constant plot (Figure 6.8), the variabilities of T_0 and T_z are much higher than the variability of $T_a \cdot Vl(fF)$. In this example, $T_a \cdot Vl(fF)$ may be more appropriate than other parameters for the assessment of absorption characteristics, since the parameter $T_a \cdot Vl(fF)$ is directly dependent on the absorption time and the extent of absorption.

Example 2: Relatively Long Second Decay Time

Bioequivalence of two formulations (tablet and suppository) of etodolac was assessed by giving 200 mg etodolac of both formulations to ten healthy subjects [10]. The mean plasma concentration profiles after dosing the two formulations are shown in Figure 6.9. Because etodolac is not noticeably subjected to the first pass effect, it can be expected that a possible difference in the bioavailability between the oral and rectal formulations may be due to a difference in the fraction absorbed but not due to the first pass effect. The concentration curves exhibit biexponential elimination phases. Therefore, Model 2 is used to estimate the pharmacokinetic parameters. The estimated

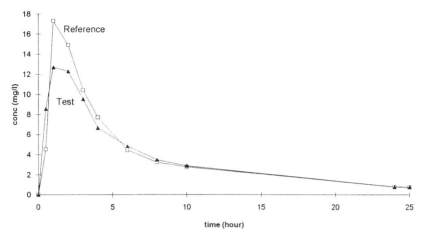

FIGURE 6.9. Mean plasma concentration profiles of etodolac in ten healthy subjects following a single dose of 200 mg etodolac of two formulations. (Reproduced from Reference [10] with permission.) The time constant plot comparing the two formulations is shown in Figure 6.10.

parameters are listed in Table 6.5, and the estimated time constants are presented in Figure 6.10.

Now let us examine the time constant plot (Figure 6.10). The second decay time constant T_{z2} is much longer than the first decay time constant T_{z1}; therefore, the terms containing the second decay exponent λ_{z2} in the numerator of Equation (6.12) are canceled out in the process of calculating $T_a \cdot V_1/(fF)$. The difference in C_{max} is much higher than the difference in AUC and the difference in $T_a \cdot V_1/(fF)$ between the two formulations. The differences in the mean residence time $\bar{t}$ and in the time constants T_0, T_{z1},

TABLE 6.5. *Pharmacokinetic Parameters of Etodolac for the Example in Figure 6.9 Estimated by the Time Constant Analysis.*

Parameter	Reference*	Test*	Percent Difference	Equation
$\bar{t}$ (hr)	8.9	9.1	1.7%	(6.8)
T_0 (hr)	0.75	0.65	13.5%	(6.3)
T_{z1} (hr)	1.61	1.72	6.9%	(6.3)
T_{z2} (hr)	11.76	10.99	6.6%	(6.3)
$T_a \cdot V_1/fF$ (hr·L)	7.04	7.58	7.6%	(6.12)
C_{max} (mg/L)	17.3	12.7	26.6%	
AUC (mg·hr/L)	105.3	100.3	4.7%	

*Estimated from the mean concentration profiles.

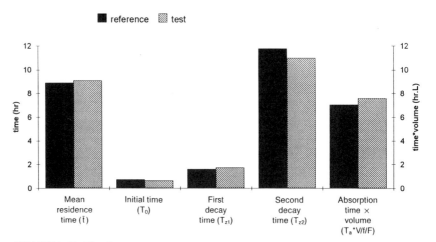

FIGURE 6.10. The time constant plot of etodolac using Model 2, comparing two different formulations. The differences in the mean residence time $\bar{t}$ and in the time constants $T_a \cdot V_1/(fF)$, T_0, T_{z1}, and T_{z2} between the two formulations are relatively small, suggesting that the elimination, distribution, and absorption time constants are similar between the two formulations.

and T_{z2} between the two formulations are also small, suggesting that the elimination, distribution, and absorption time constants are similar between the two formulations. To summarize, all the time constants and parameters, except for the maximum concentration, indicate similar performance between the two formulations. The results from the time constant analysis therefore suggest that the absorption rate is not significantly different between the two formulations, despite the fact that they are administered through two different routes (oral and rectal).

REFERENCES

1. Benko S. M., Grezal E., and Klebovich I., "Comparative bioavailability of two different rectal preparations of piroxicam in man," *Eur. J. Clin. Pharmacol.*, 1992; 43:315–317.
2. Broggini M., Benvenuti C., Botta V., and Broccali G., "Pharmacokinetics of fluocinolone acetonide in patch versus cream formulations," *Int. J. Clin. Pharm. Res.*, 1991; XI(1):17–21.
3. Chen M., "An alternative approach for assessment of rate of absorption in bioequivalence studies," *Pharmaceutical Research*, 1992; 9(11):1380–1385.
4. DeVito J. M., Kozloski G. D., Tonelli A. P., and Johnson J. B., "Bioequivalence of oral and injectable levoleucovorin and leucovorin," *Clinical Pharmacy*, Apr. 1993; 12:293–299.

5. Endrenyi L., Fritsch S., and Yan W., "C_{max}/AUC is a clearer measure than C_{max} for absorption rates in investigations of bioequivalence," *International Journal of Clinical Pharmacology, Therapy and Toxicology,* 1991; 29(10):394–399.

6. Lenhard G., Kieferndorf U., Berner G., Vogtle-Junkert U., and Wagener H. H., "The importance of pharmacokinetic data on sulpiride: Results of a bioequivalence study of two sulpiride 200 mg preparations following oral administration," *International Journal of Clinical Pharmacology, Therapy and Toxicology,* 1991; 29(6):231–237.

7. Lennernas H., Ahrenstedt O., Hallgren R., Knutson L., Ryde M., and Paalzow L. K., "Regional jejunal perfusion, a new in vivo approach to study oral drug absorption in man," *Pharmaceutical Research,* 1992; 9(10):1243–1251.

8. Li Kam Wa T. C., Freestone S., Samson R. R., Johnston N. R., and Lee M. R., "A comparison of the effects of two putative 5-hydroxytryptamine renal prodrugs in normal man," *Br. J. Clin. Pharmac.,* 1993; 36:19–23.

9. Martinez M. N. and Jackson A. J., "Suitability of various nonlinear under the plasma concentration-time curve (AUC) estimates for use in bioequivalence determinations: Relationship to AUC from zero to time infinity (AUC0–inf)," *Pharmaceutical Research,* 1991; 8(4):512–517.

10. Molina-Martinez I. T., Herrero R., Gutierrez J. A., Iglesias J. M., Fabregas J. L., Martinez-Tobed A., and Cadorniga R., "Bioavailability and bioequivalence of two formulations of etodolac (tablets and suppositories)," *Journal of Pharmaceutical Sciences,* 1993; 82(2):211–213.

11. Sauter R., Steinijans V. W., Diletti E., Bohm A., and Schulz H.-U., "Presentation of results from bioequivalence studies," *International Journal of Clinical Pharmacology, Therapy and Toxicology,* 1992; 30 suppl. (1):S7–30.

12. Schulz H. U., Dysing R., Luhrmann B., and Frercks H. J., "Investigation of the bioequivalence of two carbamazepine sustained-release formulations in healthy subjects," *International Journal of Clinical Pharmacology, Therapy and Toxicology,* 1992; 30(10):410–414.

13. Schulz H. U. and Steinijans V. W., "Striving for standards in bioequivalence assessment: A review," *International Journal of Clinical Pharmacology, Therapy and Toxicology.* 1992; 30, suppl. (1):s1–6.

14. Tsai J. J., Lai M. L., Kao Yang Y. H., and Huang J. D., "Comparison on bioequivalence of four phenytoin preparations in patients with multiple-dose treatment," *J. Clin. Pharmacol.* 1992; 32:272–276.

15. Valecha N., Gupta U., and Mehta V. L., "Comparative bioequivalence study of different brands of acetyl salicylic acid in human volunteers," *European Journal of Drug Metabolism and Pharmacokinetics,* 1993; 18(3):251–253.

16. Vigano G., Garagiola U., and Gaspari F., "Pharmacokinetic study of a new oral buffered acetylsalicylic acid (ASA) formulation in comparison with plain ASA in healthy volunteers," *Int. J. Clin. Pharm. Res.,* 1991; XI(3):129–135.

17. "Guidance: Statistical procedures for bioequivalence studies using a standard two-treatment crossover design," Division of Bioequivalence, Office of Generic Drugs, Food and Drug Administration, 1992.

18. Abdou H. M., *Dissolution, Bioavailability & Bioequivalence,* MACK Publishing Company, 1989.

CHAPTER 7

Influence of Dosage on Pharmacokinetics – Dose Proportionality

INTRODUCTION

The invariance, with respect to dose, of the time constants and bioavailability of a drug and its metabolites is determined in the dose proportionality study. If plasma concentration of a drug is proportional to dose, one can assume that the pharmacological effect also changes proportionally with dose unless the effect-concentration relationship is nonlinear. On the other hand, if drug concentration does not change proportionally with dose, caution must be taken when altering the dose. There is a distinction between linearity and proportionality. Linearity means that the relationship between two variables (for example, hepatic elimination time and dose) falls on a straight line. Proportionality means that this straight line passes through the origin.

Several factors can cause dose nonlinearity. The most common one is a saturable metabolism [11], where hepatic enzyme receptors become saturated with the drug as the plasma drug concentration increases with dose. As a result of the saturable metabolism, the drug accumulates disproportionally in the body when increasing the dose. A second factor that can lead to dose nonlinearity is active intestinal absorption, which occurs in many hydrophilic drugs such as amoxicillin [14] and cefadroxil [8]. After the administration of a dose that saturates absorption, a zero-order absorption kinetics is followed by a first-order absorption kinetics. A third factor affecting the dose linearity is active renal tubular secretion and saturable renal tubular reabsorption [8]. To summarize, the key time constants in a dose proportionality study include the hepatic elimination, the absorption, and the renal elimination time.

Common themes among the dose proportionality study and other pharmacokinetic studies can be revealed by the time constant analysis.

143

Nonlinearity in pharmacokinetics can be a common theme among different studies. If dose nonlinearity in time constants is identified in a dose proportionality study, nonlinearity in these time constants may also be observed in a sustained release versus immediate release study since different levels of drug concentrations will be produced by the two types of formulations. Nonlinearity in pharmacokinetics can also be observed in the multiple-dose study. For example, if nonlinearity in decay time is observed in a single-dose study, the time constant may also change with dosing days in a multiple dose study. A saturable protein binding can also be a common theme among different studies. A nonlinear renal elimination time may be caused by a saturable protein binding, where higher plasma drug concentration will result in a greater free fraction of drug and a shorter renal elimination time. In this case, the elimination time is susceptible to any factor affecting protein binding, such as those in renal impairment (Chapter 17), inflammatory diseases (Chapter 19), age (Chapter 15), gender (Chapter 16), and drug interaction studies (Chapter 14). Poor dissolution can be another common theme among studies. If nonlinearity in absorption time is caused by dissolution limited absorption, meal and formulation may shorten the absorption time in food (Chapter 13) and bioequivalence studies since these two factors can improve the dissolution.

Two models are discussed in this chapter: (1) the first model describes the pharmacokinetics of drugs without information about metabolism, and (2) the second model describes the pharmacokinetics of drugs with the concentration profiles of metabolites. Two simulated case studies and two literature examples are discussed to illustrate the utility of these models in dose proportionality studies. Further literature examples of dose proportionality studies can be found in References [1–16].

PHARMACOKINETIC MODELS

This section presents two models that are useful in determining dose proportionality of pharmacokinetics. The goal is to establish simple relationships between time constants and measurable parameters such as (1) mean residence time, which is the sum of input and output times, and (2) area under the curves. The derivations of these relationships are straightforward and are discussed in Chapter 2.

Model 1: Drugs without Information about Metabolism

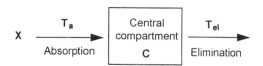

Nonlinear pharmacokinetics may be associated with almost any pharmacokinetic process: absorption, metabolism, renal excretion, renal reabsorption, plasma protein binding, tissue binding, dissolution, and distribution. All these processes may be saturable with high drug concentrations. Most commonly, metabolism is saturable because of the limited capacity of hepatic enzymes [11]. Renal elimination may be nonlinear if tubular secretion or reabsorption is involved [8]. Intestinal absorption may be nonlinear if an active absorption depends on the capacity of transport proteins in the absorbing cell [8,14]. When metabolism is not involved or metabolite concentrations are not measured in a dose proportionality study, Model 1 can be used to assess the linearity of the absorption and elimination. The key pharmacokinetic parameters can be derived from the Time Constant Approach and are listed below.

The mean residence time is simply the sum of input and output times

$$\text{Mean residence time } (\bar{t}) \ = \ \frac{\text{AUMC}}{\text{AUC}}$$

$$= \ \text{Input time } (T_{in}) \ + \ \text{Output time } (T_{out}) \ = \ T_a \ + \ T_{el} \qquad (7.1)$$

where the mean residence time can be estimated from the ratio of the area under the first moment curve to the area under the concentration curve. As shown, the mean residence time is a sum of the absorption time and the elimination time. Therefore, the mean residence time can vary with dose if either absorption or elimination follows nonlinear kinetics. Both bioavailability f (with $F = 1$ since no metabolism is involved) and renal clearance time constant T_{el}/V can be estimated from the cumulative urine recovery:

$$\text{Bioavailability } (f) \ = \ \frac{X_u}{X_0} \qquad (7.2)$$

$$\text{Renal clearance time } \left(\frac{T_{el}}{V}\right) \ = \ \frac{\text{AUC}}{X_u} \qquad (7.3)$$

where X_u is the total urine recovery of the drug. The decay time constant T_z can be estimated from a partial area under the curve as shown in the following equation (see Appendix 2):

$$\frac{1}{\text{Decay time } (T_z)} \ = \ \lambda_z \ = \ 2 \ \frac{(t_{last} \ - \ t) \ \ln (C_t) \ - \ \text{AU} \ \ln C_{t-t_{last}}}{(t_{last} \ - \ t)^2} \qquad (7.4)$$

The initial time constant T_{z0} ($1/\lambda_0$) can be estimated using a curve-stripping technique. In case of a possible flip-flop of the concentration profile, the absorption time can be more accurately characterized by $T_a \cdot V$ than by the initial time constant T_{z0} (see Chapter 6).

$$\text{Absorption time} \times \text{volume } (T_a \cdot V) = \frac{fFX_0}{A(\lambda_0 - \lambda_1)} \qquad (7.5)$$

Model 2: Drugs with the Concentration Profiles of Metabolites

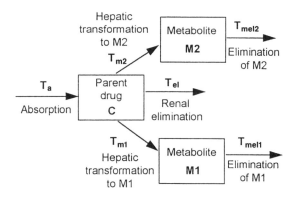

This model describes the pharmacokinetics of a drug with two metabolites. Saturable metabolism is the most common cause of nonlinearity in pharmacokinetics of drugs. The rate of metabolism frequently follows the Michaelis-Menten kinetics:

$$\text{Metabolic rate} = \frac{V_m \cdot C}{K_m + C} \qquad (7.6)$$

where the metabolic rate reaches a plateau as the drug concentration C increases. The ratio of the metabolic rate to the drug concentration $[= V_m/(K_m + C)]$ will thus drop with an increase in the concentration. Therefore, by assuming a first-order elimination kinetics for a drug with saturable metabolism, the estimated first-order rate constant will decrease with the dose.

The mean residence time of the concentration curves for the parent drug and the metabolites is the sum of input and output times:

$$\text{Mean residence time of C } (\bar{t}_C) = \frac{\text{AUMC}_C}{\text{AUC}_C}$$

$$= \text{Input time } (T_{c,in}) + \text{Output time } (T_{c,out}) = T_a + T_{el,t} \qquad (7.7)$$

$$\text{Mean residence time of } M_i \ (\bar{t}_{Mi}) \ = \ \frac{\text{AUMC}_{Mi}}{\text{AUC}_{Mi}}$$

$$= \text{ Input time } (T_{mi,in}) = \text{Output time } (T_{mi,out}) = T_a + T_{el,t} + T_{meli} \qquad (7.8)$$

where $T_{el,t} = 1/(1/T_{el} + 1/T_{ml} + 1/T_{m2})$ is the total elimination time as a result of the combination of renal elimination and hepatic elimination. The objective of the following derivation is to express elimination time constants as functions of the area under the curve or mean residence time. First, the ratio of elimination time to the formation time of a metabolite is equal to the ratio of the area under the metabolite concentration curve to the area under the parent drug concentration curve.

$$\frac{\text{Elimination clearance time of } M_i}{\text{Formation clearance time toward } M_i} = \frac{T_{meli} V_c}{T_{mi} V_{mi}} = \frac{\text{AUC}_{Mi}}{\text{AUC}_c} \qquad (7.9)$$

This ratio of area under the curve is an appropriate indicator to characterize the nonlinearity of metabolic rate in a dose proportionality study, provided the elimination time of the metabolite is constant with dose. However, if the elimination of the metabolite, either renal or hepatic, is nonlinear, this elimination time must be estimated first from the difference in the mean residence time between the metabolite and the parent drug, as seen in the following equation:

$$\text{Elimination time of } M_i \ (T_{meli}) = \bar{t}_{Mi} - \bar{t}_c \qquad (7.10)$$

Then the formation of the metabolite can be estimated according to the following expression:

$$\text{Normalized hepatic elimination time} \left(\frac{T_{mi} V_{mi}}{V_c} \right) = \frac{T_{meli} \text{AUC}_c}{\text{AUC}_{Mi}} \qquad (7.11)$$

CASE STUDIES

Case 1: Saturable Absorption and Renal Excretion

A variety of hydrophilic drugs, such as some antibiotic and chemotherapy drugs [8,14], exhibits saturable absorption and renal elimination. As the dose of these drugs increases, the absorption time and the elimination time increase. The pharmacokinetics of these drugs can be described by Model 1, and an example is shown in Figure 7.1. In this exam-

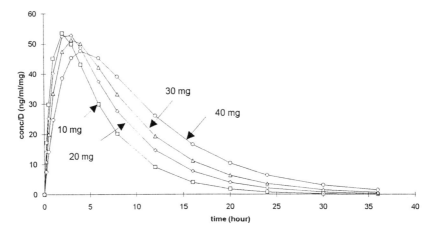

FIGURE 7.1. The simulated plasma drug concentration profiles with saturable absorption and renal excretion for four doses using Model 1. The time constant plot comparing the four doses is shown in Figure 7.2. The parameters used in this simulation are listed below.

Parameters	X_0 (mg)			
	10	20	30	40
f	0.8	0.8	0.8	0.8
F	1	1	1	1
V (L)	10	10	10	10
K_a (hr^{-1})	1.0	0.8	0.6	0.4
K_{el} (hr^{-1})	0.20	0.16	0.14	0.12

ple, the absorption and the elimination rate constants decrease with dose. The concentration profiles show that the time to reach the maximum concentration is delayed with high dose and the mean residence time increases with dose. In addition, the decay time increases with dose due to the prolonged renal elimination time.

Both saturable absorption and saturable renal excretion can affect the linearity of area under the curve, maximum concentration, and mean residence time. To determine the source of nonlinearity, time constants directly associated with the absorption and elimination must be estimated. However, if urine data are not available, as in this example, the only time constants useful for identifying nonlinear absorption and elimination are the decay time T_{z1} and the initial time constant T_{z0}. The estimated pharmacokinetic parameters using the Time Constant Approach are listed in Table 7.1. Now let us examine the time constant plot (Figure 7.2). The initial time constant T_{z0} increases with dose from 4.55 hours at 10 mg to 8.33 hours at 40 mg, indicating a saturable absorption. Since both T_{z0} and T_{z1} are

TABLE 7.1. The Estimated Pharmacokinetic Parameters Using the Time Constant Approach for the Example Shown in Figure 7.1.

Parameter	10 mg TCA	10 mg Model Value	20 mg TCA	20 mg Model Value	30 mg TCA	30 mg Model Value	40 mg TCA	40 mg Model Value	Equation
T_{z1} (hr)	4.55	5	5.88	6.25	6.67	7.14	7.69	8.33	(7.4)
T_{z0} (hr)	1.08	1.0	1.41	1.25	1.89	1.69	2.70	2.5	(7.1)
$\bar{t}$ (hr)	5.9	6	7.3	7.5	8.6	8.8	11	10.8	(7.1)
AUC (ng·hr/L)	4036	4000	10.071	10,000	17,237	17,142	26,738	26,667	
AUC/D (ng·hr/L/mg)	403	400	503	500	574	571	668	667	

TCA: Time Constant Approach.

149

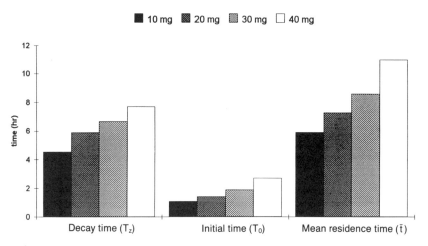

FIGURE 7.2. The time constants plot comparing four doses of the example in Figure 7.1. The initial time constant T_{z0} increases with dose from 4.55 hours at 10 mg to 8.33 hours at 40 mg, indicating a saturable absorption. At the same time the renal excretion is also saturated with a high dose, and the decay time T_{z1} increases from 1.08 hour at 10 mg to 2.7 hours at 40 mg.

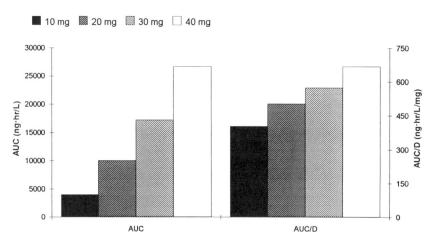

FIGURE 7.3. The area under the concentration curve and the normalized area under the curves of four doses for the example in Figure 7.1.

nonlinear, both T_a and T_{el} must be nonlinear as well. However, the assignment of T_{z0} and T_{z1} to T_a and T_{el} is uncertain due to possible flip-flop. At the same time, the renal excretion is also saturated with a high dose, and the decay time T_{z1} increases from 1.08 hour at 10 mg to 2.7 hours at 40 mg. As a result of the increase in both absorption time and elimination time, the mean residence time is prolonged from 5.9 hours to 11 hours with the increasing dose. The increase in the area under the concentration curve (AUC) is disproportional with the dose. This is revealed by the trend in the normalized area under the curve (AUC/D), which increases with the dose (Figure 7.3). To summarize, saturable absorption and elimination result in more than a proportional increase in the area under the curve with dose.

Case 2: Saturable Metabolism

When the metabolism of a drug is significant compared with the renal elimination, the dose proportionality study can be used to detect the saturable metabolic kinetics. The linearity of the parent drug with dose is determined by comparing the normalized area under the curve as discussed in Case 1. However, the saturable metabolism can be identified sometimes only by the ratio of the AUC of metabolite to that of the parent drug and not by the normalized AUC of the metabolite alone. This is especially true when one of the metabolic pathways dominates the elimination ($T_{mi} \ll T_{el}$). This is demonstrated by using Model 2 as an example, where a parent drug has two metabolites and one of the metabolites (M2) dominates the elimination. The simulated plasma concentration profiles of the parent drug and metabolites for four different doses using the model are shown in Figures 7.4–7.6. In this example, the hepatic elimination time toward M2 is much shorter than the hepatic elimination time toward M1 and the renal elimination time. As a result, hepatic metabolism toward M2 dominates the elimination.

When the disposition of a drug involves extensive metabolism, frequently, the pharmacokinetics of the drug is nonlinear due to saturable metabolic reactions. If a nonlinear metabolism is suspected, it is critical to measure the metabolite concentrations, as well as the drug concentration, in order to estimate the hepatic elimination time at different dose levels. The estimated pharmacokinetic parameters of the above example using the Time Constant Approach are listed in Table 7.2.

Now let us examine the time constant plot. Flip-flops occur with the concentration profiles of the parent drug because the elimination time is shorter than the absorption time. Therefore the decay time $T_{z,c}$ of the parent drug, which is equal to the absorption time constant due to the flip-flop, does not change with dose although the elimination time increases. The decay time of the two metabolites does not change with dose either, since the elimina-

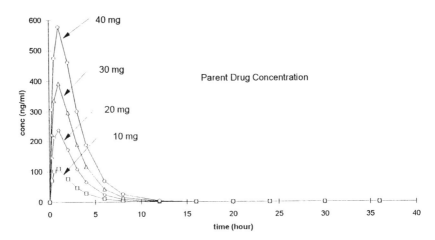

FIGURE 7.4. The simulated plasma drug concentration profiles of four doses with saturable metabolism using Model 2. The time constant plot comparing the four doses is shown in Figure 7.9. The parameters used in this simulation are listed below for each dose, X_0:

Parameters	X_0 (mg)			
	10	20	30	40
f	0.8	0.8	0.8	0.8
F	1	1	1	1
V (L)	10	10	10	10
K_a (hr^{-1})	0.5	0.5	0.5	0.5
K_{el} (hr^{-1})	0.1	0.1	0.1	0.1
K_{m1} (hr^{-1})	0.3	0.25	0.2	0.15
K_{mel1} (hr^{-1})	0.1	0.1	0.1	0.1
K_{m2} (hr^{-1})	2	1.8	1.6	1.4
K_{mel2} (hr^{-1})	0.15	0.15	0.15	0.15

152

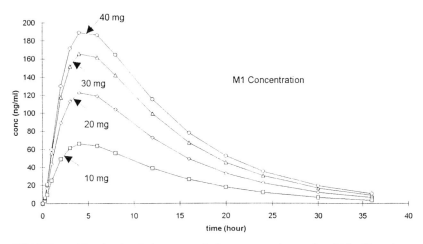

FIGURE 7.5. The simulated plasma metabolite concentration profiles (M1) of four doses using Model 2 for the example in Figure 7.4.

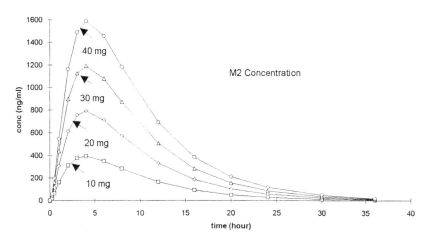

FIGURE 7.6. The simulated plasma metabolite concentration profiles (M2) of four doses using Model 2 for the example in Figure 7.4.

TABLE 7.2. The Estimated Pharmacokinetic Parameters Using the Time Constant Approach for the Example Shown in Figures 7.4–7.6.

Parameter	10 mg TCA	10 mg Model Value	20 mg TCA	20 mg Model Value	30 mg TCA	30 mg Model Value	40 mg TCA	40 mg Model Value	
$T_{z,c}$ (hr)	1.9	2 (T_a)	1.9	2 (T_s)	1.9	2 (T_a)	2.0	2 (T_a)	(7.4)
$T_{z,m1}$ (hr)	9.7	10	9.7	10	9.8	10	9.7	10	(7.4)
$T_{z,m2}$ (hr)	6.3	6.7	6.3	6.7	6.3	6.7	6.3	6.7	(7.4)
$\bar{t}_C$ (hr)	2.4	2.4	2.5	2.5	2.5	2.5	2.6	2.6	(7.7)
$\bar{t}_{M1}$ (hr)	12.3	12.4	12.4	12.5	12.4	12.5	12.5	12.6	(7.8)
$\bar{t}_{M2}$ (hr)	9	9.1	9.1	9.1	9.1	9.2	9.2	9.3	(7.8)
T_{meI1} (hr)	9.9	10.0	9.9	10.0	9.9	10.0	9.9	10.0	(7.10)
T_{meI1} (hr)	6.6	6.7	6.6	6.6	6.6	6.7	6.6	6.7	(7.10)
$T_{m1} \cdot V_{m1}/V_c$ (hr)	3.3	3.33	3.96	4.0	4.95	5.0	6.6	6.7	(7.11)
$T_{m2} \cdot V_{m2}/V_c$ (hr)	0.5	0.5	0.55	0.55	0.62	0.63	0.71	0.72	(7.11)
AUC_C (ng·hr/ml)	337	333	752	744	1275	1263	1958	1939	
AUC_{M1} (ng·hr/ml)	1002	1000	1863	1860	2530	2526	2913	2909	
AUC_{M2} (ng·hr/ml)	4469	4444	8978	8930	13,546	13,473	18,198	18,101	
AUC_C/D (ng·hr/ml/mg)	0.034	0.033	0.038	0.037	0.043	0.042	0.049	0.048	
AUC_{M1}/D (ng·hr/ml/mg)	0.1	0.1	0.093	0.093	0.084	0.084	0.073	0.073	
AUC_{M2}/D (ng·hr/ml/mg)	0.45	0.44	0.045	0.045	0.45	0.45	0.45	0.45	
AUC_{M1}/AUC_C	3	3	2.5	2.5	2.0	2	1.5	1.5	(7.9)
AUC_{M2}/AUC_C	13.3	13.3	11.9	12	10.6	10.7	9.3	9.3	(7.9)

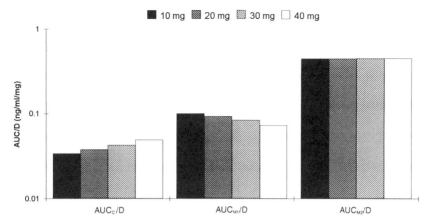

FIGURE 7.7. The normalized area under the curves for the parent drug and the metabolites of the example shown in Figures 7.4–7.6.

tion time of the metabolites (T_{mel}s) dominates the decay time of the metabolites (T_{mel1} and $T_{mel2} \gg T_{el,t}$) and T_{mel}s are not affected by the dose. The mean residence time of the drug and metabolites does not change much with the dose either, since the absorption time constant dominates the mean residence time of all three compounds. The areas under the curve for the parent drug and metabolite M1 are nonlinear with the dose, while the area under the curve for metabolite M2 is linear with the dose (Figure 7.7). How-

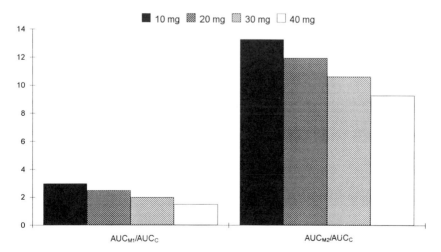

FIGURE 7.8. The ratio of the metabolite area under the curves to the parent drug area under the curve of the example shown in Figures 7.4–7.6.

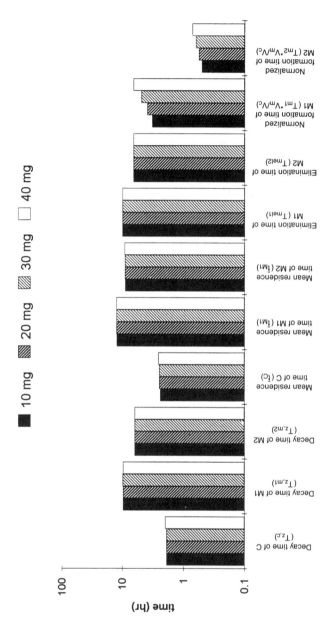

FIGURE 7.9. The time constant plot comparing four doses of the example in Figures 7.4–7.6. The nonlinear metabolism can be demonstrated by the increasing hepatic elimination times ($T_{m1} * V_m/V_c$ and $T_{m2} * V_m/V_c$) with dose.

ever, the ratios of the areas under the curves between the metabolites and the parent drug reveal the saturable kinetics for both metabolic pathways (Figure 7.8). The nonlinear metabolism can also be demonstrated by the increasing hepatic elimination time with dose, as shown in Figure 7.9.

To summarize, as a result of the nonlinearity of hepatic elimination times T_{m1} and T_{m2}, the normalized area under the drug concentration curve increases with dose; the normalized area under the metabolite M1 concentration curve decreases with dose, while the normalized area under the metabolite M2 concentration curve does not change with dose. Therefore, depending on whether the drug or the metabolites are pharmacologically active, the pharmacodynamic effect may increase, decrease, or remain unchanged with dose.

EXAMPLES

Example 1: Saturable Absorption and Saturable Tubular Reabsorption

The pharmacokinetics of cefadroxil at three dose levels were studied following the oral administration of 5, 15, and 30 mg/kg of cefadroxil to six healthy male subjects [8]. The mean plasma concentration profiles after the three different doses are shown in Figure 7.10. Based on the initial and terminal slopes of the concentration profiles, the initial time constant and the

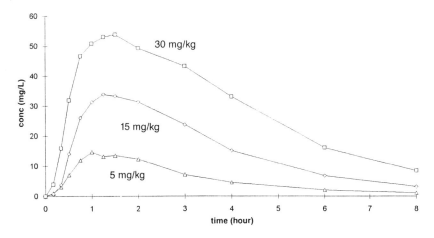

FIGURE 7.10. Mean plasma concentration of cefadroxil in healthy subjects after the oral administration of 5, 15, and 30 mg/kg of cefadroxil. (Reproduced from Reference [8] with permission.) The time constant plots comparing the three doses are shown in Figures 7.12 and 7.13.

decay time constant seem to be dose-dependent. There is no metabolism involved, and the unchanged drug is completely recovered in the urine within 24 hours. The plasma concentration curves of cefadroxil after intravenous doses are known to follow a two-compartment model; however, after the oral administration in this study, the concentration curves collapse and follow a one-compartment model.

Pharmacokinetic data of beta-lactam antibiotics in animals indicate that the drugs are actively absorbed and are subjected to active renal tubular secretion, as well as tubular reabsorption. Both active absorption and nonlinear elimination may affect the descriptive pharmacokinetic parameters, such as the area under the curve, the maximum concentration and the decay time. Therefore, key time constants must be estimated to identify the cause of nonlinearity. In this example, the key time constants are the absorption time and the renal elimination time. The pharmacokinetic parameters are estimated from Model 1, since the concentration profiles follow a one-compartmental model, and no metabolite is involved.

The absorption of cefadroxil seems to be saturable, where it follows a zero-order kinetics immediately after dosing and becomes a first-order later. Therefore, the first two time points at 0.5 and 1 hour, where the absorption follows the zero-order kinetics, are excluded from the estimation (curve-stripping technique) of the initial time constant T_{z0}. The normalized area under the concentration curve decreases with dose (Figure 7.11); however, the difference in the normalized area under the curve between the two higher doses is relatively small.

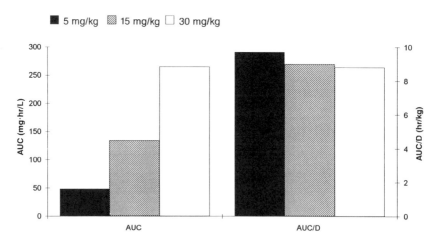

FIGURE 7.11. The area under the curve and the normalized area under the plasma concentration curve (AUC/D) of cefadroxil at three different doses in the example in Figure 7.10.

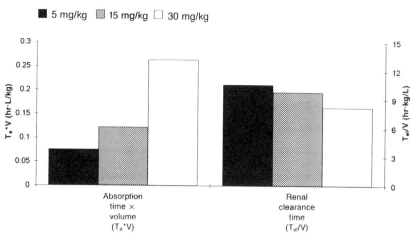

FIGURE 7.12. The absorption and elimination time of cefadroxil at three different doses in the example of Figure 7.10. The value of $T_a \cdot V$ increases significantly with the dose, indicating a saturable absorption kinetics, which is also observed in animal data. On the other hand, the renal elimination time T_{el}/V decreases slightly with the dose, reflecting a possible saturable tubular reabsorption.

Now let us examine the time constant plots (Figures 7.12 and 7.13). The mean residence time increases with doses, indicating an increase in either the absorption time or the elimination time (Figure 7.12). Both T_{z0} and T_{z1} increase with dose, and the increase is more significant in the initial time constant. Because of the possibility of flip-flop, the absorption time is further characterized by $T_a \cdot V$, and the elimination time is characterized by T_{el}/V (Figure 7.12). The value of $T_a \cdot V$ increases significantly with the dose, indicating a saturable absorption kinetics, which is also observed in animal data. On the other hand, the renal elimination time T_{el}/V decreases slightly with the dose, reflecting a possible saturable tubular reabsorption.

The decay time T_{z1} increases with the dose despite the decrease in the renal elimination time (Table 7.3); therefore, the decay time may be dominated by the distribution process instead of the elimination process, and the distribution time may also be dose-dependent, or with increasing dose the absorption time prolongs and dominates the decay time. In general, the absorption and elimination time, instead of the initial and decay time constants, should be used to characterize absorption and elimination. To summarize, the plasma concentration of cefadroxil may be less than proportional with a high dose due to saturable absorption; therefore, it may require frequent, but small, doses to effectively achieve a greater area under the concentration curve, as indicated in Reference [8].

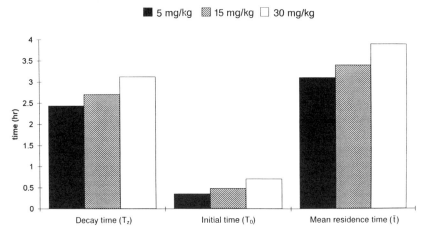

FIGURE 7.13. The decay and initial time constants and the mean residence time of cefadroxil at three different doses in the example of Figure 7.10. Both T_{z0} and T_{z1} increase with dose, and the increase is more significant in the initial time constant.

Example 2: Saturable Hepatic and Renal Eliminations

The pharmacokinetics of loperamide oxide and loperamide after oral administration of increasing dose (1 to 16 mg) of loperamide oxide were investigated in ten healthy male subjects [11]. The mean concentration profiles of loperamide oxide and loperamide after the different doses are shown in Figures 7.14 and 7.15, respectively. The concentration profiles of loperamide oxide show rapid absorption and elimination. On the other hand, loperamide concentration shows broad profiles, indicating slower elimination rates.

TABLE 7.3. *The Estimated Pharmacokinetic Parameters of Cefadroxil Using the Time Constant Approach Following Three Different Oral Doses.*

Parameter*	5 mg/kg	15 mg/kg	30 mg/kg	Equation
T_{z1} (hr)	2.44	2.70	3.13	(7.4)
T_{z0} (hr)	0.35	0.48	0.70	(7.1)
$\bar{t}$ (hr)	3.1	3.4	3.9	(7.1)
$T_a \cdot V$ (hr·L/kg)	0.075	0.122	0.263	(7.5)
T_{el}/V (hr·kg/L)	10.53	9.80	8.20	(7.3)
AUC (mg·hr/L)	48.3	134.3	264.8	
AUC/D (hr/L)	9.7	9.0	8.8	
f	0.92	0.91	1.08	(7.2)

*Estimated from the mean concentration profiles or the reported mean parameters.

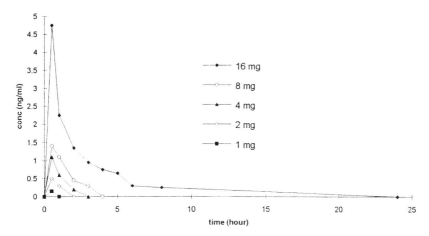

FIGURE 7.14. Mean loperamide oxide plasma concentration profiles following administration of 1 mg, 2 mg, 4 mg, 8 mg, and 16 mg of loperamide oxide. (Reproduced from Reference [11] with permission.) The time constant plot comparing the five doses is shown in Figure 7.18.

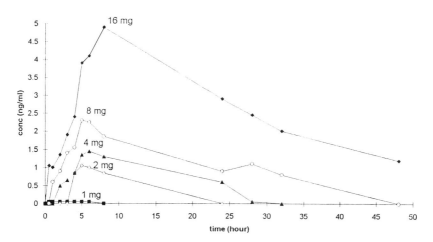

FIGURE 7.15. Mean loperamide plasma concentration profiles following administration of 1 mg, 2 mg, 4 mg, 8 mg, and 16 mg of loperamide oxide. (Reproduced from Reference [11] with permission.)

161

It is important in this example to measure plasma concentrations and urine recoveries of the drug and metabolites in order to separately determine the linearity of hepatic and renal eliminations. The key time constants in this example are hepatic and renal elimination times. The pharmacokinetic parameters are estimated using Model 2, and the results are shown in Table 7.4. The normalized area under the curve of loperamide oxide clearly shows an increasing trend with the dose, while the normalized area under the curve of loperamide increases with the smaller doses and reaches a plateau at the higher doses (Figure 7.16).

Now let us examine the time constant plot (Figure 7.18). The mean residence time of both loperamide oxide and loperamide concentration profiles increases with dose, indicating saturable elimination of both compounds. The possibility of saturable absorption is excluded because of the rapid absorption; however, the ratio of the area under the loperamide concentration curve to the area under the loperamide oxide concentration curve, with a ratio equal to $T_{mel} \cdot V_c/(T_m \cdot V_m)$, does not show any trend with the dose (Figure 7.17). This is probably because the change with dose in the formation time T_m and the elimination time T_{mel} of the metabolite cancel out each other. Therefore, it is necessary that the value of T_{mel} and $T_m \cdot V_m/V_c$ be estimated separately. Both time constants, T_m and T_{mel}, clearly increase with dose (Figure 7.18), which is also reflected by the dose-dependent increase in the mean residence time of both compounds. To summarize, the area under the drug concentration curve increases more than proportional with dose, probably due to a saturable metabolism.

TABLE 7.4. *The Estimated Pharmacokinetic Parameters of Loperamide Oxide (C) and Loperamide (M) Using the Time Constant Approach Following Five Different Oral Doses.*

Parameter*	1 mg	2 mg	4 mg	8 mg	16 mg	Equation
$\bar{t}_C$ (hr)	0.5	0.74	0.94	1.31	3.38	(7.7)
$\bar{t}_M$ (hr)	3.56	7.14	11.5	16.09	19.30	(7.8)
T_{mel} (hr)	3.06	6.41	10.53	14.71	15.87	(7.10)
$T_m \cdot V_m/V_c$ (hr)	0.52	1.15	1.45	2.94	5.00	(7.11)
AUC_C (ng·hr/ml)	0.16	0.44	1.29	3.05	10.88	
AUC_M (ng·hr/ml)	0.95	2.45	9.35	15.21	34.14	
AUC_C/D (ng·hr/ml/mg)	0.16	0.22	0.32	0.38	0.68	
AUC_M/D (ng·hr/ml/mg)	0.95	1.23	2.34	1.90	2.13	
AUC_M/AUC_C	5.9	5.6	7.2	5.0	3.1	(7.9)

*Estimated from the mean concentration profiles or the reported mean parameters.

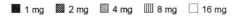

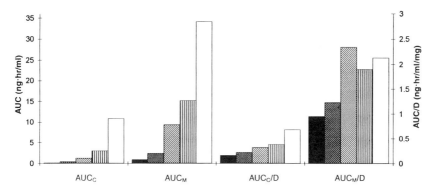

FIGURE 7.16. The area under the concentration curve and the normalized area under the plasma concentration curve of loperamide oxide (C) and loperamide (M) of five different doses.

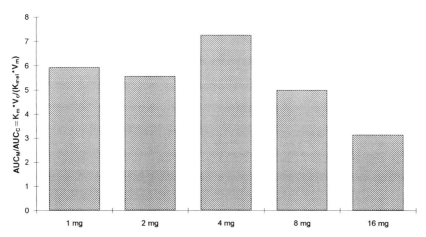

FIGURE 7.17. The ratio of the area under the loperamide concentration curve to the area under the loperamide oxide concentration curve after administration of five different doses.

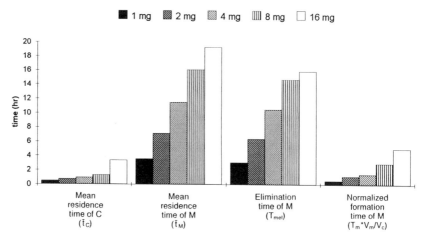

FIGURE 7.18. The time constant plot of loperamide comparing five different doses. Both hepatic elimination time constants (T_m) and elimination time of metabolite (T_{mel}) increase with dose, which is also reflected by the dose-dependent increase in the mean residence time ($\bar{t}_C$ and $\bar{t}_M$) of both compounds.

REFERENCES

1. Broggini M., Botta V., Benvenuti C., Fonio W., Congedo M., and Parini J., "Pharmacokinetics of rokitamycin after single administration to healthy volunteers," *European Journal of Drug Metabolism and Pharmacokinetics*, 1991; 16(2):137–140.

2. Chandler M. H. H., Clifon G. D., Lettieri J. T., Mazzu A. L., Allington D. R., Thieneman A. C., Foster T. S., Harrison M. R., "Multiple dose pharmacokinetics of four different doses of nisoldipine in hypertensive patients," *J. Clin. Pharmacol.*, 1992; 32:571–575.

3. Cutler N. R., Reines S. A., Mclean L. F., Sramek J. J., Porras A. G., and Hand E. L., "Pharmacokinetics and dose proportionality of D2-agonist MK-458 (HPMC) in parkinsonism," *Clin. Pharmacokinet.*, 1992; 22(3):223–230.

4. DE Caro L., Ghizzi A., and Zunino M. T., "Kinetics and pharmacodynamic effects of a novel prodrug of *N*-methyldopamine at single dose in healthy volunteers," *Drug Res.*, 1993; 43(1), Nr 6:651–655.

5. De Vries M. H., de Koning P., Floot H. L., Grahnen A., Eckernas S. A., Raghoebar M., Dahlstrom B., and Ekman L., "Dose-proportionality of eltoprazine," *Eur. J. Clin. Pharmacol.*, 1991; 41:485–488.

6. De Vries M. H., Van Harten J., Van Bemmel P., and Raghoebar M., "Pharmacokinetics of fluvoxamine maleate after increasing single oral doses in healthy subjects," *Bipharmaceutics & Drug Disposition*, 1993; 14:291–296.

7. Eldon M. A., Blake D. S., Coon M. J., Nordblom G. D., Sedman A. J., and Colburn W. A., "Clinical pharmacokinetics of procaterol: Dose proportionality after administration of single oral doses," *Biopharmaceutics & Drug Disposition*, 1992; 13:663–669.

8. Garrigues T. M., Martin U., Peris-Ribera J. E., and Prescott L. F., "Dose-dependent absorption and elimination of cefadroxil in man," *Eur. J. Clin. Pharmacol.* 1991; 41:179–183.

9. Jewell R. C., Banfield C. R., Ruggirello D. A., Huang Y. W., Noonan P. K., and Gonzalez M. A., "Dose proportionality of transdermal nitroglycerin," *Pharmaceutical Research,* 1992; 9(10):1284–1289.

10. Jonkman J. H. G., Bianchetti G., Grasmeijer G., Oosterhuis B., Thiercelin J. F., Thenot J. P., "Clinical pharmacokinetics and tolerability of alpidem in healthy subjects given increasing single doses," *Eur. J. Clin. Pharmacol.,* 1991; 41:369–374.

11. Kamali F., Adriaens L., Huang M. L., Woestenborghs R., Emanuel M., and Rawlins M. D. "Dose proportionality study of loperamide following oral administration of loperamide oxide," *Eur. J. Clin. Pharmacol.,* 1992; 42:693–694.

12. Paintaud G., Alvan G., Dahl M. L., Grahnen A., Sjovall J., and Svensson J. O., "Nonlinearity of amoxicillin absorption kinetics in human," *Eur. J. Clin. Pharmacol.,* 1992; 43:283–288.

13. Shyu W. C., Shah V. R., Campbell D. A., Wilber R. B., Pittman K. A., and Barbhaiya R. H., "Oral absolute bioavailability and intravenous dose-proportionality of cefprozil in humans," *J. Clin. Pharmacol.,* 1992; 32:798–803.

14. Sjovall J., Alvan G., and Westerlund D., "Oral cyclacillin interacts with the absorption of oral ampicillin, amoxycillin, and bacampicillin," *Eur. J. Clin. Pharmacol.,* 1985; 29:495–502.

15. Weyhenmeyer R., Mascher H., and Birkmayer J., "Study on dose-linearity of the pharmacokinetics of silibinin diastereomers using a new stereospecific assay," *International Journal of Clinical Pharmacology, Therapy and Toxicology,* 1992; 30(4):134–138.

16. Zaborny B. A., Lukacsko P., Barino-Colligon I., Ziemniak J. A., "Inhaled corticosteroids in asthma: A dose-proportionality study with triamcinolone acetonide aerosol," *J. Clin. Pharmacol.,* 1992; 32:463–469.

CHAPTER 8

Pharmacokinetics of Sustained Release and Immediate Release Formulations

INTRODUCTION

The objective of designing sustained release formulations can be one of the following: (1) to prolong the mean residence time for drugs with short elimination time, (2) to reduce the number of doses taken each day, (3) to decrease the fluctuation of the plasma drug concentration, or (4) to reduce the maximum plasma concentration for drugs with short absorption time. The objective of a clinical study of sustained release versus immediate formulations is to determine the bioavailability [6,9], absorption rate, plasma concentration fluctuation [5], time period when the plasma concentration is within the therapeutic window [6,10], saturable metabolism and protein binding [3,4], and efficacy of the sustained release formulation compared with the immediate release formulation [5]. The rate of release of drugs from a sustained release formulation can be zero-order, first-order, or a combination of the two.

Some common themes in time constant view can be observed in the sustained release versus immediate release study as well as other studies. Nonlinearity in time constants is a common theme that can be observed in both a dose proportionality study (Chapter 7) and a sustained release versus immediate release study. The absorption characteristics of a drug along the gastrointestinal tract is another common theme. The absorption characteristics of a sustained release formulation depend very much on the absorption time and bioavailability of the drug along the gastrointestinal tract, which can be determined by the gastrointestinal intubation study (Chapter 9). For example, if the intubation study determines that little absorption occurs in the colon, then the sustained release formulation will not maintain a steady plasma concentration beyond 5 hours since the average small in-

167

testinal transit time of drugs is about 4 hours [11]. In addition, if the degree of presystemic metabolism (intestinal metabolism) is found to vary along the gastrointestinal tract in the GI intubation study, a difference in metabolite to drug ratio is expected between sustained release and immediate release formulations. Flip-flop of the concentration profile usually occurs following the administration of a sustained release formulation but not following the immediate release formulation. The flip-flop occurs in the former case because the prolonged absorption time becomes longer than the elimination time. Therefore, the decay time in a sustained release study is frequently longer than the decay time in any other studies.

Three models are discussed in this chapter: (1) the first model describes formulations with a first-order release rate; (2) the second model describes formulations with a zero-order release rate; and (3) the third model describes formulations with a combined immediate release and zero-order release rate. Three simulated case studies and two literature examples are presented in this chapter to illustrate the utility of the models in the sustained release versus immediate release studies. Additional examples of sustained release versus immediate release studies can be found in the literature [1–10].

PHARMACOKINETIC MODELS

This section presents three models that are useful in describing the release of a drug from sustained release formulations. The goal is to establish simple relationships between time constants and measurable parameters such as (1) mean residence time, which is the sum of input and output times, and (2) area under the curves. The derivations of these relationships are straightforward and are discussed in Chapter 2.

Model 1: Formulations with First-Order Release Rate

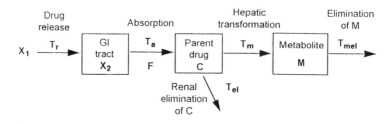

The release rate of a drug from a sustained release formulation may follow first-order kinetics as shown in Model 1. The release time constant,

T_r, is usually longer than the absorption time constant, T_a, so that the formulation can control the rate of absorption. The release time can be even longer than the elimination time constants, $T_{el,t}$, of the drug in the blood, in which case the release rate becomes the rate limiting step of the terminal phase of the plasma concentration curve. This results in a flip-flop of the concentration profile in which the decay time is equal to the release time constant rather than the elimination time constant.

The mean residence time is a key parameter to estimate for a sustained release formulation, because the long release time will prolong the mean residence time. The mean residence time is simply the sum of input and output times:

$$\text{Mean residence time of C } (\bar{t}_C) = \frac{\text{AUMC}_C}{\text{AUC}_C}$$

$$= \text{Input time } (T_{C,\text{in}}) + \text{Output time } (T_{C,\text{out}}) = T_r + T_a + T_{el,t} \quad (8.1)$$

$$\text{Mean residence time of M } (\bar{t}_M) = \frac{\text{AUMC}_M}{\text{AUC}_M}$$

$$= \text{Input time } (T_{m,\text{in}}) + \text{Output time } (T_{m,\text{out}}) = T_r + T_a + T_{el,t} + T_{\text{mel}} \quad (8.2)$$

where $T_{el,t} = 1/(1/T_{el} + 1/T_m)$. The renal elimination time of the metabolite T_{mel} is simply equal to the difference between $\bar{t}_M$ and $\bar{t}_C$: $T_{\text{mel}} = \bar{t}_M - \bar{t}_C$. The difference in the mean residence time of a sustained release formulation and an immediate release formulation gives the release time constant. If the release time constant is longer than the elimination time constant of the drug, the release time should dominate the decay time of the concentration curve (flip-flop).

$$\text{Release time } (T_r) = \bar{t}_{C,\text{sr}} - \bar{t}_{C,\text{ir}} \quad (8.3)$$

The plasma concentration of a drug following the administration of a sustained release formulation is normally lower than that following an immediate release formulation. If the metablism of the drug follows saturable nonlinear kinetics, the metabolite to drug ratio will be greater for the sustained release formulation than for the immediate release formulation. The ratio of the area under the metabolite concentration curve to the area under the drug concentration curve gives

$$\frac{\text{AUC}_M}{\text{AUC}_C} = \frac{T_{\text{mel}} V_C}{T_m V_m} = \frac{\text{Elimination clearance time of M}}{\text{Formation clearance time toward M}} \quad (8.4)$$

The decay time of the concentration profile can be estimated from a partial area under the curve (see Appendix 2):

$$\frac{1}{\text{Decay time } (T_z)} = \lambda_z = 2\frac{(t_{\text{ref}} - t_{\text{last}}) \ln (C_{t_{\text{ref}}}) - \text{AU} \ln C_{t_{\text{ref}}-t_{\text{last}}}}{(t_{\text{ref}} - t_{\text{last}})^2} \quad (8.5)$$

A sustained release formulation can reduce the fluctuation of the concentration profile. The fluctuation index can be defined as

$$\text{Fluctuation index (FI)} = \frac{C_{\text{max}} - C_{\text{min}}}{\text{AUC}/\tau} \quad (8.6)$$

where τ is the dosing interval and AUC/τ gives the average steady-state plasma concentration.

Model 2: Formulations with Zero-Order Release Rate

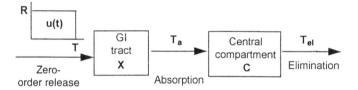

The releasing rate of a sustained release formulation may follow zero-order kinetics as in this model, where the release rate is a function of time: $u(t) = R$ as $0 < t < T$ and $u(t) = 0$ as $t > T$. The releasing rate of the drug remains constant (R) for a period of T. The total amount of dose is then equal to $R*T$. The zero-order releasing kinetics will result in a more steady concentration level than the first-order kinetics.

The mean residence time of the concentration curve is prolonged by the extended releasing time. The mean residence time is the sum of input and output times

$$\text{Mean residence time of sustained release formulation } (\bar{t}_{sr}) = \frac{\text{AUMC}}{\text{AUC}}$$

$$= \text{Input time } (T_{\text{sr,in}}) + \text{Output time } (T_{\text{sr,out}}) = T_a + T_{\text{el}} + \frac{T}{2} \quad (8.7)$$

The releasing time of a drug from a sustained release formulation can be estimated from the difference in the mean residence time of the sustained release formulation and the immediate release formulation

$$\frac{\text{Release time } (T)}{2} = \bar{t}_{sr} - \bar{t}_{ir} \tag{8.8}$$

Therefore, only half of the release time contributes to the mean residence time for a zero-order release formulation. The fluctuation index can be defined as follows:

$$\text{Fluctuation index (FI)} = \frac{C_{max} - C_{min}}{\text{AUC}/\tau} \tag{8.9}$$

Model 3: Formulations with a Combined Immediate Release and Zero-Order Release Rate

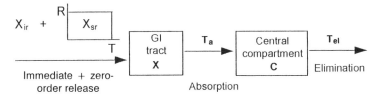

The drug plasma concentration produced from the sustained release formulation with either zero- or first-order releasing kinetics usually requires a long time to reach the maximum concentration due to the slow release of the drug. The time to reach the peak plasma concentration can be shortened by coating an immediate release layer outside the sustained release tablet. Following the administration of the coated tablet, the immediate release layer will rapidly produce a high plasma concentration, and the sustained release tablet will maintain the concentration level for a long period of time.

In this model, an immediate release layer (amount $= X_{ir}$) is coated outside a sustained release tablet (amount $= X_{sr}$). The mean residence time of the concentration curve following the administration of this formulation is simply the sum of input and output times:

$$\text{Mean residence time } (\bar{t}_{ir+sr}) = \frac{\text{AUMC}}{\text{AUC}}$$

$$= \text{Input time } (T_{ir+sr,in}) + \text{Output time } (T_{ir+sr,out}) = T_a + T_{el} + \frac{X_{sr}}{X_{ir} + X_{sr}} \frac{T}{2}$$

$$\tag{8.10}$$

The release time of the sustained release tablet can be estimated from the difference in the mean residence time between the sustained release formulation and an immediate release formulation

$$\frac{\text{Release time } (T)}{2} = \frac{X_{ir} + X_{sr}}{X_{sr}} (\bar{t}_{ir+sr} - \bar{t}_{ir}) \qquad (8.11)$$

The fluctuation index can be defined as follows

$$\text{Fluctuation index (FI)} = \frac{C_{max} - C_{min}}{\text{AUC}/\tau} \qquad (8.12)$$

CASE STUDIES

Case 1: First-Order Release

The release rate of a drug from its sustained release formulation can be a first-order process. The release process becomes the rate limiting step of the absorption if it is slower than the absorption rate. This case can be described by Model 1, and simulated plasma drug concentration profiles after dosing an immediate release formulation b.i.d. and a sustained release formulation q.d. are shown in Figure 8.1. The sustained release formulation has a release rate of 0.1 hr^{-1}, which is equivalent to a half-life of 7 hours. Therefore, 90% of the drug will be released in about 21 hours. The absorption rate (0.6 hr^{-1}) is rapid compared with the release time, and the absorption half-life is 1.15 hours. Therefore, 90% of the immediate release formulation is absorbed in 3.5 hours. Because of the fast elimination rate, the plasma concentration after dosing the immediate release formulation decreases rapidly, resulting in a long period of time between doses with relatively low plasma concentrations. On the other hand, the sustained release formulation is able to maintain a broader plasma concentration profile throughout 24 hours. Because of the slow release rate, the time to reach the maximum plasma concentration is longer with the sustained release formulation than the immediate release formulation. In addition, the maximum concentration is lower with the sustained release formulation than the immediate release formulation. The decay time of the concentration profile is longer with the sustained release formulation than the immediate release formulation because a flip-flop occurs in the sustained release formulation.

To compare a sustained release formulation (with a first-order release rate) with an immediate release formulation, the key time constant is the

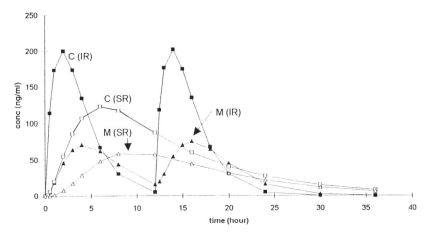

FIGURE 8.1. Simulated plasma concentration profiles of a sustained release formulation with first-order release and an immediate release formulation using Model 1. The time constant plot comparing the two formulations is shown in Figure 8.2. The parameters used in this simulation are sustained release: $X_0 = 10$ mg q.d., $f^*F = 1$, $V_c = 10$ L, $K_r = 0.1$ hr^{-1}, $K_a = 0.6$ hr^{-1}, $K_{el} = 0.2$ hr^{-1}, $V_m = 15$ L, $K_m = 0.3$ hr^{-1}, $K_{mel} = 0.35$ hr^{-1}; immediate release: $X_0 = 5$ mg b.i.d., $f^*F = 1$, $V_c = 10$ L, $K_a = 0.6$ hr^{-1}, $K_{el} = 0.2$ hr^{-1}, $V_m = 15$ L, $K_m = 0.3$ hr^{-1}, $K_{mel} = 0.35$ hr^{-1}.

release time constant to evaluate the length of time the sustained release formulation can maintain the plasma drug level. The fluctuation index is also an important parameter for the assessment of the variation of plasma concentration. The estimated pharmacokinetic parameters for the above example using the time constant analysis are listed in Table 8.1, and the estimated time constants are presented in Figure 8.2. The areas under the curve of the two formulations are similar, indicating the same extent of absorption. The ratios of area under the curve of the metabolite to that of the parent drug are the same for the two formulations, reflecting a linearity of the metabolism.

Now let us examine the time constant plot (Figure 8.2). The decay time of both the parent drug and the metabolite concentration profiles following the sustained release formulation is controlled by the release time. On the other hand, following the immediate release formulation, the decay time of the metabolite concentration profiles is longer than that of the parent drug, indicating the elimination time of the metabolite is longer than that of the parent drug. Therefore, the assignment of T_{zm} to T_{mel} or $T_{el,t}$ is uncertain. However, T_{mel} can be correctly estimated from the difference between the mean residence times of the metabolite ($\bar{t}_M$) and the parent drug ($\bar{t}_C$). The mean residence times of both the parent drug ($\bar{t}_C$) and the metabolite ($\bar{t}_M$)

TABLE 8.1. The Estimated Time Constants of Model 1 for the Example in Figure 8.1.

Parameter	Sustained Release Time Constant Analysis	Sustained Release Model Value	Immediate Release Time Constant Analysis	Immediate Release Model Value	Equation
T_{zc} (hr)	10.0	10.0 (T_r)	2.13	2.0 ($T_{el,t}$)	(8.5)
T_{zm} (hr)	10.0	10.0 (T_r)	3.13	2.86 (T_{mel})	(8.5)
$\bar{t}_C$ (hr)	13.6	13.6	9.7	9.7	(8.1)
t_M (hr)	16.7	16.6	12.5	12.5	(8.2)
$\bar{T}_{mel}$ (hr)	3.1	2.86	2.8	2.86	$T_{mel} = t_M - t_C$
$t_{C,dose}$ (hr)	13.6	13.6	3.7	3.7	
$t_{M,dose}$ (hr)	16.7	16.6	6.5	6.5	
T_r (hr)	10.2	10.0			(8.3)
$AUC_{C,dose}/\bar{t}_{C,dose}/2$ (ng/L)	74	74	137	135	
$AUC_{M,dose}/\bar{t}_{M,dose}/2$ (ng/L)	34	35	45	44	
FI_c	1.14		2.31		(8.6)
FI_m	0.78		1.14		(8.6)
AUC_C (ng·hr/L)	2022	2000	2023	2000	
AUC_M (ng·hr/L)	1143	1142	1159	1142	
AUC_M/AUC_C	0.57	0.57	0.57	0.57	(8.4)

174

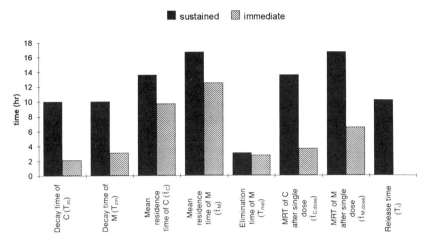

FIGURE 8.2. The time constant plot comparing a sustained release and an immediate release formulation of the example shown in Figure 8.1. The decay time of both the parent drug (T_{zc}) and the metabolite (T_{zm}) concentration profiles following the sustained release formulation are controlled by the release time (T_r). On the other hand, following the immediate release formulation, the decay time of the metabolite (T_{zm}) concentration profiles is longer than that of the parent drug (T_{zc}), indicating the elimination time of the metabolite (T_{mel}) is longer than that of the parent drug (T_{el}, not estimated).

are shorter with the sustained release formulation than the immediate release formulation. The difference in the mean residence time of the drug between the two formulations is even wider after a single dose ($\bar{t}_{C,dose}$), indicating that the sustained release formulation can maintain a broader plasma concentration profile than the immediate release formulation. The mean residence time average concentrations of the parent and the metabolite are much lower with the sustained release formulation than the immediate release formulation. The fluctuation index of the plasma concentration is smaller with the sustained release formulation than the immediate release formulation.

Case 2: Zero-Order Release

The release rate of a sustained formulation may be constant with time, following a zero-order rate. In this case, a more steady plasma concentration profile can be maintained by the zero-order release than by the first-order release. The zero-order release can be described by Model 2, and simulated plasma concentration profiles of a sustained release formulation and an immediate release formulation using the model are shown in Figure

8.3. The sustained release formulation administered q.d. releases the drug at a constant rate for 16 hours, resulting in a rather constant plasma drug level between 6 and 16 hours after dosing. The immediate release formulation administered b.i.d. produces a plasma concentration profile with two sharp peaks. The time to reach the maximum concentration is longer with the sustained release formulation than the immediate release formulation. The decay time of the sustained release formulations is the same as the immediate formulation, because the drug is completely released after 16 hours and the decay time is limited only by the elimination time.

For studying the pharmacokinetics of sustained release formulation with a zero-order release rate, the key time constant is the releasing time for the assessment of the length of time with almost steady plasma drug concentration. The estimated pharmacokinetic parameters for the above example using the time constant analysis are listed in Table 8.2, and the estimated time constants are presented in Figure 8.4. The area under the curve is the same with the two formulations, indicating the equivalence in bioavailability.

Now let us examine the time constant plot (Figure 8.4). The decay time of the plasma concentration profiles are also the same for the two formulations. The mean residence time is much longer with the sustained release formulation than the immediate release formulation, reflecting a broader concentration profile with the earlier formulation. The mean residence

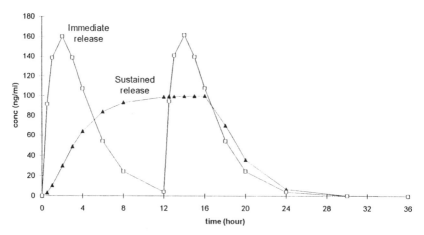

FIGURE 8.3. Simulated plasma concentration profiles of a sustained release formulation with zero-order release and an immediate release formulation using Model 2. The time constant plot comparing the two formulations is shown in Figure 8.4. The parameters used in this simulation are sustained release: $X_0 = 10$ mg q.d., $f^*F = 0.8$, $V = 10$ L, $R = 0.625$ mg/hr, $T = 16$ hr, $K_a = 0.6$ hr^{-1}, $K_{el} = 0.5$ hr^{-1}; immediate release: $X_0 = 5$ mg b.i.d., $f^*F = 0.8$, $V = 10$ L, $X_0 = 10$ mg, $T = 16$ hr, $K_a = 0.6$ hr^{-1}, $K_{el} = 0.5$ hr^{-1}.

TABLE 8.2. The Estimated Time Constants of Model 2 for the Example in Figure 8.3.

Parameter	Sustained Release		Immediate Release		Equation
	Time Constant Analysis	Model Value	Time Constant Analysis	Model Value	
$\underline{T}_z$ (hr)	2.13	2.0	2.13	2.0	(8.5)
$\underline{t}_C$ (hr)	11.8	11.7	9.7	9.7	(8.7)
$t_{C,dose}$ (hr)	11.8	11.7	3.7	3.7	
T (hr)	16.2	16.0			(8.8)
$AUC_{C,dose}/\bar{t}_{C,dose}/2$ (ng/L)	68	69	109	109	
FI_c	1.48		2.33		(8.9)
AUC_C (ng·hr/L)	1611	1600	1618	1600	

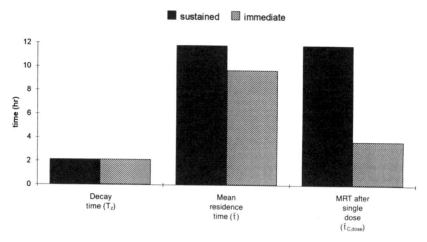

FIGURE 8.4. The time constant plot comparing a sustained release formulation and an immediate release formulation of the example shown in Figure 8.3. The mean residence time $(\bar{t}_{C,dose})$ is much longer with the sustained release formulation than the immediate release formulation, as reflected by a broader concentration profile with the earlier formulation.

time average concentration is lower, and the fluctuation index is smaller with the sustained release formulation. The releasing time of the sustained formulation is 16.2 hours, reflected by a steady plasma concentration from 6 hours up to 16 hours postdose.

Case 3: Immediate Release Plus Zero-Order Release

One of the disadvantages of the sustained release formulation in Case 2 is that it may take a long time for the plasma drug concentration to reach a therapeutic level. To accelerate the rising phase of the plasma concentration, an immediate release loading dose can be coated outside the sustained release tablet. This type of sustained release formulation can be described by Model 3, and simulated plasma concentration profiles using the model are shown in Figure 8.5. In this example, a loading dose of one-fourth of the total strength is coated in the outer layer of the sustained release formulation. The plasma concentration following the sustained release formulation increases rapidly initially and maintains a rather steady level between 2 and 16 hours. The time to reach the maximum concentration is similar with the two formulations, indicating a same initial release rate from both formulations. The decay time is the same for the two formulations, since the sustained release formulation lasts for 16 hours, after which the drug release rate is not the rate limiting step.

The concentration curve of the sustained release formulation shows rapid absorption and elimination, producing an almost rectangular-like concentration profile. Therefore, the mean residence time ($\bar{t}_c$) is a good estimate of the time length that the plasma concentration remains at the plateau. Thus, the mean residence time is the key time constant in this example. The estimated pharmacokinetic parameters for the above example using the time constant analysis are listed in Table 8.3, and the estimated time constants are presented in Figure 8.6. The area under the curve indicates an equivalence in bioavailability of the two formulations.

Now let us examine the time constant plot (Figure 8.6). The decay time is the same for the two formulations, reflecting that the release rate of the sustained release formulation is not the rate limiting step in the terminal phase. Coincidentally, the two formulations have a similar mean residence time; however, the mean residence time for a single dose is much longer with the sustained release formulation. This results in a smaller mean residence time average concentration with the sustained release formulation than with the immediate release formulation.

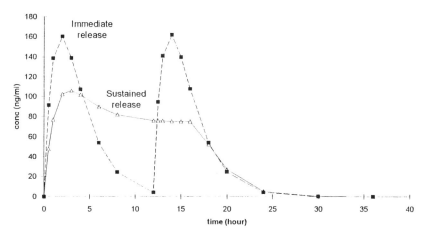

FIGURE 8.5. Simulated plasma concentration profiles of a sustained release formulation (with immediate release outside layer) and an immediate release formulation using Model 3. The time constant plot comparing the two formulations is shown in Figure 8.6. The parameters used in this simulation are sustained release: $X_1 = 2.5$ mg, $X_2 = 7.5$ mg, $f^*F = 0.8$, $V = 10$ L, $R = 0.625$ mg/hr, $T = 16$ hr, $K_a = 0.6$ hr^{-1}, $K_{el} = 0.5$ hr^{-1}; immediate release: $X_0 = 5$ mg b.i.d., $f^*F = 0.8$, $V = 10$ L, $X_0 = 10$ mg, $T = 16$ hr, $K_a = 0.6$ hr^{-1}, $K_{el} = 0.5$ hr^{-1}.

TABLE 8.3. *The Estimated Time Constants of Model 3 for the Example in Figure 8.5.*

Parameter	Sustained Release		Immediate Release		Equation
	Time Constant Analysis	Model Value	Time Constant Analysis	Model Value	
T_{zc} (hr)	2.27	2.0	2.17	2.0	(8.5)
t_C (hr)	9.7	9.7	9.7	9.7	(8.10)
$t_{C,dose}$ (hr)	9.7	9.7	3.7	3.7	
$AUC_{C,dose}/\bar{t}_{C,dose}/2$ (ng/L)	83	83	109	109	
FI_c	1.5		2.3		(8.12)
AUC_C (ng·hr/L)	1612	1600	1618	1600	

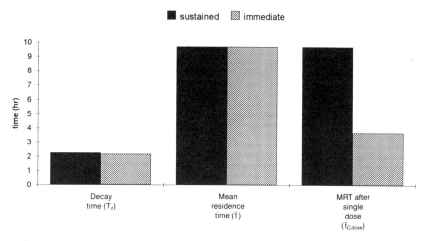

FIGURE 8.6. The time constant plot comparing a sustained release and an immediate release formulation of the example shown in Figure 8.5. The two formulations have a similar mean residence time ($\overline{t}_C$); however, the mean residence time for a single dose ($\overline{t}_{C,dose}$) is much longer with the sustained release formulation.

EXAMPLES

Example 1. Sustained Release Formulation Reduces the Fluctuation Index

Pharmacokinetics of immediate release and sustained release adinazolam were compared in fifteen healthy subjects following the administration of 40 mg immediate release (CT) and 60 mg sustained release (SR) tablets [5]. Mean plasma concentration profiles of adinazolam and its metabolite NDMAD after the two treatments are shown in Figures 8.7 and 8.8. The adinazolam and NDMAD concentrations are maintained at lower, but more steady, levels after the sustained release tablet than the immediate release tablet. The time to reach the maximum concentration after the sustained release tablet is longer than after the immediate release tablet.

Adinazolam is characterized by a short decay time, and multiple doses of the immediate release formulation of the drug give a large fluctuation index. Therefore, there is a need to develop a sustained release formulation. The key pharmacokinetic parameters are then the release time constant and the fluctuation index and are used to determine the release characteristics. The pharmacokinetic parameters of adinazolam and NDMAD are estimated using Model 1, since the metabolite is presented. The estimated pharmacokinetic parameters are listed in Table 8.4, and the estimated time

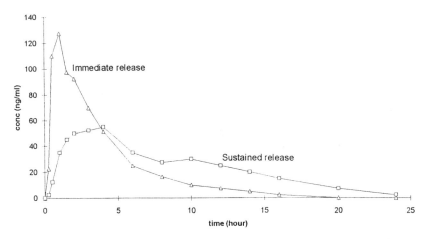

FIGURE 8.7. Mean plasma concentrations of adinazolam in fifteen healthy subjects follow-ing the administration of 40-mg immediate release (CT) and 60-mg sustained release (SR) tablets of adinazolam. (Reproduced from Reference [5] with permission.) The time constant plot comparing the two formulations is shown in Figure 8.9.

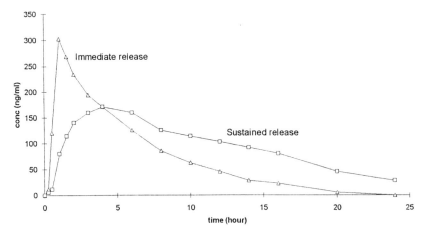

FIGURE 8.8. Mean plasma concentrations of NDMAD in fifteen healthy subjects following the administration of 40-mg immediate release (CT) and 60-mg sustained release (SR) tablets of adinazolam. (Reproduced from Reference [5] with permission.)

182

TABLE 8.4. *The Estimated Pharmacokinetic Parameter of Adinazolam and Its Metabolite NDMAD Using Models 1 and 2.*

Parameter*	C-CT 40 mg	C-SR 60 mg	M-CR 40 mg	M-SR 60 mg	Equation
$T_{\frac{1}{2}}$ (hr)	3.66	6.54	5.49	7.63	(8.5)
t_{dose} (hr)	3.95	8.16	5.67	9.67	(8.1, 8.2)
T_r (hr)		4.22			(8.3)
T (hr)		8.4			(8.8)
FI	5.98	2.31	4.16	1.79	(8.6)
AUC/X_0/$\bar{t}_{dose}$/2 (ng/ml/mg)	3.44	1.32	8.06	4.43	
AUC (ng·hr/ml)	543	647	1826	2543	
AUC/X_0 (ng·hr/ml/mg)	13.6	10.8	45.7	42.4	
AUC_M/AUC_C			4.36	4.51	(8.4)

*Parameters estimated from the mean concentration profiles or the mean reported values.
C: adinazolam, M: NDMAD, CT: immediate release, SR: sustained release.

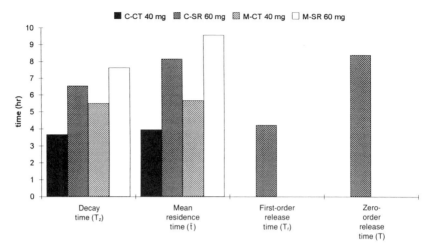

FIGURE 8.9. The time constant plot of adinazolam comparing a sustained release and an immediate release formulation using Models 1 and 2. The decay times (T_z) of the concentration curves are longer for the sustained released tablet than the immediate release tablet, probably due to a flip-flop of the concentration curve following the sustained release tablet where the drug release time (T_r or T) is the rate limiting step.

constants are presented in Figure 8.9. The normalized area (AUC/X_0) under the adinazolam and NDMAD concentration curves is similar between the sustained release tablet and the immediate release formulation, indicating similar bioavailability of the two formulations and dose linearity in this dosing range. The ratios of the area under the NDMAD concentration curve to the area under the adinazolam concentration curve are similar between the two formulations, indicating linear metabolic kinetics in this dosing range.

Now let us examine the time constant plot (Figure 8.9). The decay times of the concentration curves are longer for the sustained release tablet than the immediate release tablet, probably due to a flip-flop of the concentration curve following the sustained release tablet where the drug release is the rate limiting step. The mean residence time average concentration (AUC/X_0/$\bar{t}_{dose}$/2 normalized by dose) is lower, and the fluctuation index is smaller after the sustained release formulation than the immediate release formulation. The drug release time constant from the SR tablet, estimated from the Model 1, is 4.2 hours. The mean release time, estimated from Model 2, is about 8.4 hours. To summarize, the sustained release formulation produces a more stable, but lower, plasma concentration than the immediate release formulation. The reduction in the plasma drug level after the sustained release formulation results in smaller sedation and psychomotor performance compared with the immediate release formulation after a single-dose administration [5].

Example 2. Decay Time Increases with Sustained Release Formulation

The relative bioavailability of a sustained release (SR) oxprenolol against a regular release (RR) tablet was investigated in twelve healthy subjects following the administrations of a 160-mg q.d. sustained release tablet and an 80-mg b.i.d. regular release tablet [6]. Mean plasma concentration profiles of oxprenolol following the two doses at steady state (5 days after the first dose) are shown in Figure 8.10. due to a relatively short half-life of oxprenolol (2 hours in this example), the drug concentration drops to a very low level between doses of the regular release formulation. On the other hand, the sustained release formulation is able to maintain a higher plasma oxprenolol concentration 3 hours after dosing than can the regular release formulation.

Oxprenolol has a relatively short decay time after the regular release tablet; therefore, a sustained release formulation is needed to reduce the fluctuation of the plasma concentration. The key parameters to determine the performance of the sustained release formulation are the fluctuation

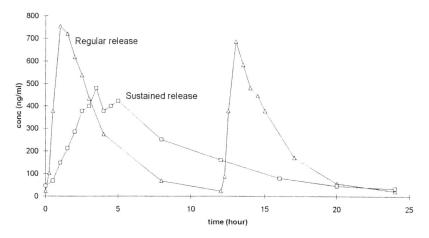

FIGURE 8.10. Mean plasma concentration of oxprenolol in twelve healthy subjects following the administration of a 160-mg q.d. sustained release tablet and an 80-mg b.i.d. regular release tablet. (Reproduced from Reference [6] with permission.) The time constant plot comparing the two formulations is shown in Figure 8.11.

TABLE 8.5. The Estimated Pharmacokinetic Parameter of
Oxprenolol Using Models 1 and 2.

Parameter*	RR	SR	Equation
T_z (hr)	3.0	6.9	(8.5)
t (hr)	8.7	7.8	(8.1)
t_{dose} (hr)	3.1	7.8	(8.1)
T_r (hr)		4.69	(8.3)
T (hr)		9.4	(8.8)
FI	3.46	2.73	(8.6)
AUC (ng·hr/ml)	4906.5	4040.7	
$AUC_{dose}/t_{dose}/2$ (ng/ml)	395	259	

*Parameters estimated from the mean concentration profiles or the mean reported values.
RR: regular release, SR: sustained release.

index and the release time constant. The pharmacokinetic parameters of
oxprenolol are estimated using both Models 1 and 2, since the in vitro dissolution profiles of the sustained release formulation are not available for
selection of the appropriate model. The estimated pharmacokinetic parameters are listed in Table 8.5, and the estimated time constants are presented
in Figure 8.11. The area under the concentration curves for the sustained
release formulation is 82% of that for the regular release formulation.

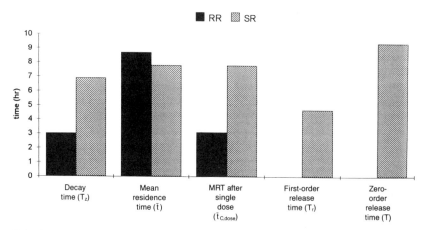

FIGURE 8.11. The time constant plot of exprenolol comparing a sustained release and a
regular release formulation using Models 1 and 2. The mean residence time of the concentration curve after a single dose ($\bar{t}_{dose}$) is longer for the sustained release formulation, reflecting the ability of the formulation to maintain higher plasma concentrations for a longer
time.

Now let us examine the time constant plot (Figure 8.11). The decay time of the concentration profile is longer after the sustained release formulation than the regulation formulation, indicating that the release rate may be the rate limiting step following the sustained release formulation. The mean residence time of the concentration curve after a single dose ($\bar{t}_{dose}$) is longer for the sustained release formulation, reflecting the ability of the formulation to maintain higher plasma concentrations for a longer time. The fluctuation index is lower for the sustained release formulation than the regular release formulation. The release time constant of the SR tablet is 4.69 hours based on Model 1, and the release time is 9.4 hours based on Model 2. Notice that the release time based on Model 2 is twice as long as that based on Model 1 because only half of the release time in Model 2 contributes to the mean residence time [see Equation (8.8)]. To summarize, the sustained release tablet reduces the fluctuation and prolongs the mean residence time of the plasma concentration curve after a single dose compared with the regular release tablet.

REFERENCES

1. Bass, J., Shepard K. V., Lee J. W., and Hulse J., "An evaluation of the effect of food on the oral bioavailability of sustained-release morphine sulfate tablets (ORAMORPH SR) after multiple doses," *J. Clin. Pharmacol.*, 1992; 32:1003–1007.

2. Betlach C. J., Straughn A. B., Meyer M. C., Bialer M., Vashi V. I., Lieberman P., and Gonzalez M. A., "The effect of raising gastric pH with ranitidine on the absorption and elimination of theophylline for a sustained-release theophylline tablet," *Pharmaceutical Research*, 1991; 8(12):1516–1519.

3. Bruno R., Santoni Y., Iliadis A., Djiane P., Serradimigni A., and Cano J. P., "Simultaneous modeling of mexiletine and hydroxy-methyl-mexiletine data after single- and multiple-dose administration of a sustained-release mexiletine formulation," *Biopharmaceutics & Drug Disposition*, 1992; 13:481–493.

4. Davies R. F., Siddoway L. A., Shaw L., Barbey J. T., Roden D. M., and Woosley R. L., "Immediate- versus controlled-release disopyramide: Importance of saturable binding," *Clinical Pharmacology & Therapeutics*, 1993; 54(1):16–22.

5. Fleishaker J. C. and Wright C. E., "Pharmacokinetics and pharmacodynamic comparison of immediate-release and sustained-release adinazolam mesylate tablet after single- and multiple-dose administration," *Pharmaceutical Research*, 1992; 9(4):457–463.

6. Gupta P. K., Lim J. K. C., Zoest A. R., Lam F. C., and Hung C. T., "Relative bioavailability of oral sustained-release and regular-release oxprenolol tablets at steady-state,"*Biopharmaceutics & Drug Disposition*, 1991; 12:493–503.

7. Hussey E. K., Donn K. H., Powell J. R., Lahey A. P., and Pakes G. E., "Albuterol extended-release products: Effect of food on the pharmacokinetics of single oral doses of volmax and proventil repetabs in healthy male volunteers," *J. Clin. Pharmacol.*, 1991; 31:561–564.

8. Meyer M. C., Straughn A. B., Jarvi E. J., Wood G. C., Vashi V. I., Hepp P., and Hunt

J., "The effect of gastic pH on the absorption of controlled-release theophylline dosage forms in humans," *Pharmaceutical Research*, 1993; 10(7):1037–1045.

9. Neuvonen P. J., Roivas L., Laine K., and Sundholm O., "The bioavailability of sustained release nicotinic acid formulation," *Br. J. Clin. Pharmac.*, 1991; 32:473–476.

10. Shrikant V. D. and Wallace P. A., "Bioavailability and bioequivalence of oral controlled release products: A regulatory perspective," in *Pharmacokinetics, Regulatory/Industrial/Academic Perspectives*, edited by Welling P. G. and Tse F. L. S., Marcel Dekker, Inc., New York and Basel, 1988.

11. Davis S. S., Hardy J. G., and Fara J. W., "Transit of pharmaceutical dosage forms through small intestine," *Gut*, 1986; 27:886–892.

ABSORPTION, DISTRIBUTION, METABOLISM, AND PHARMACODYNAMICS

CHAPTER 9

Absorption of Drugs in the Gastrointestinal Tract

INTRODUCTION

The absorption of drugs along the gastrointestinal tract can be characterized in a gastrointestinal intubation study, which determines the permeability of a drug at certain gastrointestinal sites [7]; compares absorption at different gastrointestinal sites [2–4], investigates intestinal metabolism [9]; determines the relationship between gastrointestinal motility, pH, and drug absorption [3]; or evaluates effects of different factors such as glucose and osmolarity on absorption [6]. The gastrointestinal tract is intubated with specially designed tubes in the GI absorption study, and then solutions of drugs are infused or perfused via the lumens within the tube. In a perfusion study, the perfusate exiting the intestine is collected and assayed for drug and metabolite concentrations, and the permeability of the drug across the intestinal wall or the extent of metabolism within the intestine is determined [6,7]. In an infusion study, drugs are typically dosed to several sites along the gastrointestinal tract, and pharmacokinetics are determined by analyzing the plasma concentration profiles of the drugs [3,9]. Several factors influence the pharmacokinetics of drugs in the infusion study, which include gastric emptying time constant, intestinal pH, absorption time constant, intestinal metabolism, first pass metabolism, intestinal transit time, and intestinal secretion. Each of these factors has different degrees of importance at different intestinal sites. The key time constants and pharmacokinetic parameters affected by these factors include gastric emptying time, the absorption time, the fraction absorbed, and the first pass metabolism.

Some common themes in the time constant view can be observed in the gastrointestinal absorption study as well as other studies. The different ab-

191

sorption characteristics at different gastrointestinal sites determined in a GI absorption study will also be reflected in a sustained release formulation study. For example, if the absorption at the colon site is minimal, then the plasma concentration profile following the administration of a sustained release formulation will not be able to maintain a steady concentration after 2–6 hours, which is the approximate small intestinal transit time of drugs [12]. If a site-specific metabolism in the intestine is identified in the GI absorption study, a difference in metabolite to drug ratio in the plasma may also be observed between the sustained release formulation and the immediate release formulation.

Three models are discussed in this chapter to determine the pharmacokinetics in a gastrointestinal absorption study: (1) the first model describes the effect of gastric emptying on the plasma concentration profile; (2) the second model describes constant intraintestinal infusions; and (3) the third model describes the first pass effects. Three simulated case studies and two literature examples are presented in this chapter to illustrate the utilities of these models in GI absorption studies. Additional literature examples of GI absorption studies can be found [1–11].

PHARMACOKINETIC MODELS

This section presents three models that are useful in determining pharmacokinetics in a gastrointestinal absorption study. The goal is to establish simple relationships between time constants and measurable parameters such as (1) mean residence time, which is the sum of input and output times, and (2) area under the curves. The derivations of these relationships are straightforward and are discussed in Chapter 2.

Model 1: Effect of Gastric Emptying on the Plasma Concentration Profile

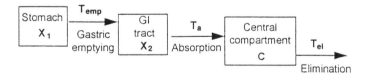

In gastrointestinal intubation studies, drugs can be given through oral administration, infusion into the stomach, or infusion into different sites along the gastrointestinal tract. The mean residence time and the time to reach the maximum concentration after the oral and gastric administrations are usually longer than after the intraintestinal administration because of the delay of absorption by gastric emptying after the oral and gastric administrations [3]. This can be described by Model 1, in which the drug is emptied from the stomach with a time constant T_{emp} and then absorbed from the intestine with a time constant T_a. The amount of the drug in the stomach is represented by X_1 and the amount in the intestine by X_2.

The mean residence time of C is simply the sum of input and output times:

$$\text{Mean residence time } (\bar{t}) = \frac{\text{AUMC}}{\text{AUC}}$$

$$= \text{Input time } (T_{in}) + \text{Output time } (T_{out}) = T_{emp} + T_a + T_{el} \quad (9.1)$$

The mean residence following the oral or gastric administration is longer than that following the intraintestinal administration due to the delay of the gastric emptying. The decay time of the plasma concentration profile can be estimated from a partial area under the curve:

$$\frac{1}{\text{Decay time } (T_z)} = \lambda_z = 2 \frac{(t_{ref} - t_{last}) \ln (C_{t_{ref}}) - \text{AU} \ln C_{t_{ref} - t_{last}}}{(t_{ref} - t_{last})^2} \quad (9.2)$$

Model 2: Constant Intraintestinal Infusions

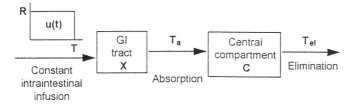

In an intestinal intubation study, the drug can be administered as a constant rate infusion instead of a bolus to prolong the rising phase of the plasma concentration profile and to obtain better absorption characteristics at different intestinal sites. The constant intestinal infusion can be described by Model 2, in which the drug is administered at a constant rate R for a time period T and the total dose is $R \cdot T$. Therefore, the infusion rate $u(t) = R$ when $0 < t \leq T$, and $u(t) = 0$ when $t > T$. The absorption rate is assumed to be first-order with a time constant T_a.

The mean residence time depends on the absorption time constant, elimination time constant, and the infusion time:

$$\text{Mean residence time following infusion } (\bar{t}_{inf}) = \frac{\text{AUMC}}{\text{AUC}}$$

$$= \text{Input time } (T_{\text{inf,in}}) + \text{Output time } (T_{\text{inf,out}}) = T_a + T_{el} + \frac{T}{2} \quad (9.3)$$

and the mean residence after a bolus administration is

$$\text{Mean residence time following bolus dose } (\bar{t}_{\text{bolus}})$$

$$= \text{Input time } (T_{\text{bolus,in}}) + \text{Output time } (T_{\text{bolus,out}}) = T_a + T_{el} \quad (9.4)$$

The absorption time may change along the gastrointestinal tract, and Equations (9.3) and (9.4) can be used to estimated T_a from T_{el}, T, $\bar{t}_{\text{inf}}$, and $\bar{t}_{\text{bolus}}$. The difference in the mean residence time of plasma concentration curve between an intestinal infusion and a bolus is equal to half of the infusion time:

$$\frac{\text{Infusion time } (T)}{2} = \bar{t}_{\text{inf}} - \bar{t}_{\text{bolus}} \quad (9.5)$$

Equation (9.5) can be served as a verification of the accuracy of the estimated $\bar{t}_{\text{inf}}$ and $\bar{t}_{\text{bolus}}$ since the infusion time is already known from the experimental setting.

Model 3: The First Pass Effects

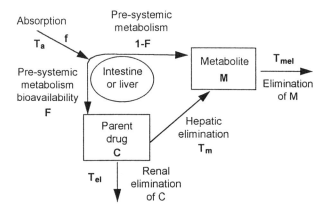

The presystemic first pass effect, especially the intestinal metabolism, of drugs may be different at different intestinal sites. Model 3 can be used to describe the first pass effect following the intestinal infusion, in which the drug is absorbed at a first-order rate with a fraction absorbed f and a first pass effect of $(1 - F)$.

The area under the parent drug concentration will increase with a decrease in the first pass effect, while the area under the metabolite concentration curve will decrease with a decrease in the first pass effect (Chapter 5). However, a change in the first pass effect will not affect the elimination time constant of the drug in the plasma. Therefore, the ratio of the area under the metabolite concentration curve to the area under the drug concentration curve is an indicator for detecting a change in the first pass effect at various gastrointestinal sites. This ratio will decrease with a decrease in the first pass effect.

$$\frac{\text{AUC}_M}{\text{AUC}_C} = \frac{V_C}{V_M}\frac{T_{mel}}{T_m} + \frac{V_C}{V_M}\frac{1 - F}{F}\frac{T_{mel}(T_m + T_{el})}{T_m T_{el}}$$

$$= \frac{V_C}{V_M}\frac{1}{F}\frac{T_{mel}(T_m + T_{el})}{T_m T_{el}} - \frac{V_C}{V_M}\frac{T_{mel}}{T_{el}} \qquad (9.6)$$

The mean residence time of the drug and its metabolite is the sum of input and output times (see Chapter 2)

$$\text{Mean residence time of C } (\bar{t}_C) = \frac{\text{AUMC}_C}{\text{AUC}_C}$$

$$= \text{Input time } (T_{c,in}) + \text{Output time } (T_{c,out}) = T_a + T_{el,t} \qquad (9.7)$$

$$\text{Mean residence time of M } (\bar{t}_M) = \frac{\text{AUMC}_M}{\text{AUC}_M}$$

$$= \text{Input time } (T_{m,in}) + \text{Output time } (T_{m,out})$$

$$= \frac{FT_m T_{el}^2}{(T_m + T_{el})(T_{el} + T_m - FT_m)} + T_a + T_{mel} \qquad (9.8)$$

where $T_{el,t} = 1/(1/T_m + 1/T_{el})$. The above equation can be simplified under extreme conditions:

$$\text{as } F \to 0 \qquad \bar{t}_M \to T_a + T_{mel} \qquad (9.9)$$

$$\text{as } F \to 1 \qquad \bar{t}_M \to T_{el,t} + T_a + T_{mel} \qquad (9.10)$$

CASE STUDIES

Case 1: Difference in Absorption at Various Gastrointestinal Sites

To determine the absorption characteristics of a drug at different sites along the gastrointestinal tract, the drug can be administered through a gastrointestinal tube directly to these sites. In this example, a drug is infused as a bolus into the stomach, duodenum, and ileum. A lower bioavailability is expected at the ileum sites because of a shorter intestinal transit time and a smaller absorption surface area. Other physiological factors affecting the rate and extent of absorption include the change in pH along the GI tract, the secretion of bile salt, possible metabolism by intestinal enzymes, transit velocity in the gut, and the compactness and mixability of the intestinal contents. The absorption of the drug after dosing into the stomach may be delayed, compared with intraintestinal administrations because the drug stays in the stomach for a period of time before it is emptied into the intestine for absorption. In this example, it is assumed that no metabolism is involved with this drug. Therefore, the key pharmacokinetic parameters in this case are the gastric emptying time constant, the fraction absorbed, and the absorption time constant. Model 1 is used to describe the absorption at different gastrointestinal sites in this example. Simulated plasma drug concentration profiles using the model are shown in Figure 9.1. The differences in pharmacokinetic parameters between the three sites are as follows: a gastric emptying rate constant is assumed for the stomach site but not at the intestinal sites; the rate constant and extent of absorption are the same at the stomach and the duodenum sites but smaller at the ileum site. The plasma concentration profile after dosing at the stomach site is delayed relative to the other two sites due to the slow gastric emptying. The maximum concentration after dosing at the stomach site is slightly lower than at the duodenum site, but the extent of absorption is the same at the two sites. The maximum concentration and the area under the curve after dosing at the ileum site are much lower than those at the two proximal sites, indicating a lower bioavailability at the distal site.

The objective of this simulated study is to determine the extent of absorption at various gastrointestinal sites and assess the effect of gastric emptying on the absorption. Therefore, the key pharmacokinetic parameters are the area under the curve and the mean residence time. The estimated pharmacokinetic parameters using the time constant analysis are listed in Table 9.1, and the estimated time constants are presented in Figure 9.2.

Now let us examine the time constant plot (Figure 9.2). The decay time T_z, representing the elimination time, is not different between the three

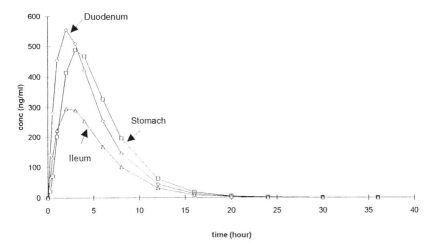

FIGURE 9.1. Simulated plasma drug concentration profiles using Model 1 for administration at three different sites: stomach, duodenum, and ileum, with different absorption at the three sites. The time constant plot comparing the three absorption sites is shown in Figure 9.2. The parameters used in this simulation are stomach: $X_0 = 10$ mg, $f = 1$, $F = 1$, $V = 10$ L, $K_{emp} = 1$ hr^{-1}, $K_a = 0.8$ hr^{-1}, $K_{el} = 0.3$ hr^{-1}; duodenum: $X_0 = 10$ mg, $f = 1$, $F = 1$, $V = 10$ L, $K_{emp} = 20$ hr^{-1}, $K_a = 0.8$ hr^{-1}, $K_{el} = 0.3$ hr^{-1}; ileum: $X_0 = 10$ mg, $f = 0.6$, $F = 1$, $V = 10$ L, $K_{emp} = 20$ hr^{-1}, $K_a = 0.6$ hr^{-1}, $K_{el} = 0.3$ hr^{-1}.

sites. The mean residence time after dosing at the stomach site is longer than the duodenum site due to a long gastric emptying time at the stomach site, while the mean residence time after dosing at the ileum site is longer than the duodenum site because of a longer absorption time at the distal site. However, the difference in mean residence time between the ileum and duodenum sites is quite small and may not be detectable when data variability is pronounced. The initial time constant ($T_{emp} + T_a$) at the stomach site is not comparable to those of the other two sites because the gastric emptying time constant is incorporated into the initial time constant at the stomach site. The absorption time at the duodenum site is shorter than the ileum site by comparing the mean absorption time ($T_{emp} + T_a$). The extent of absorption is the same at the stomach and duodenum sites, while the mean residence time is longer and the maximum concentration is slightly lower at the stomach site. The extent of absorption at the ileum is less than the other two sites; however, the absorption at the ileum site (about 60% of the proximal sites) cannot be ignored when designing a controlled release formulation of the drug.

TABLE 9.1. *The Estimated Pharmacokinetic Parameters Using Time Constant Analysis for the Example Shown in Figure 9.1.*

Parameter	Stomach		Duodenum		Ileum		Equation
	TCA	Model Value	TCA	Model Value	TCA	Model Value	
T_z (hr)	3.33	3.33	3.33	3.33	3.33	3.33	(9.2)
$\bar{t}_c$ (hr)	5.6	5.6	4.6	4.6	5	5	(9.1)
$T_{emp} + T_a$ (hr)	2.3	2.3	1.3	1.3	1.7	1.7	(9.1)
AUC (ng·hr/L)	3379	3333	3375	3333	2025	2000	

TCA: Time constant analysis.

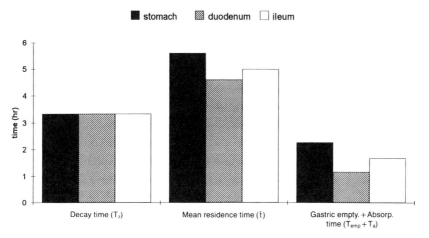

■ stomach   ▨ duodenum   ☐ ileum

FIGURE 9.2. The time constant plot comparing administrations at three different sites: stomach, duodenum, and ileum in the example shown in Figure 9.1. The mean residence time $(\bar{t})$ after dosing at the stomach site is longer than the duodenum site due to a long gastric emptying time (T_{emp}) at the stomach site, while the mean residence time after dosing at the ileum site is longer than the duodenum site because of a longer absorption time (T_a) at the distal site.

Case 2: Identify Difference in Absorption Rate at Various Intestinal Sites by Intraintestinal Infusion

The rate of absorption of a drug at different gastrointestinal sites can also be compared by continuously infusing the drug into the various sites. The advantage of the continuous infusion over the bolus infusion (as in Case 1) is that the number of data points in the absorption phase is greater with the continuous infusion so that the estimation of the absorption time is more accurate. The continuous infusion to different gastrointestinal sites can be described by Model 2, and simulated plasma concentration profiles using the model as shown in Figure 9.3. A bolus dose is given at the stomach site, while 5-hour infusions are given to both duodenum and ileum sites. The rate and extent of absorption at the stomach and duodenum sites are the same, and those at the ileum are less. The plasma concentration profiles after dosing at the duodenum and ileum sites show a longer time to reach the maximum concentration than the stomach site due to the long infusion time at the two distal sites. The maximum concentration after infusion at the duodenum site is greater than the ileum site, indicating a slower and less extensive absorption at the latter site. The number of data points during the absorption phase is reasonably large compared with the bolus infusion in

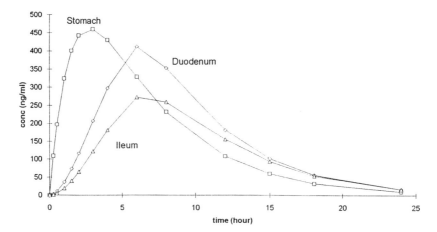

FIGURE 9.3. Simulated plasma drug concentration profiles using Model 2 for bolus dose to the stomach and continuous infusion at two intestinal sites: duodenum and ileum. The time constant plot comparing the absorption at the three sites is shown in Figure 9.4. The parameters used in this simulation are stomach: $X_0 = 10$ mg, $f = 0.8$, $F = 1$, $V = 10$ L, $K_a = 0.6$ hr^{-1}, $K_{el} = 0.2$ hr^{-1}; duodenum: $X_0 = 10$ mg, $T = 5$ hr, $f = 0.8$, $F = 1$, $V = 10$ L, $t = 5$ hr, $K_a = 0.6$ hr^{-1}, $K_{el} = 0.2$ hr^{-1}; ileum: $X_0 = 10$ mg, $T = 5$ hr, $f = 0.6$, $F = 1$, $V = 10$ L, $t = 5$ hr, $K_a = 0.4$ hr^{-1}, $K_{el} = 0.2$ hr^{-1}.

Case 1, and the absorption time at the duodenum site is clearly shorter than the ileum site.

Since the initial rising phase of the concentration profile is prolonged by the slow infusion, the number of time points along the rising phase is sufficient for a good estimation of the initial time constant T_0, which is the key time constant useful for the assessment of the absorption rate in this example. The pharmacokinetic parameters of the above example are estimated from the time constant analysis and listed in Table 9.2, and the estimated time constants are presented in Figure 9.4.

Now let us examine the time constant plot (Figure 9.4). The mean residence time of the concentration profile after dosing at the stomach site is significantly shorter than the other two sites because a bolus, instead of an infusion, is given at the stomach site. The mean residence time is slightly longer at the ileum site than the duodenum site due to a longer absorption time at the distal site, but the difference may be too small to be detected. Another way to compare the absorption time is to examine the initial time constant T_0 since a large number of data points are located in the absorption phase. Based on T_0, the absorption time is shorter at the duodenum site than the ileum site, which may be due to the larger surface area, lower pH, or bile secretion at the proximal site. The fraction absorbed can be de-

TABLE 9.2. The Estimated Pharmacokinetic Parameters Using Time
Constant Analysis for the Example Shown in Figure 9.3.

Parameter	Stomach		Duodenum		Ileum		Equation
	TCA	Model Value	TCA	Model Value	TCA	Model Value	
T_{z1} (hr)	5.0	5.0	5.0	5.0	5.0	5.0	(9.2)
$\bar{t}_C$ (hr)	6.5	6.7	9.1	9.2	9.4	10	(9.1)
T_0 (hr)	1.61	1.67	2.70	na	3.23	na	(9.2)
AUC (ng·hr/L)	4028	4000	3929	4000	3009	3000	

TCA: Time constant analysis; na: not available; the theoretical initial slope is 0.

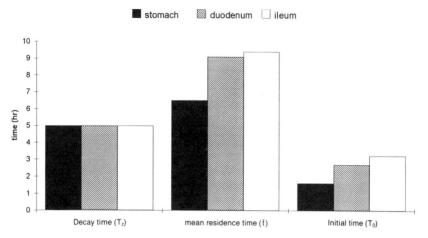

FIGURE 9.4. The time constant plot comparing bolus dose to the stomach and continuous infusion at two intestinal sites: duodenum and ileum in the example in Figure 9.3. The mean residence time $(\bar{t})$ is slightly longer at the ileum site than the duodenum site due to a longer absorption time (T_a) at the distal site. Based on T_0, the absorption time is shorter at the duodenum site than the ileum site, which may be due to the larger surface area, lower pH, or bile secretion at the proximal site.

termined from the area under the concentration curve AUC, since there is no hepatic or gut wall metabolism involved. The extent of absorption is similar at the stomach and duodenum site, but significantly smaller at the ileum site. It is not surprising that the bioavailability at the two proximal sites is similar, since the only difference in the absorption process between the two sites is the gastric emptying after dosing at the stomach.

Case 3: Different Degrees of Presystemic Metabolism at Various Intestinal Site

If a drug is subjected to an extensive first pass metabolism, the bioavailability may be improved by dosing the drug directly to an intestinal site where presystemic metabolism (gut wall or hepatic) is relatively low. However, if such a site is at a distal position along the intestine, the transit time of the drug in the intestine will be short, and the surface area will be small, which may result in a small fraction absorbed. Therefore, the effect of reduced presystemic metabolism on the bioavailability may be compensated by the decreased fraction absorbed at the distal site. This case can be described by Model 3, and simulated plasma drug concentration profiles after dosing at three sites along the intestine are shown in Figure 9.5. In this example, the fraction absorbed decreases from 0.8 at the duodenum and 0.6 at ileum to 0.4 at the colon. The extent of first pass effects is the same for the duodenum and ileum sites but is reduced at the colon site.

To evaluate the presystemic metabolism at various intestinal sites, the key pharmacokinetic parameter is the ratio of the area under the metabolite concentration curve to the area under the drug concentration curve. The estimated pharmacokinetic parameters using the time constant analysis is shown in Table 9.3, and the estimated time constants are present in Figure 9.6.

Now let us examine the time constant plot (Figure 9.6). The mean residence time of the parent drug is the same after dosing at the three different sites, which indicates the absorption time is similar at all three sites. The mean residence time of metabolite is the same after dosing at the duodenum and ileum sites but is longer at the colon site due to the decrease in the presystemic metabolism [Equation (9.8)]. Based on the mean residence time of the metabolite, an erroneous conclusion may be made that a delay in absorption occurs at the colon site, while the actual cause for the prolonged mean residence time is a reduction in the presystemic metabolism. There-

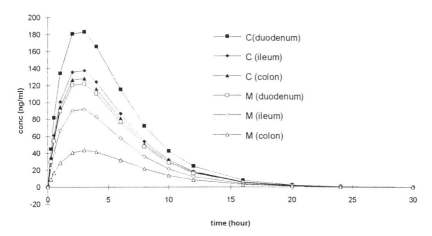

FIGURE 9.5. Simulated plasma drug concentration profiles using Model 3 for continuous infusion with different presystemic metabolism at three different sites: duodenum, ileum, and colon. The time constant plot comparing the three absorption sites is shown in Figure 9.6. The parameters used in this simulation are duodenum: $X_0 = 10$ mg, $f = 0.8$, $F = 0.5$, $V = 10$ L, $V_m = 15$ L, $K_a = 0.5$ hr^{-1}, $K_{el} = 0.2$ hr^{-1}, $K_m = 0.1$ hr^{-1}, $K_{mel} = 0.4$ hr^{-1}; ileum: $X_0 = 10$ mg, $f = 0.6$, $F = 0.5$, $V = 10$ L, $V_m = 15$ L, $K_a = 0.5$ hr^{-1}, $K_{el} = 0.2$ hr^{-1}, $K_m = 0.1$ hr^{-1}, $K_{mel} = 0.4$ hr^{-1}; colon: $X_0 = 10$ mg, $f = 0.4$, $F = 0.7$, $V = 10$ L, $V_m = 15$ L, $K_a = 0.5$ hr^{-1}, $K_{el} = 0.2$ hr^{-1}, $K_m = 0.1$ hr^{-1}, $K_{mel} = 0.4$ hr^{-1}.

TABLE 9.3. The Estimated Pharmacokinetic Parameters Using
Time Constant Analysis for the Example Shown in Figure 9.5.

Parameter	Duodenum		Ileum		Colon		Equation
	TCA	Model Value	TCA	Model Value	TCA	Model Value	
$T_{z,c}$ (hr)	3.33	3.33	3.33	3.33	3.33	3.33	(9.2)
$T_{z,m}$ (hr)	3.33	3.33	3.33	3.33	3.33	3.33	(9.2)
$\bar{t}_C$ (hr)	5.3	5.3	5.3	5.3	5.3	5.3	(9.7)
$\bar{t}_M$ (hr)	5.3	5.3	5.3	5.3	6.0	6.0	(9.8)
AUC_C (ng·hr/L)	1338	1333	1003	1000	936	933	
AUC_M (ng·hr/L)	892	888	669	667	356	355	
AUC_M/AUC_C	0.67	0.67	0.67	0.67	0.38	0.38	(9.6)

TCA: Time constant analysis.

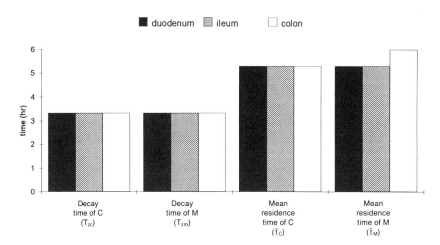

FIGURE 9.6. The time constant plot comparing continuous infusion at three different sites: duodenum, ileum, and colon in the example shown in Figure 9.5. The mean residence time of metabolite $(\bar{t}_m)$ is the same after dosing at the duodenum and ileum sites but is longer at the colon site due to the decrease in the presystemic metabolism.

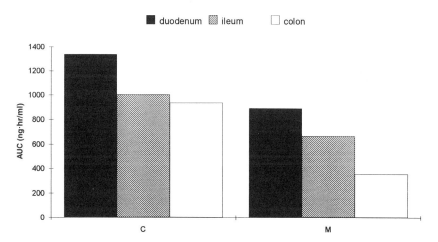

FIGURE 9.7. The area under the concentration curve of the parent drug and the metabolite of the example in Figure 9.5.

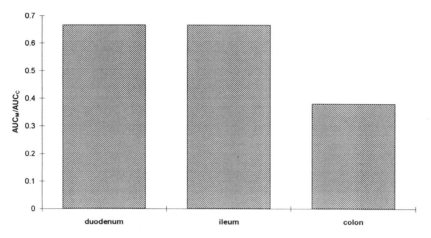

FIGURE 9.8. The ratio of the area under the metabolite concentration curve to the area under the parent drug concentration curve of the example in Figure 9.5.

fore, the comparison of the absorption time should be based on the mean residence time of the parent drug instead of the metabolite. The area under the concentration curve (Figure 9.7) of the parent drug is similar at the ileum and the colon sites, while that at the duodenum site is 30% greater than the two distal sites. Based on the similarity in AUC between the ileum and colon sites, another erroneous conclusion may be made that the fraction absorbed is similar at the two sites. However, from the ratio of the area under the curve of the metabolite to that of the parent drug (Figure 9.8), it is revealed that the presystemic metabolism is significantly reduced at the colon site. The fraction absorbed at the colon site is less than the fraction absorbed at the ileum site, but because of the less extent of the presystemic metabolism at the colon site, the bioavailability is similar at the two sites.

EXAMPLES

Example 1: Extent of Absorption Varies along the Intestine

The absorption of danazol after oral or intraintestinal administration to the proximal jejunum or proximal ileum was studied in healthy female subjects by gastrointestinal intubation [3]. The mean plasma concentration profiles of danazol following the administration of 100 mg danazol at the three different sites along the gastrointestinal tract are shown in Figure 9.9. The plasma concentration of danazol following the oral administration is higher than those after the intraintestinal administrations. This is probably because the longer the transit time of the drug in the intestine, the greater is the extent of the absorption. The time to reach the maximum concentration is prolonged after the oral administration, compared with the intraintestinal administration, probably because the gastric emptying delays the oral dose absorption.

The objective of this study is to evaluate the extent of absorption at three gastrointestinal sites and to assess the effect of gastric emptying on the absorption. Therefore, the key pharmacokinetic parameters are the area under the curve for the assessment of bioavailability and the mean residence time for the assessment of gastric emptying and absorption times. Each plasma concentration profile exhibits a monoexponential terminal phase, and gastric emptying may affect the oral absorption; therefore, Model 1 can be used to interpret the pharmacokinetic parameters. The estimated pharmacokinetic parameters are listed in Table 9.4, and the estimated time constants are presented in Figure 9.10. The area under the plasma concentration curve decreases as the dosing site moves down the gastrointestinal tract, probably due to a decreased transit time of the drug after the administration in the lower intestine. As shown in the time constant plot (Figure 9.10), the mean residence time following the oral administration is longer than that following the administration in the jejunum, probably delayed by gastric emptying. There is no evidence of difference in ab-

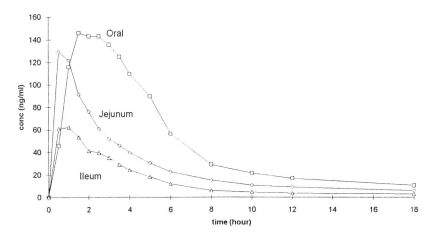

FIGURE 9.9. The mean plasma concentration profiles of danazol following the administration of 100 mg of danazol emulsion to healthy female subjects through three different gastrointestinal sites: oral, proximal jejunum, and proximal ileum. (Reproduced from Reference [3] with permission.) The time constant plot comparing the three absorption sites is shown in Figure 9.10.

TABLE 9.4. The Estimated Pharmacokinetic Parameters of Danazol (Model 1) after Administration of 100 mg Danazol to Different Gastrointestinal Sites.

Parameter*	Oral	Jejunum	Ileum	Equation
T_z (hr)	5.26	5.88	5.0	(9.2)
$\bar{t}$ (hr)	5.1	4.4	4.2	(9.1)
AUC (ng·hr/ml)	999	543	264	

*Parameters estimated from the mean concentration curves or the reported mean values.

sorption time or elimination time between the two intestinal sites, since the decay time and mean residence time of the two sites are similar. To summarize, the absorption after the oral administration is delayed, compared with the intraintestinal administrations, probably due to a slow gastric emptying rate. The extent of absorption decreases in the distal part of the intestine, as a result of several possible reasons: (1) the intestinal surface area decreases in the distal part, and (2) bile salt excretion in the proximal intestine may help solubilize the drug.

Example 2: Difference in the Presystemic Metabolism at Various Intestinal Sites

The bioavailability of gepirone was studied following the administration of 20 mg gepirone to seven healthy male subjects at three gastrointestinal

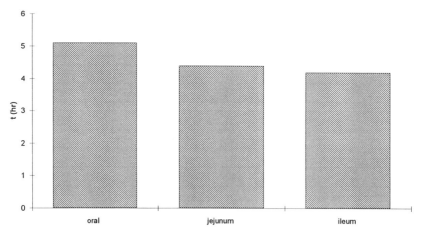

FIGURE 9.10. The time constant plot of danazol after the administration at three different sites: oral, proximal jejunum, and proximal ileum.

sites by gastrointestinal intubation and one multiple oral dose treatment: (1) oral, (2) distal small intestinal, (3) proximal small intestine, and (4) four consecutive 5-mg oral doses at hourly interval [9]. The mean plasma concentration profiles following the four treatments are shown in Figure 9.11. The plasma concentration of gepirone is slightly higher after dosing at the distal intestine than at the proximal site. The time to reach the maximum concentration is prolonged after the four consecutive oral doses, compared with the other three treatments, simply because of the extended administration time.

The objective of this study is to find the window of absorption along the gastrointestinal tract that is especially important for the sustained released formulation. Therefore, one key parameter in this example is the area under the curve. In addition, to identify a potential difference in the presystemic metabolism, the key parameter is the ratio of the area under the metabolite concentration curve to the area under the drug concentration curve. Gepirone is subjected to significant metabolism, and Model 3 is used to estimate the pharmacokinetic parameters of the drug. The estimated parameters of gepirone and its metabolite are listed in Table 9.5, and the estimated mean residence times are presented in Figure 9.12. The area under the curve and the mean residence times are greater following the multiple oral dose than following the single oral dose, simply because of the prolonged

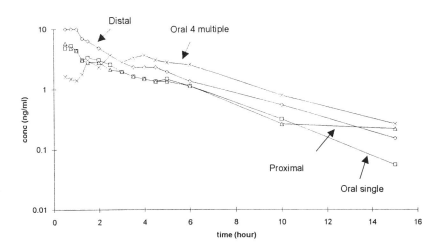

FIGURE 9.11. The mean concentration profiles of gepirone following the administration of 20 mg gepirone to seven healthy male subjects at three gastrointestinal sites and one multiple oral dose treatment: oral, distal small intestinal, proximal small intestine, and four consecutive 5-mg oral doses at hourly intervals. (Reproduced from Reference [9] with permission.) The time constant plot comparing the three absorption sites is shown in Figure 9.12.

TABLE 9.5. The Estimated Pharmacokinetic Parameters of Gepirone Using Model 3 Following Four Different Treatments Shown in Figure 9.11.

Parameter*	Oral (single)	Distal	Proximal	Oral (four multiple)	Equation
T_{zc} (hr)	3.98	4.57	4.69	4.37	(9.2)
T_{zm} (hr)	6.99	7.09	8.06	9.80	(9.2)
$\bar{t}_C$ (hr)	3.53	3.28	3.70	5.13	(9.7)
AUC_C (ng·hr/ml)	18.07	29.83	17.74	26.17	
AUC_M (ng·hr/ml)	83.99	102.38	97.49	108.63	
AUC_M/AUC_C	4.65	3.43	5.50	4.15	(9.6)

*Parameters estimated from the mean concentration curves or the reported mean values.

administration time period in the multiple dose treatment. The area under the gepirone concentration curve is much higher following the administration at the distal intestine than those following oral single-dose administration and the administration at the proximal intestine. The ratios of the area under the metabolite concentration curve to the area under the gepirone concentration curve are smaller after the administration at the distal intestinal site than after the oral dose and the administration at the proximal intestinal site, indicating a possible site of metabolism before the distal intestine. However, the difference in the ratios is not statistically significant [9]. The site-specific metabolism is slower at the distal intestine than at the

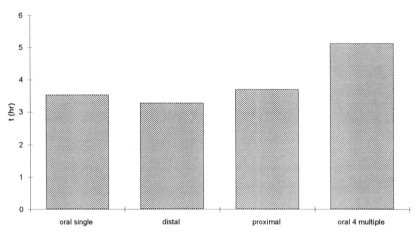

FIGURE 9.12. The time constant plot of gepirone comparing gastrointestinal sites: oral, distal small intestinal, proximal small intestine, and four consecutive 5-mg oral doses at hourly intervals, using Model 3.

proximal intestine, and it is likely to occur presystemically since the decay time and the mean residence time indicate no difference in the systemic elimination of gepirone. To summarize, the extent of absorption of gepirone is greater at the distal site than the proximal site, probably due to a decrease in the presystemic metabolism along the intestinal tract.

REFERENCES

1. Borgstrom L., Kennedy B. M., Nilsson B., and Angelin B., "Relative absorption of two enantiomers of terbutaline after duodenal administration," *Eur. J. Clin. Pharmacol.,* 1990; 38:621–623.

2. Brockmeier D., Grigoleit H. G., and Leonhardt H., "Absorption of benclamide from different sites of the gastrointestinal tract," *Eur. J. Clin. Pharmacol.,* 1985; 29:193–197.

3. Charman W. N., Rogge M. C., Boddy A. W., Barr W. H., and Berger B. M., "Absorption of danazol after administration to different sites of the gastrointestinal tract and the relationship to single- and double-peak phenomena in the plasma profiles," *J. Clin. Pharmacol.,* 1993; 33:1207–1213.

4. d'Agay-Abensour L., Fjellestad-Paulsen A., Ngo Y., Paulsen O., and Rambaud J. C., "Absolute bioavailability of an aqueous solution of 1-deamino-8-D-arginine vasopressin from different regions of the gastrointestinal tract in man," *Eur. J. Clin. Pharmacol.,* 1993; 44:473–476.

5. Jobin J., Cortot A., Godbillon J., Duval M., Scholler J. P. Hirtz J., and Bernier J. J., "Investigation of drug absorption from the gastrointestinal tract of man. I. Metoprolol in the stomach, duodenum and jejunum," *Br. J. Clin. Pharmacol.,* 1985; 19:97S–105S.

6. Lennernas H., Nilsson D., Aquilonius S. M., Ahrenstedt O., Knutson L., and Paalzow L. K., "The effect of L-leucine on the absorption of levodopa, studied by regional jejunal perfusion in man," *Br. J. Clin. Pharmac.,* 1993; 35:243–250.

7. Lennernas H., Ahrenstedt O., Hallgren R., Knutson L., Ryde M., and Paalzow L. K., "Regional jejunal perfusion, a new in vivo approach to study oral drug absorption in man," *Pharmaceutical Research*, 1992; 9(10):1243–1251.

8. Modigliani R., Rambaud J. C., and Bernier J. J. "The method of intraluminal perfusion of the human small intestine: Principle and technique," *Digestion,* 1973; 9:176–192.

9. Tay L. K., Dixon Jr. F., Sostrin M. B., Barr W. H., Farmen R. H., and Pittman K. A., "The site of gastrointestinal absorption of gepirone in humans," *J. Clin. Pharmacol.,* 1992; 32:827–832.

10. Vidon J., Evard D., Godbillion J., Rongier M., Duval M., Schoeller J. P., Bernier J. J., and Hirtz J., "Investigation of drug absorption from the gastrointestinal tract of man. I. Metoprolol in the jejunum and ileum," *Br. J. Clin. Pharmacol.,* 1985; 19:107S–112S.

11. Vidon N., Palma R., Godbillon J., Franchisseur C., Gosset G., Bernier J. J., and Hirtz J. J., "Gastric and intestinal absorption of oxprenolol in humans," *J. Clin. Pharmacol.,* 1986; 26:611–615.

12. Hardy J. G., Davis S. S., Wilson C. G., *Drug Delivery to the Gastrointestinal Tract,* Ellis Horwood Limited Publishers, 1990.

CHAPTER 10

Drug Distribution into Tissue – Tissue Penetration

INTRODUCTION

If the action of a drug takes place in a particular tissue or organ, it is important to determine if the drug concentration in the tissue or organ reaches the therapeutic ranges in a timely manner. The correlation of drug concentrations in the tissue and the plasma can be determined in a tissue penetration study. The descriptive pharmacokinetic parameters of interest in a tissue penetration study include the ratio of area under the concentration curve in the tissue to that in the plasma, the delay of the peak concentration in the tissue relative to the peak plasma concentration, the duration of the drug concentration in the tissue that is within the therapeutic range, and the clearance and the half-life of the drug in the tissue. Concentrations of drugs have been measured in many tissues and organs in humans, including saliva [16], lung [7,14,17], sputum [6,13,18], bone [1,10,19], synovial fluid [11], brain [4], peritoneum, urine, tears [21], blister fluid [2,3,9], gynecological tissue [5,8], heart [15], liver [15], kidney [15], pancreas [15], spleen [15], cerebrospinal fluid, and milk. The relationship between the concentrations in the tissue and the blood can be reversible or irreversible. If the relationship between the plasma and tissue concentrations is reversible, the ratio of the two concentrations will reach an equilibrium with time. The key time constants determining the tissue concentration profile in a tissue penetration study are the penetration time into the tissue and elimination time from the tissue. The penetration time of a drug into the tissue and the elimination time from the tissue depend on many factors, for example, ionization of the drug, lipophilicity of the drug, protein binding with the drug, tissue binding with the drug, pH in the blood and tissue, blood flow, capillary permeability, perfusion within tissue, interface area between blood and tissue, volume of distribution, and tissue metabolism.

Some common themes in the time constant view can be observed in the tissue penetration study as well as other studies. For drugs with biexponential decay, a common factor in many studies is whether the second decay time represents the total elimination time or the redistribution time. This factor can be determined in a tissue distribution study by determining whether the second decay time matches the redistribution time from the tissue compartment or the total elimination time from the plasma compartment. If the second decay time represents the redistribution time, then factors affecting the distribution will alter the half-life of the drug, such as those factors in an age study (Chapter 15), gender study (Chapter 16), and drug interaction study (Chapter 14) involving a protein binding displacer. A relatively long redistribution time will also be reflected by large apparent volume of distribution in all these studies. Lipophilicity of drugs is another common factor affecting time constants in many pharmacokinetics studies, including the tissue penetration study. Lipophilic drugs usually have short tissue distribution times and long redistribution times; they also tend to have large apparent volumes of distribution because of easy tissue penetration, and this will be reflected by long mean residence times in all studies. Lipophilic drugs may show a long dissolution time in the bioequivalence study due to their low water solubility. Some of the basic lipophilic drugs are susceptible to the first pass effect, which can be identified in a bioavailability or food study (Chapter 13). For lipophilic drugs, the mean residence time (influenced by the tissue distribution time) will be a key time constant in age (Chapter 15) and gender (Chapter 16) studies, since tissue binding of lipophilic drugs depends on the body mass content of fat, which is different between these groups of different age or gender.

Four models are discussed in this chapter for pharmacokinetic parameter estimation in tissue distribution studies: (1) the first model describes an irreversible distribution; (2) the second model describes a reversible distribution; (3) the third model is an isolated multi-compartment model with an irreversible distribution; and (4) the fourth model is an isolated multi-compartment model with a reversible distribution. Three simulated case studies and three literature examples are presented in this chapter to illustrate the utility of these models in tissue distribution studies. Additional literature examples can be found [1–21].

PHARMACOKINETIC MODELS

This section presents four models that are useful in estimating pharmacokinetic time constants in tissue penetration studies. The goal is to establish simple relationships between time constants and measurable parameters such as (1) mean residence time, which is the sum of input and output times, and (2) area under the curves. The derivations of these relationships are straightforward and are discussed in Chapter 2.

Model 1: Irreversible Distribution

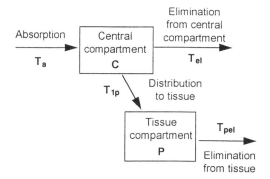

The distribution kinetics of a drug into a peripheral compartment can be irreversible, where the metabolism may be responsible for the elimination of the drug in the tissue compartment. In this case, the decay time of the concentration profile in the peripheral compartment may be longer than or equal to that in the central compartment, depending on the elimination time from the tissue compartment. On the other hand, if the distribution is reversible, the decay time of the drug in the tissue compartment is likely the same as the decay time in the plasma.

The mean residence time of the concentration profiles in the central and peripheral compartments is simply the sum of input and output times

$$\text{Mean residence time in central compartment } (\bar{t}_C) = \frac{\text{AUMC}_C}{\text{AUC}_C}$$

$$= \text{Input time } (T_{c,in}) + \text{Output time } (T_{c,out}) = T_a + T_{el,t} \quad (10.1)$$

$$\text{Mean residence time in peripheral compartment } (\bar{t}_P) = \frac{\text{AUMC}_P}{\text{AUC}_P}$$

$$= \text{Input time } (T_{p,in}) + \text{Output time } (T_{p,out}) = T_a + T_{el,t} + T_{pel}$$

$$(10.2)$$

where $T_{el,t} = 1/(1/T_{el} + 1/T_{lp})$. The elimination time constant of the drug in the peripheral compartment can be estimated from the difference in the mean residence time of the peripheral and central compartments.

$$\text{Elimination time from the peripheral compartment } (T_{pel}) = \bar{t}_P - \bar{t}_C$$

$$(10.3)$$

The decay time of the concentration profiles can be estimated from a partial area under the curve (see Appendix 2).

$$\frac{1}{\text{Decay time } (T_z)} = \lambda_z = 2\frac{(t - t_{last}) \ln C_t - AU \ln C_{t-t_{last}}}{(t - t_{last})^2} \qquad (10.4)$$

The ratio of the area under the tissue concentration curve to the area under the plasma concentration curve gives the ratio of clearance time from the tissue to the penetration clearance time to the tissue.

$$\frac{AUC_P}{AUC_C} = \frac{T_{pel}V_c}{T_{lp}V_p} = \frac{\text{Elimination clearance time from peripheral}}{\text{Distribution clearance time from central to peripheral}}$$

$$(10.5)$$

Then the penetration clearance time can be estimated as follows:

$$\text{Normalized distribution time } \left(T_{lp}\frac{V_p}{V_c}\right) = \frac{AUC_C}{AUC_P} T_{pel} \qquad (10.6)$$

Model 2: Reversible Distribution

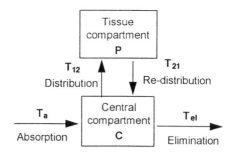

The distribution kinetics of a drug between the central and tissue compartments can also be reversible as in this model. In this case, the decay time of the tissue and plasma concentration curves will be similar, and the terminal phases of the tissue and plasma concentration profiles will be parallel to each other if the sampling time is long enough for the equilibrium to be established.

The mean residence time is the sum of input and output times (see Chapter 2)

$$\text{Mean residence time in central compartment } (\bar{t}_\text{C}) = \frac{\text{AUMC}}{\text{AUC}}$$

$$= \text{Input time } (T_{\text{c,in}}) + \text{Output time } (T_{\text{c,out}}) = T_\text{a} + T_\text{el} + T_\text{el}\frac{T_{21}}{T_{12}}$$

$$(10.7)$$

$$\text{Mean residence time in peripheral compartment } (\bar{t}_\text{P}) = \frac{\text{AUMC}}{\text{AUC}}$$

$$= \text{Input time } (T_{\text{p,in}}) + \text{Output time } (T_{\text{p,out}}) = T_\text{a} + T_\text{el} + T_\text{el}\frac{T_{21}}{T_{12}} + T_{21}$$

$$(10.8)$$

and can be estimated from the ratio of the area under the first moment curve to the area under the concentration curve. The distribution time constant from the peripheral compartment back to the central compartment can be estimated from the difference in the mean residence time of the peripheral and central compartments.

$$\text{Redistribution time } (T_{21}) = \bar{t}_\text{P} - \bar{t}_\text{C} \qquad (10.9)$$

The ratio of the area under the peripheral concentration to the area under the plasma concentration gives

$$\frac{\text{AUC}_\text{P}}{\text{AUC}_\text{C}} = \frac{T_{21}V_\text{c}}{T_{12}V_\text{p}} = \frac{\text{Redistribution clearance time}}{\text{Distribution clearance time}} \qquad (10.10)$$

As a result, the distribution time constant to the peripheral compartment can be estimated as follows:

$$\text{Normalized distribution time }\left(T_{12}\frac{V_\text{p}}{V_\text{c}}\right) = \frac{\text{AUC}_\text{C}}{\text{AUC}_\text{P}}T_{21} \qquad (10.11)$$

Model 3: Isolated Multi-Compartment Model with an Irreversible Distribution

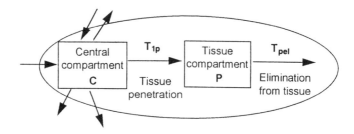

If the pharmacokinetics of a drug are too complicated or the data from the clinical study are not sufficient to determine all the parameters of the full pharmacokinetic model, an isolated multi-compartment model can be used to describe the distribution part of the pharmacokinetics. (The theories regarding local models versus global models are discussed in Chapter 3.)

The ratio of the area under the peripheral concentration curve to the area under the plasma concentration curve gives

$$\frac{AUC_P}{AUC_C} = \frac{T_{pel} C_c}{T_{1p} V_p} = \frac{\text{Elimination clearance time from peripheral}}{\text{Distribution clearance time from central to pheripheral}}$$

$$(10.12)$$

The difference in the mean residence time of the peripheral and plasma concentration curves gives the elimination time constant from the peripheral compartment.

$$\text{Elimination time from peripheral } (T_{pel}) = \bar{t}_P - \bar{t}_C \quad (10.13)$$

The peripheral concentration can be estimated from the plasma concentration by a convolution

$$C_p = C * \frac{V_c}{T_{1p} V_p} e^{-t/T_{pel}} \quad (10.14)$$

Additional discussions of the multi-compartmental model have been presented in Chapter 2.

Model 4: Isolated Multi-Compartment Model with a Reversible Distribution

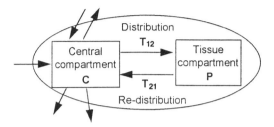

This is an isolated multi-compartmental model and reversible distribution kinetics. The difference in the mean residence time of the peripheral and central compartments gives the distribution time constant from the peripheral to the central compartments.

$$\text{Redistribution time } (T_{21}) = \bar{t}_{\text{P}} - \bar{t}_{\text{C}} \qquad (10.15)$$

The ratio of the area under the peripheral concentration to the plasma concentration curve gives the ratio of the distribution time constants:

$$\frac{\text{AUC}_{\text{P}}}{\text{AUC}_{\text{C}}} = \frac{T_{21}V_{\text{c}}}{T_{12}V_{\text{p}}} = \frac{\text{Redistribution clearance time}}{\text{Distribution clearance time}} \qquad (10.16)$$

The distribution time constant from the central to the peripheral compartments can be estimated as follows:

$$\text{Normalized distribution time } \left(T_{12}\frac{V_{\text{p}}}{V_{\text{c}}}\right) = \frac{\text{AUC}_{\text{C}}}{\text{AUC}_{\text{P}}} T_{21} \qquad (10.17)$$

The concentration in the peripheral compartment can be estimated from the plasma concentration by a convolution method

$$C_{\text{p}} = C* \frac{V_{\text{c}}}{T_{12}V_{\text{p}}} e^{-t/T_{21}} \qquad (10.18)$$

CASE STUDIES

Case 1: Irreversible Tissue Penetration

The relationship between the tissue concentration and the plasma concentration can be irreversible. One possible scenario is that, once the drug enters the tissue, it may be eliminated by metabolic enzymes in the tissue and not return to the blood. This case can be described by Model 1, and simulated plasma and tissue concentration profiles are shown in Figure 10.1. In this example, a drug is irreversibly distributed into the tissue with a rate constant of 0.3 hr^{-1}, and the elimination rate constant from the tissue is 0.25 hr^{-1}. The peak tissue drug concentration is lower than the peak plasma drug concentration, which can be due to a slow tissue penetration or fast elimination from the tissue. There is an approximate 4-hour delay in the peak tissue concentration relative to the peak plasma concentration, which corresponds to the elimination time (4 hours) from the tissue compartment. The relationship between the tissue concentration and the plasma concentration is irreversible, reflected by the fact that the tissue to plasma concentration ratio increases with time (Figure 10.2). The ratio of tissue concentration to plasma concentration reaches 200 after 36 hours postdose, suggesting the irreversible nature of the tissue distribution. The lag time between the tissue and plasma concentrations can be demonstrated by the tissue versus plasma concentration plot (Figure 10.3), which results in a hysteresis loop.

The key time constant in this example is the elimination time of the tissue concentration, which determines the lag time between the tissue and plasma concentration and the decay time of the tissue concentration. The

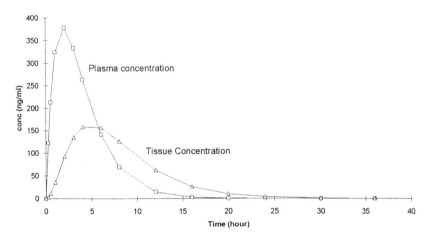

FIGURE 10.1. Simulated plasma and tissue concentration profiles with irreversible tissue penetration using Model 1. The time constant plot comparing pharmacokinetics in tissue and plasma is shown in Figure 10.4. The parameters used in this simulation are $X_0 = 10$ mg, f*F = 0.8, $V_c = 10$ L, $K_a = 0.7$ hr^{-1}, $K_{el} = 0.1$ hr^{-1}, $K_{1p} = 0.3$ hr^{-1}, $K_{pel} = 0.25$ hr^{-1}, $V_p = 15$ L.

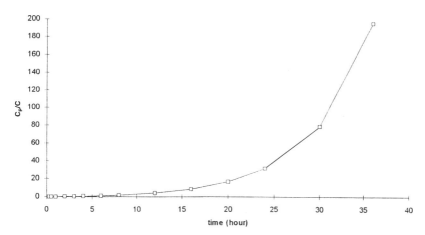

FIGURE 10.2. The ratio of the tissue drug concentration to the plasma drug concentration as a function of time for the example in Figure 10.1.

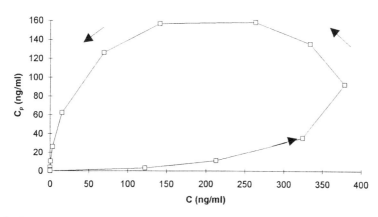

FIGURE 10.3. The tissue concentration versus plasma concentration plot for the example in Figure 10.1.

TABLE 10.1. Estimated Time Constants of Model 1
for the Example Shown in Figure 10.1.

| Parameter | Central Cmpt. | | Tissue Cmpt. | | Equation |
	Time Constant Analysis	Model Value	Time Constant Analysis	Model Value	
$T_{pel}*V_c/T_{1p}/V_p$ (AUC$_P$/AUC$_C$)			0.8	0.8	(10.5)
T_z (hr)	2.5	2.5 ($T_{el,t}$)	4.17	4.0 (T_{pel})	(10.4)
$\bar{t}$ (hr)	3.9	3.9	7.9	7.9	(10.1, 10.2)
T_{pel} (hr)			4.0	4.0	(10.3)
AUC (ng·hr/L)	2026	2000	1612	1600	

ratio of the tissue concentration clearance time, T_{pel}/V_p, to the penetration clearance time, T_{1p}/V_c, is an indicator of the ratio of steady-state tissue concentration to steady-state plasma concentration. The estimated pharmacokinetic parameters of the above example using the time constant analysis are listed in Table 10.1, and the estimated time constants are presented in Figure 10.4. The ratio of the area under the curve in the tissue to that in the plasma is less than one, which indicates that the clearance time from the tissue is less than penetration clearance time into the tissue. The clearance times represent the concentration-average time required to move the drug from one unit volume in a compartment. Now let us examine the time constant plot (Figure 10.4). The decay time of the tissue concentration is longer than that of the plasma concentration, reflecting a slower elimination in the tissue than the plasma. The mean residence time of the tissue concentration is 4 hours longer than that of the plasma concentration, corresponding to the value of T_{pel}.

Case 2: Reversible Tissue Distribution

The relationship between the tissue and plasma concentrations can be reversible, especially for drugs that are freely perfused into and out of the tissue. A reversible distribution can be described by Model 2, and simulated plasma and tissue concentration profiles using the model are shown in Figure 10.5. The distribution rate constant from the tissue to the plasma is 0.2 hr^{-1}, resulting in a 4 to 5-hour delay of the peak tissue concentration relative to the peak plasma concentration. The tissue concentration is lower than the plasma concentration, indicating that the ratio of

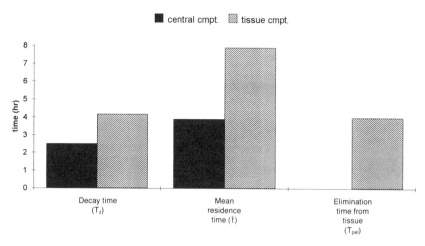

FIGURE 10.4. The time constant plot for pharmacokinetics in tissue and plasma with irreversible tissue penetration in the example shown in Figure 10.1. The mean residence time ($\bar{t}$) of the tissue concentration is 4 hours longer than that of the plasma concentration, corresponding to the value of elimination time from the tissue (T_{pel}).

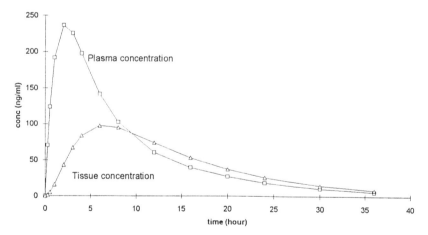

FIGURE 10.5. Simulated plasma and tissue concentration profiles with reversible tissue distribution using Model 2. The time constant plot comparing the pharmacokinetics in tissue and plasma is shown in Figure 10.7. The parameters used in this simulation are $X_0 = 10$ mg, $f^*F = 0.8$, $V_c = 10$ L, $V_p = 20$ L, $K_a = 0.4$ hr^{-1}, $K_{el} = 0.35$ hr^{-1}, $K_{12} = 0.3$ hr^{-1}, $K_{21} = 0.2$ hr^{-1}.

223

distribution clearance time, T_{12}/V_c, to the redistribution clearance time, T_{21}/V_p, is less than one. The ratio of tissue concentration to the plasma concentration reaches an equilibrium (Figure 10.6), indicating a possible reversible relationship between the two concentrations.

The key time constants in this example are the penetration time into the tissue (T_{12}) and the redistribution time (T_{21}) from the tissue. These time constants determine the time required to establish the quasi-equilibrium between the tissue and plasma concentrations. The estimated pharmacokinetic parameters of the above example using the time constant analysis are listed in Table 10.2, and the estimated time constants are presented in Figure 10.7. The ratio of the area under the tissue concentration curve to the area under the plasma concentration curve is less than one, indicating that the penetration clearance time into the tissue is longer than the elimination clearance time from the tissue.

Now let us examine the time constant plot (Figure 10.7). The decay time of the plasma concentration is the same as the decay time of the tissue concentration, suggesting that a quasi-equilibrium between the tissue and plasma drug concentrations may be achieved at the terminal phase. The mean residence time of the tissue concentration profile is 5 hours longer than that of the plasma concentration, corresponding to the elimination time from the tissue (T_{21}). To summarize, based on the penetration time and the redistribution time, it may require 14.6 hours ($2 \times$ the larger of T_{21} or $T_{12}*V_p/V_c$) to reach a quasi-equilibrium (90%) between plasma and tissue concentration.

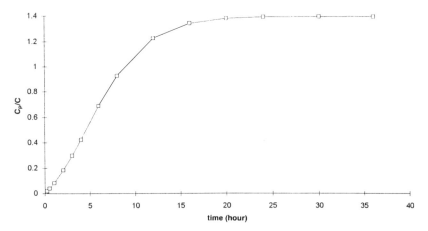

FIGURE 10.6. The ratio of the tissue drug concentration to the plasma drug concentration as a function of time for the example in Figure 10.5.

TABLE 10.2. *Estimated Time Constants of Model 2
for the Example Shown in Figure 10.5.*

Parameter	Central Cmpt.		Tissue Cmpt.		Equation
	Time Constant Analysis	Model Value	Time Constant Analysis	Model Value	
$T_{21}*V_c/T_{12}/V_p$ (AUC$_P$/AUC$_C$)			0.75	0.75	(10.10)
T_z (hr)	10.4	10.9 (T_{z2})	10.4	10.9 (T_{z2})	(10.4)
$\bar{t}$ (hr)	9.5	9.6	14.5	14.6	(10.7, 10.8)
T_{21} (hr)			5.0	5.0	(10.9)
$T_{12}*V_p/V_c$ (hr)			7.3	7.3	(10.11)
AUC (ng·hr/L)	2296	2285	1711	1714	

Case 3: Isolated Multi-Compartmental Model

The pharmacokinetics of a drug may involve more than one peripheral compartment, multiple metabolites, and multiple elimination routes. However, the relationship between the drug concentration in a tissue and the plasma concentration can be determined without the detailed knowledge of the rest of the pharmacokinetics. (The model-independent estimation of time constants is discussed in Chapter 2.) This is achieved by using the isolated multi-compartment model (Model 3 or 4). Simulated plasma and tissue concentration profiles using Model 4 are shown in Figure 10.8. In this example, a drug is reversibly distributed into the tissue, and the full pharmacokinetic model of the drug has not been determined. As indicated in Figure 10.9, the relationship between the plasma and tissue concentrations is likely to be reversible, since the ratio of the tissue concentration to the plasma concentration reaches an equilibrium. It is also possible that the distribution is irreversible (following Model 3) and the elimination time from the tissue compartment is shorter than that from the central compartment. The lag time between the peak tissue concentration and the peak plasma concentration is 5 hours, which corresponds to the value of T_{21}.

In a multi-compartmental model, the key time constants to be estimated are the penetration time (T_{12}) and the redistribution time (T_{21}). The estimated pharmacokinetic parameters of the above example using the time constant analysis are listed in Table 10.3, and the estimated time constants are presented in Figure 10.10. The ratio of the area under the tissue concen-

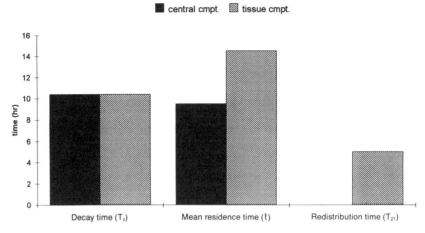

FIGURE 10.7. The time constant plot comparing the pharmacokinetics in tissue and plasma with reversible tissue penetration in the example shown in Figure 10.5. The mean residence time ($\bar{t}$) of the tissue concentration profile is 5 hours longer than that of the plasma concentration, corresponding to the elimination time from the tissue (T_{21}).

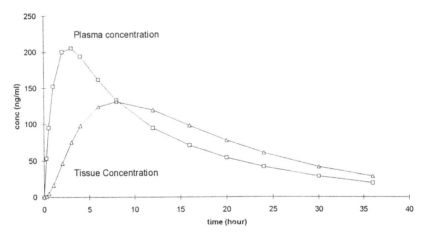

FIGURE 10.8. Simulated plasma and tissue concentration profiles with reversible tissue distribution using isolated multi-compartment Model 4. The time constant plot comparing the pharmacokinetics in tissue and plasma is shown in Figure 10.10. The parameters used in this simulation are: $X_0 = 10$ mg, $f^*F = 0.8$, $V_1 = 10$ L, $V_2 = 20$ L, $K_{12} = 0.3$ hr^{-1}, $K_{21} = 0.2$ hr^{-1}. (Published originally in Reference [6]; reprinted courtesy of Bioscience Ediprint.)

226

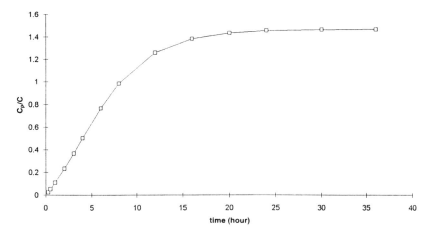

FIGURE 10.9. The ratio of the tissue drug concentration to the plasma drug concentration as a function of time for the example in Figure 10.8.

tration curve to the area under the plasma concentration curve is one, indicating an equivalent penetration clearance time into the tissue and elimination clearance time from the tissue compartment. However, the ratio of the tissue concentration to the plasma concentration at the equilibrium does not equal one (Figure 10.9). As shown in the time constant plot (Figure 10.10), the mean residence time of the tissue concentration is 5 hours longer than that of the plasma concentration, corresponding to the value of T_{21}.

TABLE 10.3. Estimated Time Constants of Model 3 for the Example Shown in Figure 10.8.

Parameter	Central Cmpt. Time Constant Analysis	Central Cmpt. Model Value	Tissue Cmpt. Time Constant Analysis	Tissue Cmpt. Model Value	Equation
$T_{21}*V_1/T_{12}/V_2$ (AUC_P/AUC_C)			1	1	(10.16)
T_z (hr)	15.4	15.4	15.4	15.4	(10.4)
$\bar{t}$ (hr)	15.1	15.3	20.3	20.3	
T_{21} (hr)			5.3	5.0	(10.15)
AUC (ng·hr/L)	3199	3200	3191	3200	

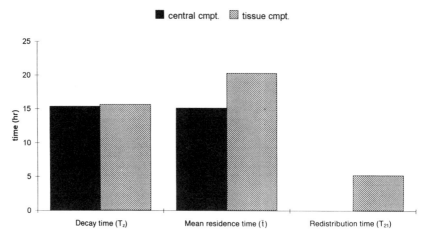

FIGURE 10.10. The time constant plot comparing the pharmacokinetics in tissue and plasma with reversible distribution in the example shown in Figure 10.8. The mean residence time ($\bar{t}$) of the tissue concentration is 5 hours longer than that of the plasma concentration, corresponding to the value of the redistribution time from tissue (T_{21}).

EXAMPLES

Example 1: Penetration into Sputum

The pharmacokinetics of mezlocillin were determined in serum and sputum following the treatment with 1 g/i.m./12 hr in patients suffering from bronchopulmonary infections [6]. The mean mezlocillin concentrations in serum and sputum following the treatment are shown in Figure 10.11. There is a lag time between the mezlocillin concentrations in sputum and the serum, indicating a slow elimination from the sputum. The concentration in sputum is ten times lower than the concentration in the serum, reflecting a slow penetration of the drug into the respiratory tract.

To determine how fast mezlocillin penetrates into the respiratory tract (sputum), the key time constant to be estimated is the penetration time T_{lp}. The elimination time of the drug from the sputum provides information about the lag time between the sputum and plasma concentrations and the time length of the drug concentration that can be maintained in the sputum. The pharmacokinetic parameters of mezlocillin in serum and sputum were estimated using Model 1, since the sputum/serum concentration ratio does not reach an equilibrium. It is also possible that a redistribution time is too long to be observed in this sampling time scale. The estimated parameters are listed in Table 10.4, and the estimated time constants are presented in

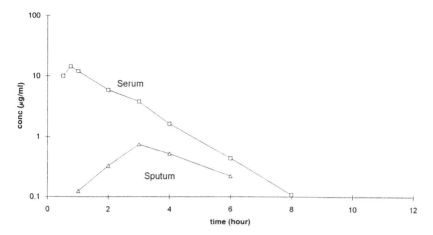

FIGURE 10.11. Mean mezlocillin concentration profiles in serum and sputum following the treatment with 1 g/i.m./12 hr in patients suffering from bronchopulmonary infections. (Reproduced from Reference [6] with permission.) The time constant plot comparing the pharmacokinetics in sputum and plasma is shown in Figure 10.12.

Figure 10.12. The area under the concentration curve in the sputum is ten times smaller than that in the serum, indicating a slow penetration of the drug.

Now let us examine the time constant plot (Figure 10.12). The decay time of the concentration curve in sputum is longer than that in the serum, indicating that the elimination time is slower in sputum than in serum. The

TABLE 10.4. The Estimated Pharmacokinetic
Parameters of Mezlocillin in Serum
and Sputum Using Model 1.

Parameter*	Serum	Sputum	Equation
$T_{pel}*V_c/T_{1p}/V_p$ (AUC_P/AUC_C)		0.103	(10.5)
T_z (hr)	1.41	1.85	(10.4)
$\bar{t}$ (hr)	1.88	3.63	(10.1, 10.2)
T_{pel} (hr)		1.75	(10.3)
$T_{1p} \cdot V_p/V_c$ (hr)	16.95		(10.6)
AUC (μg·hr/ml)	25.14	2.6	

*Parameters estimated from the mean concentration curves or the
reported mean values.

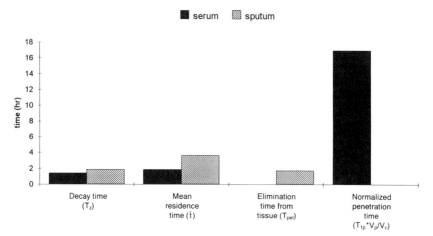

FIGURE 10.12. The time constant plot comparing the pharmacokinetics in sputum and plasma of mezlocillin using Model 1. The elimination time constant (T_{pel}) is similar to the decay time (T_z) of the concentration curve in sputum, indicating that the elimination time from sputum is the rate limiting step of the concentration in sputum. The penetration time constant ($T_{1p}*V_p/V_c$) is relatively long, resulting in a low sputum drug concentration.

elimination time constant (T_{pel}) is similar to the decay time of the concentration curve in sputum, indicating that the elimination from sputum is the rate limiting step of the concentration in sputum. The penetration time constant ($T_{1p}*V_p/V_c$) is relatively long, resulting in a low sputum drug concentration. To summarize, there is a short lag time (1.75 hour) between the sputum concentration and plasma concentration, and the decay time of the sputum and plasma concentrations are similar. Therefore, there may be a slight delay of the pharmacological effect in the respiratory tract, if the pharmacodynamic effect is directly correlated to the tissue drug concentration. The sputum concentration is lower than the plasma concentration; however, the former exceeds the MIC for most common bacteria responsible to respiratory tract infection for a sufficient length of time [6].

Example 2: Penetration into Saliva

The pharmacokinetics of metronidazole in serum and saliva were studied in eight healthy subjects following an oral treatment with 500 mg metronidazole [16]. The mean serum and saliva concentrations of metronidazole after the treatment are shown in Figure 10.13. The log concentration profiles in serum and saliva are parallel to each other, indicating a reversible distribution kinetics. The saliva to serum concentration ratio (Figure 10.14) remains almost constant throughout 48 hours.

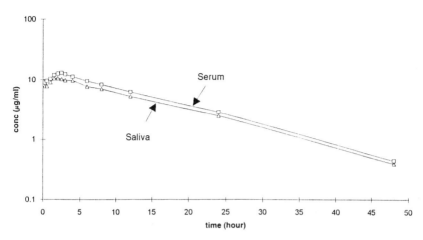

FIGURE 10.13. Mean serum and saliva concentration profiles of metronidazole in eight healthy subjects following the oral treatment of 500 mg metronidazole. (Reproduced with permission from Reference [16].) The time constant plot comparing the pharmacokinetics in saliva and plasma is shown in Figure 10.15.

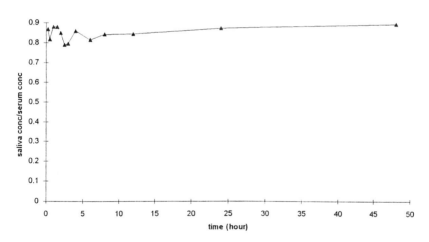

FIGURE 10.14. The saliva to serum metronidazole concentration ratio as a function of time. (Reproduced from Reference [16] with permission.)

TABLE 10.5. The Estimated Pharmacokinetic
Parameters of Metronidazole in
Serum and Saliva Using Model 2.

Parameter*	Serum	Saliva	Equation
$T_{21}*V_c/T_{12}/V_p$			
$\quad$(AUC$_P$/AUC$_C$)		0.854	(10.10)
T_z (hr)	11.5	11.6	(10.4)
$\bar{t}$ (hr)	12.31	12.50	(10.7, 10.8)
T_{21} (hr)		0.18	(10.9)
$T_{12}*V_p/V_c$ (hr)	0.21		(10.11)
AUC (μg·hr/ml)	179.8	153.6	

*Parameters estimated from the mean concentration curves or the
reported mean values.

The objective of this study is to determine whether the saliva concentration of metronidazole can replace the plasma concentration in pharmacokinetic studies. To ensure all time constants derived from the saliva concentrations are similar to those of plasma concentration, a rapid equilibrium must be established between the two concentrations. Therefore, the key time constants are the penetration time (T_{12}) and redistribution time (T_{21}). The pharmacokinetic parameters of metronidazole in the serum and saliva are determined using Model 2. The estimated pharmacokinetic parameters are listed in Table 10.5, and the estimated time constants are presented in Figure 10.15. The area under the concentration curve in serum and saliva is comparable, indicating a good penetration.

Now let us examine the time constant plot (Figure 10.12). The decay time and the mean residence time are similar in serum and saliva. The short distribution time (T_{21} and $T_{12}*V_p/V_c$) results in the rapid equilibrium between serum and saliva. To summarize, the saliva concentration can be used in place of plasma concentration in pharmacokinetic studies because of the similarity between the two concentration profiles, as suggested in Reference [16]. The good penetration of metronidazole into saliva is probably due to several properties of the drug: low molecular weight, being un-ionized at physiological pH, and minimal protein binding.

Example 3: Penetration into Blister Fluid

The pharmacokinetics and tissue penetration of cefprozil were examined in twelve healthy subjects following the oral administration of 250 and 500 mg of cefprozil [2]. The mean cefprozil concentrations in serum and blister

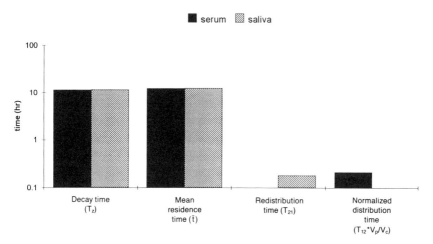

FIGURE 10.15. The time constant plot comparing the pharmacokinetics in saliva and plasma of metronidazole using Model 2. The short distribution times (T_{21} and $T_{12} {}^{*} V_p / V_c$) result in the rapid equilibrium between serum and saliva.

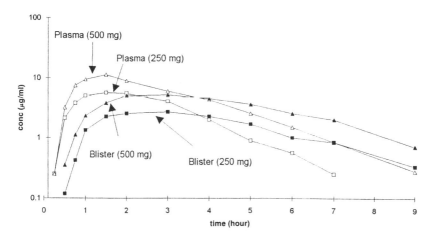

FIGURE 10.16. Mean concentration of cefprozil in serum and blister fluid in twelve healthy subjects following the oral administration of 250 and 500 mg of cefprozil. (Reproduced from Reference [2] with permission.) The time constant plot comparing pharmacokinetics in blister and serum is shown in Figure 10.17.

TABLE 10.6.   The Estimated Pharmacokinetic Parameters of Cefprozil in Serum and Blister Fluid Using Model 4.

Parameter*	Plasma (250 mg)	Plasma (500 mg)	Blister (250 mg)	Blister (500 mg)	Equation
$T_{21}*V_c/T_{12}/V_p$ (AUC$_P$/AUC$_C$)			0.82	0.85	(10.16)
T_z (hr)	2.04	1.89	3.45	3.13	(10.4)
$\bar{t}$ (hr)	2.6	2.7	5	4.8	
T_{21} (hr)			2.38	2.08	(10.15)
$T_{12}*V_p/V_c$ (hr)	2.94	2.44			(10.17)
AUC (μg·hr/ml)	16.3	32.0	13.4	27.3	

*Parameters estimated from the mean concentration curves or the reported mean values.

fluid following the treatments are shown in Figure 10.16. There is a delay in the penetration of the drug into blister. The concentration of cefprozil in the blister fluid is lower than that in the plasma.

The blister fluid can communicate with the intravascular fluid such that the blister concentration of cefprozil may represent the tissue concentration. The pharmacokinetic parameters of cefprozil in serum and blister fluid are estimated using Model 4. However, an equilibrium between the plasma and tissue concentrations has not been reached within the 9 hours of

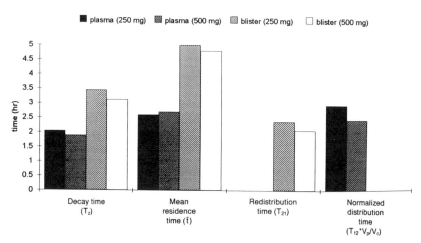

FIGURE 10.17. The time constant plot comparing pharmacokinetics in blister and serum of cefprozil using Model 4. The decay time (T_z) of the concentration in blister fluid is longer than that in the serum, reflecting a slower elimination from blister than from serum.

observation time. The estimated pharmacokinetic parameters are listed in Table 10.6, and the estimated time constants are presented in Figure 10.17. The area under the concentration curve in blister fluid is 82 to 85% of that in serum, indicating a good penetration of the drug.

Now let us examine the time constant plot (Figure 10.17). The decay time of the concentration in blister fluid is longer than that in the serum, reflecting a slower elimination rate in blister than in serum. The normalized penetration time, $T_{12}*V_p/V_c$, into the blister is 2.4 to 3 hours, and the elimination time, T_{21}, from the blister is 2 to 2.4 hours. There is not much difference between the two doses in the penetration time into the blister and elimination time from the blister. To summarize, the blister concentration is lower than the plasma concentration of cefprozil (probably due to a 45% plasma protein binding of the drug [2]). The maximum concentration of cefprozil in the blister is delayed, compared with the plasma concentration due to a 2- to 2.4-hour redistribution time constant.

REFERENCES

1. Adam D., Heilmann H. D., and Weismeier K., "Concentrations of ticarcillin and clavulanic acid in human bone after prophylactic administration of 5.2 g of timentin," *Antimicrobial Agents and Chemotherapy,* 1987; 31(6):935–939.

2. Barbhaiya R. H., Shukla U. A., Gleason C. R., Shyu W. C., Wilber R. B., and Pittman K. A., "Comparison of cefprozil and cefaclor pharmacokinetics and tissue penetration," *Antimicrobial Agents and Chemotherapy,* 1990; 34(6):1204–1209.

3. Blaser J., Rieder H. L., and Luthy R., "Interface-area-to-volume ratio of interstitial fluid in humans determined by pharmacokinetic analysis of netilmicin in small and large skin blisters," *Antimicrobial Agents and Chemotherapy,* 1991; 35(5):837–839.

4. Bossuyt A., Morgan G. F., Deblaton M., Pirotte R., Chirico A., Clemens P., Vandenbroeck P., and Thornback J. R., "Technetium-99m-MRP20, a potential brain perfusion agent: In vivo biodistribution and SPECT studies in normal male volunteers," *The Journal of Nuclear Medicine,* 1991; 32(3):399–403.

5. Bouver O., Bressolle F., Courtieu C., and Galtier M., "Penetration of pefloxacin into gynecological tissues," *Journal of Antimicrobial Chemotherapy,* 1992; 29:579–587.

6. Braga P. C., Marchi E., Scaglione F., Scarpazza G., Faravelli M., and Fraschini F., "Kinetics of penetration and clearance of mezlocillin in the bronchopulmonary tract," *Int. J. Clin. Pharm. Res.,* 1984; IV(5):361–365.

7. Coates G., Firnau G., Meyer G. J., and Gratz K. F., "Noninvasive measurement of lung carbon-11-serotonin extraction in man," *The Journal of Nuclear Medicine,* 1991; 32(4):729–732.

8. Fraschini F., Scaglione F., Proto M., Braga P. C., and Ciampini M., "Kinetics of cefatrizine penetration into gynaecological tissues after oral administration," *Chemotherapy,* 1987; 33:93–96.

9. Frongillo R. F., Galuppo L., and Moretti A., "Suction skin blister, skin window, and skin chamber techniques to determine extravascular passage of cefotaxime in humans," *Antimicrobial Agents and Chemotherapy,* 1981, 19(1):22–28.

10. Graziani A. L., Lawson L. A., Gibson G. A., Steinberg M. A., and MacGregor R. R., "Vancomycin concentrations in infected and noninfected human bone," *Antimicrobial Agents and Chemotherapy*, 1988; 32(9):1320–1322.

11. Grimer R. J., Karpinski M. R. K., Andrews J. M., and Wise R., "Penetration of amoxycillin and clavulanic acid into bone," *Chemotherapy*, 1986; 32:185–191.

12. Kavi J., Andrews J. M., Ashby J. P., Hillman G., and Wise R., "Pharmacokinetics and tissue penetration of cefpirome, a new cephalosporin," *Journal of Antimicrobial Chemotherapy*, 1988; 22:911–916.

13. Kovarik J. M., Hoepelman A. I. H., Smit J. M., Sips P. A., Rozenberg-Arska M., Glerum J. H., and Verhoef J., "Steady-state pharmacokinetics and sputum penetration of lomefloxacin in patients with chronic obstructive pulmonary disease acute respiratory tract infections," *Antimicrobial Agents and Chemotherapy*, 1992; 36(11):2458–2461.

14. MacFadyen R. J., Lees K. R., Gemmill K. R., Gemmill J. D., Hillis W. S., and Reid J. L., "Transpulmonary pharmacokinetics of an ACE inhibitor (perindoprilat) in man," *Br. J. Clin. Pharmac.*, 1991; 32:193–199.

15. Mejia A. A., Nakamura T., Masatoshi I., Hatazawa J., Masaki M., and Watanuki S., "Estimation of absorbed doses in humans due to intravenous administration of fluorine-18-fluorodeoxyglucose in PET studies," *The Journal of Nuclear Medicine*, 1991; 32(4):699–706.

16. Mustofa, Suryawati S., and Santoso B., "Pharmacokinetics of metronidasole in saliva," *International Journal of Clinical Pharmacology, Therapy and Toxicology*, 1991; 29(12):474–478.

17. Naline E., Sanceaume M., Toty L., Bakdach H., Pays M., and Advenier C., "Penetration of minocycline into lung tissues," *Br. J. Clin. Pharmac.*, 1991; 32:402–404.

18. Nightingale C. H., "Penetration and concentration of cefadroxil in sputum, lung and pleural fluid," *Drugs*, 1986; 32(suppl 3):17–20.

19. Roncoroni A. J., Manuel C., Nedjar C., Bauchet J., and Mariani D., "Cefamandole bone diffusion in patients undergoing total hip replacement," *Chemotherapy*, 1981; 27:166–172.

20. Schwiersch U., Lang N., and Wildfeuer D. A., "Concentration of sulbactam and ampicillin in serum and the myometrium," *Drugs*, 1986; 31(suppl. 2):26–28.

21. Tang-Liu D. D., Schwob D. L., Usansky J. I., and Gordon J. G., "Comparative tear concentrations over time of ofloxacin and tobramycin in human eyes," *Clinical Pharmacology & Therapeutics*, 1994; 55(3):284–292.

Pharmacokinetics of Metabolites

INTRODUCTION

Hepatic metabolism plays an important role in the disposition of drugs, not only because it affects the plasma levels of the parent drugs, but also because the metabolites may be pharmacologically active or toxic. Therefore, it is important to understand the pharmacokinetics and pharmacodynamics of the metabolites. The objective of a metabolism study is to identify and quantify the major metabolites of a drug in the plasma, urine, and feces [13,14]; study the pharmacokinetics of the metabolites [3,11]; identify subpopulations that have different metabolic rates [1,12]; or determine the potency of the metabolites [15]. The pharmacokinetics of metabolites can be much more complicated than that of the parent drug, since there may be more than one metabolite involved and the metabolic pathways can be complex. The metabolic pathways may include irreversible or reversible reactions arranged in parallel or in series. If several metabolites derive from a parent drug through different pathways parallel to one another [11], the plasma levels of a metabolite will depend on its rate of formation relative to the other metabolites since all metabolites compete concurrently for the parent drug. If several metabolites are formed in series [5], then the metabolite that has the longest elimination time (the rate limiting step) will likely have the highest plasma level among all, assuming the same volume of distribution for all metabolites and the parent drug. In a metabolism study, urine samples, as well as plasma samples, should be harvested in order to analyze the complicated pharmacokinetics. Radiolabeled drugs can be used to account for all metabolites in the plasma, urine, feces, and breath [3]. Metabolites, instead of parent drugs, can be administered to subjects to identify the sequence of reactions in the metabolic pathways and determine

237

the reversibility of metabolic reactions. The key pharmacokinetic parameters in a metabolism study are the hepatic elimination time toward the metabolitse and the elimination time of the metabolites.

Some common themes in the time constant view can be observed in the metabolism study as well as other studies. The predominant route of elimination is a common factor influencing the outcomes of many pharmacokinetic studies. Clinical factors affecting the predominant route of elimination will have a great impact on the total elimination time. Either the metabolism or the renal excretion can dominate the elimination, and the metabolism study can determine which one does. Examples of factors that may affect metabolism are hepatic impairment (Chapter 18), gender (Chapter 16), age (Chapter 15), and drug interaction (Chapter 14). Examples of factors that may affect renal elimination time are renal impairment (Chapter 17) and age (Chapter 15). If a metabolite is the pharmacologically active compound, the mean resaidence time of the effect curve in a pharmacokinetic/pharmacodynamic study (Chapter 12) will correlate better with the mean residence time of the metabolite than with the parent drug. Another common factor in many studies is the order of magnitude of the total elimination times of the metabolite and the parent drug; whichever is longer will limit the decay time of the metabolite. If the elimination time of the metabolite limits the decay time of the metabolite, then factors, such as renal impairment (Chapter 17), affecting the elimination of the metabolite will alter the decay time of the metabolite. On the other hand, if the elimination time of the parent drug limits the decay time of the metabolite, then factors affecting the elimination of the parent drug will alter the decay time of the metabolite, such as hepatic impairment (Chapter 18), age (Chapter 15), and drug interaction (Chapter 14).

Based on the estimated first pass effect [from bioavailability (Chapter 5) or food studies (Chapter 13)] and the estimated hepatic elimination time (from the metabolism study), one can qualitatively determine the size of the central compartment volume of distribution. If the first pass effect is extensive and the hepatic elimination time is long, then the central compartment volume of distribution is likely to be relatively large. The large volume of distribution dilutes the drug concentration, attenuates the rate at which the drug is eliminated by the liver, and thus prolongs the elimination time. On the other hand, if the first pass effect is small and the hepatic elimination time is short, the central compartment volume of distribution is likely to be small. Another integrated conclusion can be obtained from the bioavailability and metabolism studies: if the first pass effect is insignificant but the metabolites dominate the urine recovery, the renal elimination time of the parent drug must be relatively long compared with the hepatic elimination time. The long renal elimination time may be due to either (1) an extensive protein binding resulting in a very small free fraction in the blood or (2) a high lipophilicity resulting in complete tubular reabsorption.

Models of six different types of metabolic pathways are discussed in this chapter to describe some of the typical drug metabolisms. Four simulated case studies and four literature examples are presented in this chapter to illustrate the utility of these models in metabolism studies. Additional examples of metabolism studies can be found in the literature [1–12].

PHARMACOKINETIC MODELS

This section presents six models that are useful in describing different metabolic pathways. The goal is to establish simple relationships between time constants and measurable parameters such as (1) mean residence time, which is the sum of input and output times, and (2) area under the curves. The derivations of these relationships are straightforward and are discussed in Chapter 2.

Model 1: Parallel Metabolic Pathway

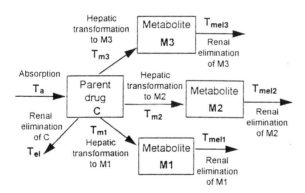

The simplest model for drug metabolism consists of irreversible metabolic kinetics as in Model 1. Several metabolites can be produced from the parent drug, and the metabolic pathways are parallel to each other.

The mean residence time of the drug and the metabolites is simply the sum of input and output times:

$$\text{Mean residence time of C } (\bar{t}_C) = \frac{\text{AUMC}_C}{\text{AUC}_C}$$

$$= \text{Input time } (T_{c,\text{in}}) + \text{Output time } (T_{c,\text{out}}) = T_a + T_{el,t} \quad (11.1)$$

$$\text{Mean residence time of M}_i \ (\bar{t}_{Mi}) = \frac{\text{AUMC}_{Mi}}{\text{AUC}_{Mi}}$$

$$= \text{Input time} \ (T_{mi,in}) + \text{Output time} \ (T_{mi,out}) = T_a + T_{el,t} + T_{meli} \quad (11.2)$$

where $T_{el,t} = 1/(1/T_{el} + 1/T_m)$ is the total elimination time constant. The elimination time of the metabolites can be estimated from the difference in the mean residence time between the metabolite and the parent drug:

$$\text{Elimination time of metabolite M}_i \ (T_{meli}) = \bar{t}_{Mi} - \bar{t}_c \quad (11.3)$$

The decay time of the concentration curve can be estimated from a partial area under the curve (see Appendix 2):

$$\frac{1}{\text{Decay time} \ (T_z)} = \lambda_z = 2 \frac{(t - t_{last}) \ln (C_t) - \text{AU} \ln C_{t-t_{last}}}{(t - t_{last})^2} \quad (11.4)$$

The ratio of the area under a metabolite concentration curve to the area under the parent drug concentration curve gives the ratio of renal clearance time of the metabolite to the hepatic clearance time from the parent drug to the metabolite.

$$\frac{\text{AUC}_{Mi}}{\text{AUC}_c} = \frac{T_{meli} V_c}{T_{mi} V_{mi}} = \frac{\text{Elimination clearance time of M}_i}{\text{Formation clearance time toward M}_i} \quad (11.5)$$

Then the hepatic clearance time toward a metabolite can be estimated as follows:

$$\text{Formation clearance time toward M}_i \left(\frac{T_{mi}}{V_c}\right) = \frac{T_{meli}}{V_{mi}} \frac{\text{AUC}_c}{\text{AUC}_{Mi}} \quad (11.6)$$

The metabolite that is formed with a short hepatic clearance time will appear earlier in the blood than the other metabolites. The renal clearance time can be estimated from the cumulative urine recovery:

$$\text{Renal clearance time} \left(\frac{T_{el}}{V}\right) = \frac{\text{AUC}}{X_u} \quad (11.7)$$

The above equation can be applied to the parent drug and the metabolites. The apparent total clearance time is defined as the area under the curve divided by dose

$$\text{Apparent total clearance time} \left(\frac{T_{el,t}}{V_c} fF \right) = \frac{\text{AUC}_C}{X_0} \qquad (11.8)$$

The apparent volume of distribution can be defined as the ratio of the decay time to the total clearance time:

$$\text{Apparent volume of distribution } (V_z) = \frac{T_z V_c}{T_{el,t} fF} \qquad (11.9)$$

The bioavailability of an oral dose can be estimated from the urine recovery assuming the renal excretion is the predominant route of elimination:

$$\text{Bioavailability } (f) = \frac{X_{uc} + X_{um}}{X_0} \qquad (11.10)$$

Equations (11.4), (11.7), (11.8), (11.9), and (11.10) are not model specific and can be used in all other models described below.

Model 2: Metabolic Pathway in Series

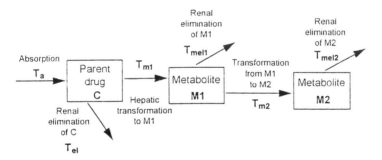

The metabolism of a drug may consist of several metabolic reactions arranged in series as in this model. In the model, the drug is converted to metabolite M1 and then to M2. Therefore, M1 will appear in the blood earlier than M2. The parent drug and both metabolites can be excreted by the kidney.

The mean residence time is simply the sum of input and output times:

$$\text{Mean residence time of C } (\bar{t}_C) = \frac{\text{AUMC}_C}{\text{AUC}_C}$$

$$= \text{Input time } (T_{c,in}) + \text{Output time } (T_{c,out}) = T_a + T_{el,t} \qquad (11.11)$$

$$\text{Mean residence time of M}_1 \; (\bar{t}_{M1}) = \frac{\text{AUMC}_{M1}}{\text{AUC}_{M1}}$$

$$= \text{Input time } (T_{m1,in}) + \text{Output time } (T_{m1,out}) = T_a + T_{el,t} + T_{mel1,t}$$

$$(11.12)$$

$$\text{Mean residence time of M}_2 \; (\bar{t}_{M2}) = \frac{\text{AUMC}_{M2}}{\text{AUC}_{M2}}$$

$$= \text{Input time } (T_{m2,in}) + \text{Output time } (T_{m2,out}) = T_a + T_{el,t} + T_{mel1,t} + T_{mel2}$$

$$(11.13)$$

where $T_{el,t} = 1/(1/T_{el} + 1/T_{m1})$ and $T_{mel1,t} = 1/(1/T_{mel1} + 1/T_{m2})$. The mean residence time can be calculated from the ratio of the area under the first moment curve to the area under the curve. The hepatic clearance time toward metabolite M1 can be estimated from the combined urine recoveries of metabolites M1 and M2.

$$\text{Hepatic clearance time toward M}_1 \left(\frac{T_{m1}}{V_c}\right) = \frac{\text{AUC}_c}{X_{um1} + X_{um2}} \qquad (11.14)$$

The hepatic clearance time toward metabolite M2 can be estimated from the urine recovery of M2:

$$\text{Hepatic clearance time toward M}_2 \left(\frac{T_{m2}}{V_{m1}}\right) = \frac{\text{AUC}_{M1}}{X_{um2}} \qquad (11.15)$$

Model 3: Reversible Metabolism with Elimination from the Parent Drug

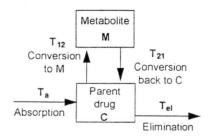

A metabolic reaction can be reversible, as shown in this model, in which only the parent drug is eliminated from the body. When the ratio of the metabolite concentration to the drug concentration is plotted against time, the ratio will reach a constant after a long enough observation time if the metabolism is reversible as in this example. However, the opposite is not true: if the ratio of metabolite to drug reaches a constant with time, the metabolism can be reversible (as in this model) or irreversible (as in Model 1), with an elimination rate of the metabolite faster than the parent drug. In this case, the reversibility of the metabolism can be verified by administering the metabolite and determining if the reverse reaction occurs.

The following are the key pharmacokinetic parameters derived from this model. The mean residence time is the sum of input and output times (see Appendix 1):

$$\text{Mean residence time of C } (\bar{t}_C) = \frac{\text{AUMC}_C}{\text{AUC}_C}$$

$$= \text{Input time } (T_{c,in}) + \text{Output time } (T_{c,out}) = T_a + T_{el} + T_{el}\frac{T_{21}}{T_{12}}$$

$$(11.16)$$

$$\text{Mean residence time of M } (\bar{t}_M) = \frac{\text{AUMC}_M}{\text{AUC}_M}$$

$$= \text{Input time } (T_{m,in}) + \text{Output time } (T_{m,out}) = T_a + T_{el} + T_{12} + T_{el}\frac{T_{21}}{T_{12}}$$

$$(11.17)$$

$$\text{Reconversion time from metabolite } (T_{21}) = \bar{t}_M - \bar{t}_C \quad (11.18)$$

Model 4: Reversible Metabolism with Elimination from the Metabolite

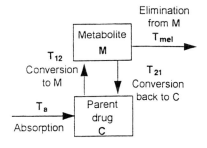

This model is similar to Model 3, but only the metabolite is eliminated from the body; therefore, only the metabolite will appear in the urine. The key pharmacokinetic parameters derived from this model are listed below. The mean residence time is the sum of input and output times (see Appendix 1):

$$\text{Mean residence time of C } (\bar{t}_C) = \frac{\text{AUMC}_C}{\text{AUC}_C}$$

$$= \text{Input time } (T_{c,in}) + \text{Output time } (T_{c,out})$$

$$= -T_{mel,t} + T_a + T_{mel} + T_{12} + T_{mel}\frac{T_{12}}{T_{21}} \qquad (11.19)$$

$$\text{Mean residence time of M } (\bar{t}_M) = \frac{\text{AUMC}_M}{\text{AUC}_M}$$

$$= \text{Input time } (T_{m,in}) + \text{Output time } (T_{m,out}) = T_a + T_{mel} + T_{12} + T_{mel}\frac{T_{12}}{T_{21}}$$

$$(11.20)$$

$$\text{Total elimination time of metabolite } (T_{mel,t}) = \bar{t}_M - \bar{t}_C \quad (11.21)$$

where $T_{mel,t} = 1/(1/T_{mel} + 1/T_{21})$.

Model 5: Reversible Metabolism with Elimination from Both Parent Drug and Metabolite

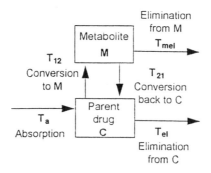

This model is similar to Models 3 and 4, with elimination of both the drug and the metabolite. The mean residence time is the sum of input and output times.

$$\text{Mean residence time of C } (\bar{t}_C) = \frac{\text{AUMC}_C}{\text{AUC}_C}$$

$$= \text{Input time } (T_{c,in}) + \text{Output time } (T_{c,out})$$

$$= -T_{mel,t} + T_a + \frac{(T_{mel,t} + T_{el,t})T_{el}T_{mel}}{T_{el}T_{21} + T_{21}T_{12} + T_{mel}T_{12}} \tag{11.22}$$

$$\text{Mean residence time of M } (\bar{t}_M) = \frac{\text{AUMC}_M}{\text{AUC}_M}$$

$$= \text{Input time } (T_{m,in}) + \text{Output time } (T_{m,out})$$

$$= T_a + \frac{(T_{mel,t} + T_{el,t})T_{el}T_{mel}}{T_{el}T_{21} + T_{21}T_{12} + T_{mel}T_{12}} \tag{11.23}$$

where $T_{el,t} = 1/(1/T_{12} + 1/T_{el})$ and $T_{mel,t} = 1/(1/T_{21} + 1/T_{mel})$. The total elimination time constant of the metabolite can be estimated from the difference in the mean residence time between the drug and the metabolite.

$$\text{Total elimination time of metabolite } (T_{mel,t}) = \bar{t}_M - \bar{t}_C \tag{11.24}$$

The ratio of the area under the metabolite concentration curve to the area under the drug concentration curve is equal to the ratio of the total clearance time of the metabolite to the hepatic clearance time toward the metabolite.

$$\frac{\text{AUC}_M}{\text{AUC}_C} = \frac{T_{mel,t}V_c}{T_{12}V_m} = \frac{\text{Total elimination clearance time of metabolite}}{\text{Formation clearance time toward metabolite}} \tag{11.25}$$

The normalized hepatic elimination time can then be estimated from the following equation:

$$\text{Normalized hepatic elimination time}\left(T_{12}\frac{V_m}{V_c}\right) = T_{mel,t}\frac{\text{AUC}_C}{\text{AUC}_M} \tag{11.26}$$

Model 6: Combination of Irreversible and Reversible Metabolic Pathways

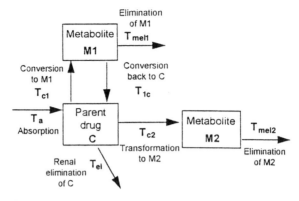

The metabolism of a drug may consist of both reversible and irreversible pathways as in this model. The reversibility can be tested by plotting the ratio of the metabolite to the drug concentrations versus time. If a pathway is reversible, the ratio will reach a constant with a long enough observation time. When a pathway is irreversible, it is also possible for the metabolite to drug ratio to reach a constant with time, provided that the elimination rate of the metabolite is much faster than the elimination of the drug.

The mean residence time is the sum of input and output times

$$\text{Mean residence time of C } (\bar{t}_C) = \frac{\text{AUMC}_C}{\text{AUC}_C}$$

$$= \text{Input time } (T_{c,in}) + \text{Output time } (T_{c,out}) = -T_{mel1,t} + T_a + \frac{1}{\lambda_1} + \frac{1}{\lambda_2}$$

$$(11.27)$$

$$\text{Mean residence time of M}_1 \ (\bar{t}_{M1}) = \frac{\text{AUMC}_{M1}}{\text{AUC}_{M1}}$$

$$= \text{Input time } (T_{m1,in}) + \text{Output time } (T_{m1,out}) = T_a + \frac{1}{\lambda_1} + \frac{1}{\lambda_2} \quad (11.28)$$

$$\text{Mean residence time of M}_2 \ (\bar{t}_{M2}) = \frac{\text{AUMC}_{M2}}{\text{AUC}_{M2}}$$

$$= \text{Input time } (T_{m2,in}) + \text{Output time } (T_{m2,out})$$

$$= -T_{mel1,t} + T_a + \frac{1}{\lambda_1} + \frac{1}{\lambda_2} + T_{mel2} \quad (11.29)$$

where $T_{\text{mel1},t} = 1/(1/T_{\text{mel1}} + 1/T_{\text{lc}})$ and λ_1 and λ_2 are defined by Equations (11.a28) and (11.a29) in Appendix 3. The ratios of the area under the metabolite concentration to the area under the drug concentration are equal to the ratios of the total clearance time of the metabolite to the hepatic clearance time toward the metabolite

$$\frac{\text{AUC}_{M1}}{\text{AUC}_C} = \frac{T_{\text{mel1},t} V_c}{T_{c1} V_{m1}} = \frac{\text{Total elimination clearance time from M}_1}{\text{Formation clearance time toward M}_1} \quad (11.30)$$

$$\frac{\text{AUC}_{M2}}{\text{AUC}_C} = \frac{T_{\text{mel2},t} V_c}{T_{c2} V_{m2}} = \frac{\text{Total elimination clearance time from M}_2}{\text{Formation clearance time toward M}_2} \quad (11.31)$$

The hepatic clearance time toward the metabolites can then be estimated as follows:

$$\text{Normalized hepatic elimination time toward M}_1 \left(T_{c1} \frac{V_{m1}}{V_c}\right)$$

$$= T_{\text{mel1},t} \frac{\text{AUC}_C}{\text{AUC}_{M1}} \quad (11.32)$$

$$\text{Normalized hepatic elimination time toward M}_2 \left(T_{c2} \frac{V_{m2}}{V_c}\right)$$

$$= T_{\text{mel2}} \frac{\text{AUC}_C}{\text{AUC}_{M2}} \quad (11.33)$$

The hepatic elimination times can be estimated from the difference in mean residence time between the metabolites and the drug:

$$\text{Total elimination time of M}_1 \ (T_{\text{mel1},t}) = \bar{t}_{M1} - \bar{t}_C \quad (11.34)$$

$$\text{Total elimination time of M}_2 \ (T_{\text{mel2},t}) = \bar{t}_{M2} - \bar{t}_C \quad (11.35)$$

CASE STUDIES

Case 1: Parallel Metabolic Pathways

The metabolism of a drug may consist of several parallel pathways, such as those metabolites that are produced from the parent drug through different hepatic enzymes [11]. The plasma concentrations of the metabolites depend on the formation and elimination times of the metabolites. Since several metabolic pathways compete for the parent drug, the formation time of a metabolite determines the percentage of the parent drug that will convert to the metabolite. If the renal elimination time of a metabolite is long, the metabolite will accumulate in the body. The urine recovery of a metabolite, on the other hand, depends only on the formation time and not on the elimination time of the metabolite, assuming the metabolite is solely eliminated by the kidney. As long as a metabolite is formed through an irreversible pathway and no further metabolism occurs beyond the metabolite (i.e., the end product of a pathway), the whole amount of the metabolite should be excreted in the urine regardless of the renal elimination time (assuming no bile secretion). The elimination time of a metabolite influences two important aspects of the pharmacokinetics of the metabolite: first, it affects the plasma levels of the metabolite, and second, it determines the lag time between the plasma concentration profiles of the metabolite and its parent drug. The longer the renal elimination time of the metabolite, the greater is the area under the curve and the longer the lag time.

The parallel metabolism can be described by Model 1, and a simulated example of plasma concentration profiles of a drug and its metabolites using the model is shown in Figure 11.1. The parent drug is rapidly absorbed in

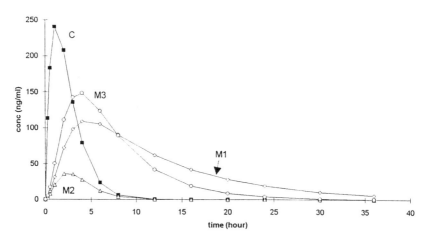

FIGURE 11.1. Simulated plasma concentrations of a drug and its metabolites with parallel metabolic pathways using Model 1. The time constant plot comparing pharmacokinetics of the drug and its metabolites is shown in Figure 11.2. The parameters used in this simulation are $X_0 = 10$ mg, $f^*F = 0.8$, $V_c = 10$ L, $V_{m1} = 10$ L, $V_{m2} = 12$ L, $V_{m3} = 15$ L, $K_a = 0.7$ hr^{-1}, $K_{el} = 0.1$ hr^{-1}, $K_{m1} = 0.2$ hr^{-1}, $K_{mel1} = 0.1$ hr^{-1}, $K_{m2} = 0.2$ hr^{-1}, $K_{mel2} = 0.8$ hr^{-1}, $K_{m3} = 0.5$ hr^{-1}, $K_{mel3} = 0.2$ hr^{-1}.

the intestine after dosing and eliminated mostly through hepatic metabolism. The formation rates of metabolites M1 and M2 are the same, and that of metabolite M3 is faster. Nonrenal elimination of the metabolites is not involved. The rate of renal elimination of metabolite M1 is the slowest among all, that of metabolite M3 the fastest, and that of metabolite M2 intermediate. The plasma concentration of the parent drug reaches a maximum and quickly disappears, indicating fast absorption and elimination rates. The concentration profiles of metabolites M1 and M3 are much broader than that of the parent drug, and the peak concentrations of the two metabolites also appear much later than the parent drug, all indicating longer elimination times of the two metabolites than the parent drug. On the other hand, metabolite M2 seems to have a comparable elimination time as the parent drug. The decay time of the concentration profiles also shows that elimination of M1 and M3 is slower than M2 and the parent drug. Metabolite M3 appears first in the plasma, indicating its faster formation rate than the others.

Since the metabolic pathways are parallel to each other, the hepatic elimination time toward each pathway will determine the timing of appearance of each metabolite in the plasma and the amount excreted of each metabolite in the urine. In addition, the elimination time of each metabolite will affect the accumulation and thus the area under the curve of each metabolite. Therefore, the key time constants in this example are the hepatic elimination time toward the metabolites and the elimination time of the metabolites. The estimated pharmacokinetic parameters for the above example using the time constant analysis are listed in Table 11.1, and the estimated time constants are presented in Figure 11.2. The areas under the curves of metabolites M1 and M3 are much larger than that of M2, indicating large ratios of renal clearance time of the metabolite to the hepatic clearance time $[(T_{mel} V_c)/(T_m V_m)]$ for M1 and M3. Now let us examine the time constant plot (Figure 11.2). The decay time of the parent drug and metabolite M2 exhibits flip-flops; therefore, the decay times are not good estimates of the elimination times in this case. The mean residence times of metabolites M1 and M3 are much longer than that of the parent drug, reflecting that the elimination times of the two metabolites are relatively long and cause the prolonged accumulation of the metabolites. The mean residence time for metabolite M2 is comparable to that of the parent drug, indicating a shorter elimination time of M2 than M1 and M3. The urine recoveries, X_us, of the metabolites are greater than that of the parent drug, indicating that metabolism dominates the elimination of the parent drug. The percentages of the metabolites $X_u\%$ in the total urine recovery reflect the order of magnitude of the metabolic formation times. The hepatic clearance time T_m/V_c toward the metabolites is proportional to the urine recovery data. The renal clear-

TABLE 11.1. The Estimated Pharmacokinetic Parameters Using Time Constant Analysis for the Example Shown in Figure 11.1.

Parameter	C TCA	C Model Value	M1 TCA	M1 Model Value	M2 TCA	M2 Model Value	M3 TCA	M3 Model Value	Equation
T_z (hr)	1.43	1.43 (T_a)	10.0	10.0 (T_{mel1})	1.47	1.43 (T_a)	5.0	5.0 (T_{mel3})	(11.4)
$\bar{t}$ (hr)	2.4	2.4	12.4	12.4	3.7	3.7	7.3	7.4	(11.1, 11.2)
T_{el}/V (hr/L)	1	1	1	1	0.104	0.104	0.333	0.333	(11.7)
T_m/V_c (hr/L)			0.5	0.5	0.5	0.5	0.2	0.2	(11.6)
T_{mel} (hr)			10.0	10.0	1.2	1.25	4.9	5.0	(11.3)
$f*F$	0.81	0.8							(11.10)
AUC (ng·hr/L)	806	800	1604	1600	169	166	1346	1333	
AUC_M/AUC_C			1.99	2.0	0.21	0.21	1.68	1.67	(11.5)
X_u (μg)	806	800	1604	1600	1624	1600	4038	4000	
X_u %	10%	10%	20%	20%	20%	20%	50%	50%	
X_u/D	0.08	0.08	0.16	0.16	0.16	0.16	0.4	0.4	

TCA: Time constant analysis.

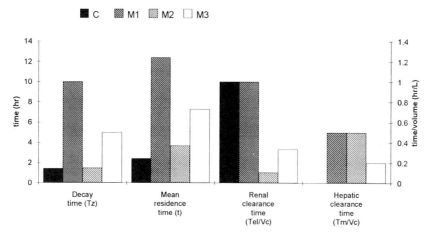

FIGURE 11.2. The time constant plot comparing pharmacokinetics of the drug and its metabolites with parallel metabolic pathways in the examples shown in Figure 11.1. The hepatic clearance time (T_m/V_c) toward the metabolites is shorter for metabolite M3 than for the other two metabolites, producing a greater amount of urinary recovery of M3 than the others. The renal clearance time (T_{el}/V) of metabolite M2 is much shorter than those of the other metabolites, resulting in a small area under the curve and a short mean residence time of M2.

ance time of metabolite M2 is much shorter than those of the other metabolites, resulting in a small area under the curve and a short mean residence time of M2. The lag time between the metabolites and the parent drug can be illustrated by plotting the metabolite concentration against the parent drug concentration (Figure 11.3). The metabolite versus parent plots show hysteresis loops. The longer the lag time between a metabolite and the parent drug, the larger the area within the loop. Since the lag time is controlled solely by the renal elimination time of the metabolites, the hysteresis loop will collapse with a short elimination time. When the hysteresis loop collapses, the slope of the collapsed line will be equal to $T_m V_m / T_{mel} V_c$, and there will be a linear relationship between the metabolite and parent drug concentrations.

Case 2: Metabolic Reactions in Series

The metabolic pathway of a drug may consist of several reactions in series [5]. In this case, an accumulation will occur to the metabolite of which the elimination is the rate limiting step in the pathway. The plasma levels of the metabolites depend on two factors: first, the formation to elimination ratio and, second, the volume of distribution. If the volume of distribution of a

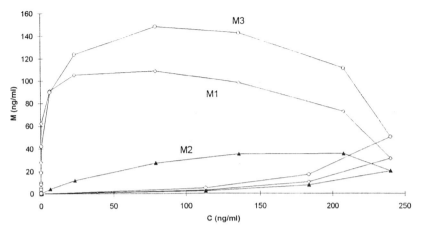

FIGURE 11.3. The concentrations of the metabolites versus the parent drug of the example in Figure 11.1.

metabolite is small compared with its precursors, then once the metabolite is formed, it will be displaced from the tissue to the blood and exhibit a high concentration relative to the precursors. The mean residence time of a later metabolite is always longer than an earlier metabolite along a pathway, if there is no significant first pass effect. Therefore, the sequence of formation of the metabolites in a serial pathway can be determined from the mean residence time. The urine recovery of a metabolite depends not only on the formation rate of the metabolite itself but also on the formation rate of its precursors. The pharmacokinetics of a drug with a serial metabolic pathway can be described by Model 2. Simulated plasma concentration profiles using the model are shown in Figure 11.4. In this example, the parent drug has fast absorption and elimination rates. The elimination rates of the two metabolites are slower than that of the parent drug. The peak concentrations of the metabolites appear in a sequence corresponding to the position of the metabolites in the pathway. The area under the curve of metabolite M2 is much greater than that of metabolite M1, indicating either a large formation to elimination ratio or a small volume of distribution of M2. The radiolabeled drug is given in this case to account for all metabolites. The total radioactivity in the plasma shows double peaks because of the pronounced profile of metabolite M2 (Figure 11.5). The double peaks of radioactivity occur because of the fact that the parent drug is rapidly absorbed and eliminated, that a significant lag time exists between the metabolite and the parent drug, and that the volume of distribution of the metabolite is much smaller than that of the parent drug.

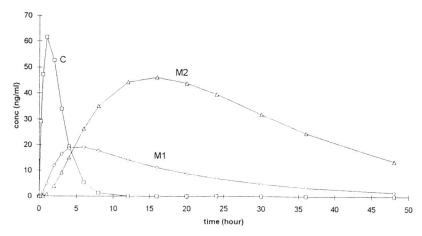

FIGURE 11.4. Simulated plasma concentrations of a drug and its metabolites with metabolic pathways in series using Model 2. The time constant plot comparing the pharmacokinetics of the drug and its metabolites is shown in Figure 11.6. The parameters used in this simulation are $X_0 = 10$ mg, $f^*F = 0.8$, $V_c = 50$ L, $V_{m1} = 40$ L, $V_{m2} = 5$ L, $K_a = 0.9$ hr^{-1}, $K_{el} = 0.7$ hr^{-1}, $K_{m1} = 0.1$ hr^{-1}, $K_{mel1} = 0.01$ hr^{-1}, $K_{m2} = 0.05$ hr^{-1}, $K_{mel2} = 0.1$ hr^{-1}.

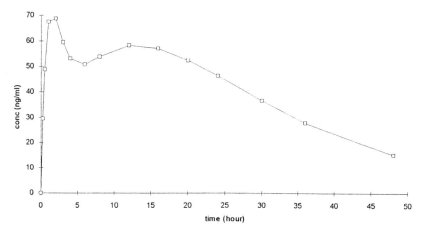

FIGURE 11.5. The total concentration of the parent and metabolites in the example in Figure 11.3 measured by radioactivity.

253

TABLE 11.2. The Estimated Pharmacokinetic Parameters Using Time Constant Analysis for the Example Shown in Figure 11.4.

Parameter	C		M1		M2		Equation
	TCA	Model Value	TCA	Model Value	TCA	Model Value	
T_z (hr)	1.25	1.25 $(T_{el,t})$	16.67	16.67 $(T_{mel1,t})$	16.67	16.67 $(T_{mel1,t})$	(11.4)
$\bar{t}$ (hr)	2.4	2.4	19	19	32	29	(11.11, 11.13)
T_{el}/V_c (hr/L)	0.029	0.029	2.5	2.5	2.0	2.0	(11.7)
T_m/V_c (hr/L)			0.19	0.2	0.45	0.5	(11.14, 11.15)
$f*F$	0.81	0.8					(11.10)
AUC (ng·hr/L)	201	200	418	416	1749	1666	
X_u (µg)	7057	7000	167	166	874	833	
X_u%	87%	88%	2%	2%	10%	10%	
X_u/X_0	0.71	0.7	0.017	0.017	0.087	0.083	

TCA: Time constant analysis.

When metabolites are pharmacologically active or produce a toxic effect, it is important to determine their mean residence time or decay time. In a metabolic pathway with metabolites produced in series, the metabolites after a rate limiting step will have longer decay times than those of the metabolites before the rate limiting step. Therefore, the key time constant in this example is the total elimination time of the metabolites to determine the rate limiting step. The estimated pharmacokinetic parameters of the above example using the time constant analysis are listed in Table 11.2, and the estimated time constants are presented in Figure 11.6. The area under the curve of metabolite M2 is much greater than those of metabolite M1 and the parent drug. Based solely on the size of the area under the curve of M2, an erroneous conclusion may be made that the hepatic elimination toward metabolite M2 dominates the elimination of the parent drug, while the fact is that the large area under the curve is due to a long renal elimination time of M2.

Now let us examine the time constant plot (Figure 11.6). The decay times of the two metabolites are longer than that of the parent drug. The mean residence time is longer for the metabolites that appear later in the pathway. The difference in the mean residence between metabolite M1 and the parent drug corresponds to the elimination time of M1. Similarly, the difference in the mean residence between metabolites M1 and M2 corresponds to the elimination time of M2. The urine data indicate that the metabolism only

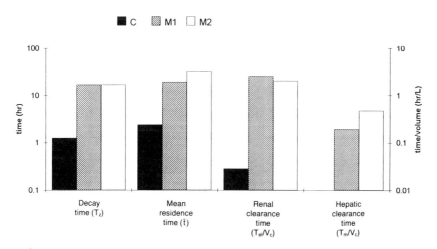

FIGURE 11.6. The time constant plot comparing the pharmacokinetics of the drug and its metabolites with metabolic pathways in series in the examples shown in Figure 11.4. The renal clearance time (T_{el}/V) of the parent drug is much shorter than the hepatic clearance time (T_m/V) toward M1, which explains the high recovery of the parent drug in the urine.

occurs to a small extent. The renal clearance time is much shorter than the hepatic clearance time of the parent drug, which explains the high recovery of the parent drug in the urine. The renal clearance times are similar between the two metabolites. The hepatic clearance time toward M1 is shorter than that toward M2; however, this is not reflected proportionally by the area under the curve because the elimination time (renal + hepatic) of M1 is also shorter than the elimination time (renal) of M2. To summarize, the rate limiting step of the metabolite pathway is at the elimination of metabolite M1, since the decay times of M1 and M2 are similar and longer than that of the parent drug. As a result, the mean residence time of the two metabolites is much longer than that of the parent drug.

Case 3: Reversible Metabolic Reactions

The metabolic reactions can be reversible. A quasi-equilibrium can be established between a metabolite and the parent drug, and the ratio between the two becomes constant with time. Model 5 describes a reversible metabolic pathway. Simulated plasma concentrations of two different drugs and their metabolites using the model are shown in Figure 11.7. In the two ex-

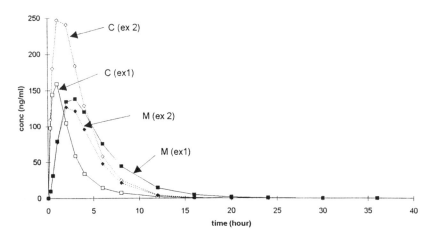

FIGURE 11.7. Simulated plasma concentrations of two drugs and their metabolites with reversible metabolism and elimination from both the drug and metabolite using Model 5. The elimination rate of the parent drug is faster than that of the metabolite in example 1, while the elimination rate of the metabolite is faster than that of the parent drug in example 2. The time constant plot comparing the two examples is shown in Figure 11.9. The parameters used in this simulation are example 1: $X_0 = 10$ mg, $f^*F = 0.8$, $V_c = 15$ L, $V_m = 10$ L, $K_a = 1$ hr^{-1}, $K_{el} = 1$ hr^{-1}, $K_{12} = 0.5$ hr^{-1}, $K_{21} = 0.3$ hr^{-1}, $K_{mel} = 0.1$ hr^{-1}; example 2: $X_0 = 10$ mg, $f^*F = 0.8$, $V_c = 15$ L, $V_m = 10$ L, $K_a = 1$ hr^{-1}, $K_{el} = 0.1$ hr^{-1}, $K_{12} = 0.5$ hr^{-1}, $K_{21} = 0.3$ hr^{-1}, $K_{mel} = 1$ hr^{-1}.

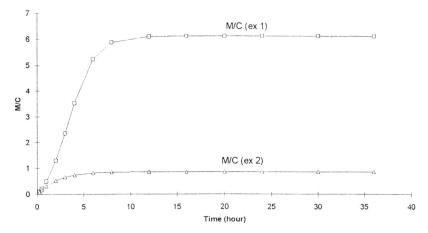

FIGURE 11.8. The ratio of metabolite to parent drug concentrations of both drugs in Figure 11.5 as functions of time.

amples, the rate constants of the reversible reactions are comparable in both directions. The elimination rate of the parent drug is faster than that of the metabolite in example 1, while the elimination rate of the metabolite is faster than that of the parent drug in example 2. The parent drug appears in the blood earlier than the metabolite in both examples, corresponding to the sequence in the pathway. The ratios of metabolite to the parent concentration reach constant levels after 8 hours for both drugs, when the quasi-equilibrium between the drugs and their metabolites is established (Figure 11.8). If the time constants of the reversible reactions are much shorter than any other time constant in the model, then the ratio of the metabolite concentration to the parent drug concentration will be $(T_{21} V_c)/(T_{12} V_m)$. In this example, however, this is not the case, so the ratio does not equal $(T_{21} V_c)/(T_{12} V_m)$ ($= 2.5$ in both examples).

The accumulation of the metabolite depends on the total elimination time of the metabolite, the renal elimination time of the drug, and the distribution time, which are then the key time constants in this example. The estimated pharmacokinetic parameters of the above examples using the time constant analysis are listed in Table 11.3, and the estimated time constants are presented in Figure 11.9. The ratio of the area under the curve of the metabolite to that of the parent drug reflects the ratio of $(T_{mel,t} V_1)/(T_{12} V_2)$ ($= 1.88$ and 0.58 in examples 1 and 2, respectively).

Now let us examine the time constant plot (Figure 11.9). The mean residence time of the metabolite is longer than that of the parent drug in both examples since the parent drugs appear in the blood earlier than the metabolites. The mean residence time of the parent drug and metabolite does not

TABLE 11.3. The Estimated Pharmacokinetic Parameters Using Time Constant Analysis for the Example Shown in Figure 11.7.

Parameter	C (ex 1) TCA	C (ex 1) Model Value	M (ex 1) TCA	M (ex 1) Model Value	C (ex 2) TCA	C (ex 2) Model Value	M (ex 2) TCA	M (ex 2) Model Value	Equation
T_z (hr)	3.57	3.57	3.57	3.57	2.33	2.33	2.33	2.33	(11.4)
$\bar{t}$ (hr)	2.7	2.7	5.2	5.2	3.3	3.2	4.0	4.0	
$T_{mel,r}$ (hr)			2.5	2.5			0.77	0.77	(11.22, 11.23)
$T_{el}V$ (hr)	0.067	0.067	1	1	0.67	0.67	0.1	0.1	(11.7)
X_u (μg)	7171	7111	899	888	1669	1650	6436	6349	(11.24)
X_u/D	0.71	0.71	0.09	0.09	0.17	0.17	0.64	0.64	
AUC (ng·hr/L)	478	474	899	888	1113	1100	643	634	
$f*F$	0.8	0.8			0.8	0.8			(11.10)

TCA: Time constant analysis.

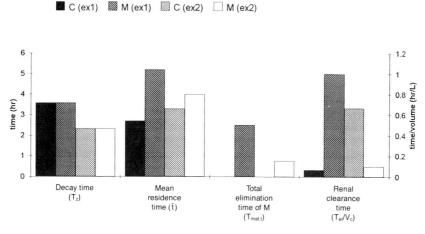

FIGURE 11.9. The time constant plot comparing the two drugs with reversible metabolic pathways and eliminations from both the drug and the metabolite in the examples in Figure 11.9. The mean residence time ($\bar{t}$) of the parent drug and metabolite does not differ much between the examples, in spite of tenfold difference in the renal clearance times (T_{el}/V).

differ much between the examples, in spite of a tenfold difference in the renal clearance times. This is because the renal excretion does not dominate the elimination of the drug in either example, and a difference in the renal elimination time does not significantly influence the mean residence time.

Case 4: Polymorphism

Polymorphism of metabolism occurs when the activity of a hepatic enzyme in one subpopulation is different from that of another subpopulation. This results in a bimodal distribution of metabolite levels in the population. An example is illustrated here using Model 6, and simulated plasma concentration profiles of a drug and its metabolites in two subjects with different metabolic rates are shown in Figure 11.10. In this example, the only difference in the pharmacokinetic parameters between the two subjects is the formation rate of metabolite M2. The time to reach the maximum concentration of the parent drug does not differ much between the two subjects, indicating that the formation of metabolite M2 does not dominate the elimination of the parent drug. Both metabolites appear later in the blood than does the parent drug corresponding to the sequence in the metabolic pathways. The ratio of the maximum concentrations of M1 to that of M2 is smaller in subject 2 than in subject 1, indicating a difference in metabolic rates between the two subjects. The ratios of metabolite M1 to the parent drug reach equilibria after 8 hours, while the ratio of metabolite M2 to the

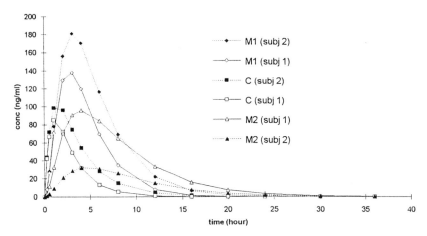

FIGURE 11.10. Simulated plasma concentrations of a drug and its metabolites in two subjects with polymorphism using Model 6. The time constant plot comparing the pharmacokinetics in the two subjects with polymorphism is shown in Figure 11.12. The parameters used in this simulation are subj 1: $X_0 = 10$ mg, $f^*F = 0.8$, $V_c = 30$ L, $V_{m1} = 10$ L, $V_{m2} = 20$ L, $K_a = 0.8$ hr^{-1}, $K_{el} = 0.2$ hr^{-1}, $K_{c1} = 0.5$ hr^{-1}, $K_{1c} = 0.3$ hr^{-1}, $K_{mel1} = 0.3$ hr^{-1}, $K_{c2} = 0.4$ hr^{-1}, $K_{mel2} = 0.2$ hr^{-1}; subj 2: $X_0 = 10$ mg, $f^*F = 0.8$, $V_c = 30$ L, $V_{m1} = 10$ L., $V_{m2} = 20$ L, $K_a = 0.8$ hr^{-1}, $K_{el} = 0.2$ hr^{-1}, $K_{c1} = 0.5$ hr^{-1}, $K_{1c} = 0.3$ hr^{-1}, $K_{mel1} = 0.3$ hr^{-1}, $K_{c2} = 0.1$ hr^{-1}, $K_{mel2} = 0.2$ hr^{-1}.

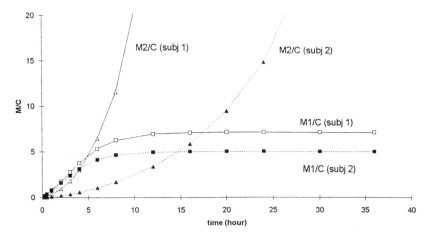

FIGURE 11.11. The ratios of metabolites M1 and M2 to the parent drug in the example shown in Figure 11.7.

TABLE 11.4. The Estimated Pharmacokinetic Parameters Using Time Constant Analysis for the Example Shown in Figure 11.10.

Parameter	C TCA	C Model Value	M1 TCA	M1 Model Value	M2 TCA	M2 Model Value	Equation
Subject 1							
T_z (hr)	2.56	2.56 (T_{z1})	2.56	2.56 (T_{z1})	5.0	5.0 (T_{mel2})	(11.4)
$\bar{t}$ (hr)	2.9	2.9	4.6	4.6	7.9	7.9	(11.27–11.29)
T_{el}/V_c (hr/L)	0.167	0.167	0.333	0.333	0.5	0.5	(11.7)
T_m/V_c (hr/L)					0.083	0.083	(11.32, 11.33)
$f*F$	0.81	0.8					
AUC (ng·hr/L)	316	313	796	784	948	941	(11.10)
X_u (μg)	1900	1882	2388	2352	3794	3764	
X_u/D	0.19	0.19	0.24	0.24	0.38	0.38	
Subject 2							
T_z (hr)	3.33	3.33 (T_{z1})	3.33	3.33 (T_{z1})	5.0	5.0 (T_{mel2})	(11.4)
$\bar{t}$ (hr)	3.8	3.8	5.5	5.5	8.8	8.8	(11.7)
T_{el}/V_c (hr/L)	0.167	0.167	0.333	0.333	0.5	0.5	(11.32, 11.33)
T_m/V_c (hr/L)					0.333	0.333	(11.27–11.29)
$f*F$	0.81	0.8					
AUC (ng·hr/L)	489	484	1228	1212	365	363	(11.10)
X_u (μg)	2939	2909	3686	3636	1463	1454	
X_u/D	0.29	0.29	0.37	0.36	0.15	0.15	

TCA: Time constant analysis.

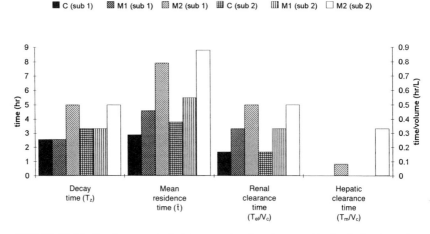

FIGURE 11.12. The time constant plot comparing the pharmacokinetics in the two subjects with polymorphism in the examples shown in Figure 11.10. The hepatic clearance time (T_m/V) toward metabolite M2 is longer in subject 1 than in subject 2, suggesting polymorphism.

parent drug increases continuously (Figure 11.11). This is consistent with the nature of the formation of the two metabolites, which is reversible for M1 and irreversible for M2.

To determine a difference in metabolic rates between the two subjects, the key time constants are the hepatic elimination times toward the metabolites. The estimated pharmacokinetic parameters in Model 6 for the above example using the time constant analysis are listed in Table 11.4, and the estimated time constants are presented in Figure 11.12. The ratio of area under the curve of metabolite M2 to M1 is greater in subject 1 than in subject 2, which is consistent with the longer hepatic clearance time toward metabolite M2 in subject 1 than in subject 2. As shown in the time constant plot (Figure 11.12), the mean residence time of the parent drug is only slightly longer in subject 2 than in subject 1, indicating the hepatic clearance toward metabolite M2 does not dominate the elimination of the parent drug. The urine recovery of M2 is much higher in subject 2 than in subject 1, also reflecting that the formation of M2 is faster in subject 2.

EXAMPLES

Example 1: Irreversible Metabolic Reaction

The pharmacokinetics of triflusal and its main metabolite HTB were

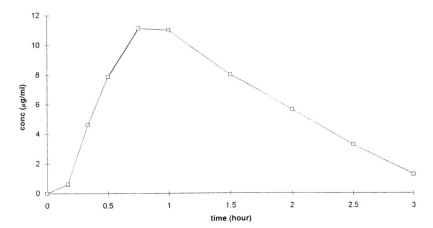

FIGURE 11.13. Mean concentration profiles of triflusal following an oral administration of 900 mg triflusal in eight healthy subjects. (Reproduced with permission from Reference [9].) The time constant plot illustrating the pharmacokinetics of triflusal is shown in Figure 11.15.

studied in eight healthy subjects following an oral administration of 900 mg triflusal [9]. The mean plasma concentration profiles of triflusal and HTB following the dose are shown in Figures 11.13 and 11.14. Triflusal is rapidly absorbed and its plasma concentration reaches a maximum within an hour. The metabolite HTB appears in the blood immediately following the administration, indicating a fast metabolic rate. The metabolite stays in the blood for a much longer time than triflusal.

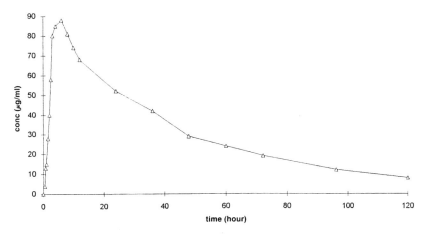

FIGURE 11.14. Mean concentration profiles of HTB following an oral administration of 900 mg triflusal in eight healthy subjects. (Reproduced with permission from Reference [9].)

TABLE 11.5. The Estimated Pharmacokinetic Parameters of
Triflusal Using Model 1.

Parameter*	Triflusal	HTB	Equation
T_z (hr)	0.75	47.6	(11.4)
$\bar{t}$ (hr)	1.4	50.1	(11.1, 11.2)
T_{mel} (hr)		47.6	(11.3)
$T_m*/V_m/V_c$ (hr)	0.233		(11.6)
$T_{el,t}*f*F/V$ (hr/L)	0.022		(11.8)
AUC (μg·hr/ml)	20.3	4227.8	
AUC_M/AUC_C		208.6	(11.5)
$V_z/f/F$ (L)	34.0		(11.9)

*Parameters estimated from the mean concentration profiles or the mean reported values.

The decay time of the triflusal and HTB is clearly different; therefore, no apparent equilibrium is established between triflusal and its metabolite. The key time constant is the elimination time of the metabolite for the assessment of the accumulation of the metabolite in the body and the hepatic elimination time to determine the extent of metabolism. The pharmacokinetic parameters of triflusal are estimated using Model 1 since there is no indication of reversible metabolism. The estimated parameters are listed in Table 11.5, and the estimated time constants are presented in Figure 11.15.

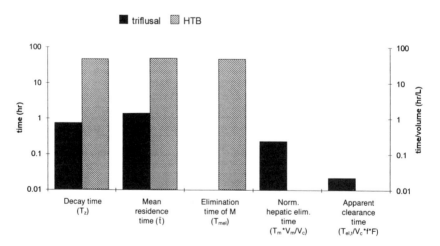

FIGURE 11.15. The time constant plot illustrating the pharmacokinetics of triflusal using Model 1 (note the logarithmic scale). The decay time (T_z) of the concentration curves indicates that the elimination of HTB is much slower than triflusal, resulting in a much longer mean residence time ($\bar{t}$) of HTB than triflusal. The hepatic clearance time (T_m*V_m/V_c) is relatively short, resulting in a rapid appearance of the metabolite in the blood.

Now let us examine the time constant plot (Figure 11.15). The decay time of the concentration curves indicates that the elimination of HTB is much slower than triflusal, resulting in a much longer mean residence time of HTB than triflusal. The estimated elimination time of HTB (T_{mel}) is equal to its decay time (T_z). The hepatic clearance time (T_m*V_m/V_c) is relatively short, resulting in a rapid appearance of the metabolite in the blood. The large ratio of the area under the HTB concentration curve to the area under the triflusal concentration curve is due to the long renal clearance time of the metabolite and the short hepatic clearance time toward the metabolite [Equation (11.5)]. To summarize, triflusal exhibits a long-lasting anti-aggregative effect [9], which may be due to the long elimination time of HTB (which is also pharmacologically active), causing the accumulation of the metabolite.

Example 2: Reversible Metabolic Reaction

The pharmacokinetics of flumazenil and its metabolite were studied in nine healthy subjects following the intravenous administration of radiolabeled flumazenil [2]. The mean plasma concentrations of flumazenil and the metabolite following the intravenous dose are shown in Figure 11.16. There is a 15-minute lag time before the metabolite concentration reaches a maximum. After 15 minutes postdose, the concentration profile of flumazenil seems to be parallel to that of its metabolite. The ratio of the metabolite concentration to flumazenil concentration reaches a constant level after

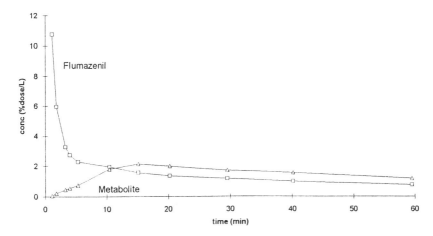

FIGURE 11.16. Mean concentration profiles of flumazenil and its metabolite following an intravenous administration of radiolabeled flumazenil in nine healthy subjects. (Reproduced with permission from Reference [2].) The time constant plot comparing the pharmacokinetics of the drug and metabolite is shown in Figure 11.18.

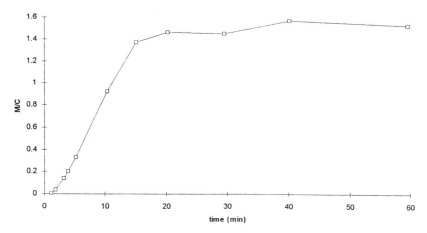

FIGURE 11.17. The ratio of metabolite to flumazenil as a function of time.

20 minutes (Figure 11.17). This can be due to a reversible metabolism between flumazenil and its metabolite (Model 5) or a fast elimination rate of the metabolite so that the elimination of flumazenil dominates the terminal slope of the metabolite (Model 1). Therefore, the elimination time constant of the metabolite must be estimated to determine whether Model 1 or 6 applies to the pharmacokinetics of flumazenil.

The mean residence time and decay time of flumazenil and its metabolite are first estimated independently of a model, and the elimination time constant of the metabolite is estimated from the difference in the mean residence time between the metabolite and the drug. The elimination time constant of the metabolite is one-third of the decay time of flumazenil. Therefore, one cannot rule out the possibility that the metabolism is irreversible and the elimination time of flumazenil dominates the decay time of the metabolite. Further studies of the metabolic pathway, such as administering the metabolite to determine if the reverse pathway exists, must be conducted to verify the reversibility of the metabolism. For now, a reversible metabolism is assumed (Model 5) for the purpose of illustration. The estimated pharmacokinetic parameters are listed in Table 11.6, and the estimated time constants are presented in Figure 11.18.

Now let us examine the time constant plot (Figure 11.18). The hepatic elimination time $(T_{12}*V_m/V_c)$ and total elimination time of the metabolite $(T_{mel,t})$ are relatively short (within minutes), reflected also by the short decay time of the drug and the metabolite $(T_z s)$. The concentration profile of flumazenil clearly shows biexponential phases (Figure 11.16), which may be explained either by the reversible metabolism or a reversible tissue distribution. The first decay time of the biexponential phase is about 2.2

TABLE 11.6. The Estimated Pharmacokinetic Parameters of Flumazenil Using Model 5.

Parameter*	C	M	Equation
T_z (min)	62.5	79.9	(11.4)
$\bar{t}$ (min)	58.6	83.9	(11.22, 11.23)
$T_{mel,t}$ (min)		25.0	(11.24)
$T_{12}*V_m/V_c$ (min)	18.5		(11.26)
$T_{el,t}/V_c$ (min/L)	1.33		(11.8)
V_z (L)	46.9		(11.9)
AUC (min/L)	133.6	180.8	
AUC_M/AUC_C		1.35	(11.25)

minutes, which does not correspond to the hepatic elimination time (T_{12}) or the total elimination time $(T_{el,t})$, assuming the values of both V_m and V_c are equal to V_z. Therefore, it is likely that a distribution occurs in the first 5 minutes after the intravenous administration. The short distribution phase may explain the rapid clinical effects of flumazenil and easy intracerebral penetration observed in earlier studies [2].

Example 3: Metabolic Reactions in Series

The pharmacokinetics of nicomorphine and its metabolites were studied in eight patients scheduled for minor lower abdominal surgery after an in-

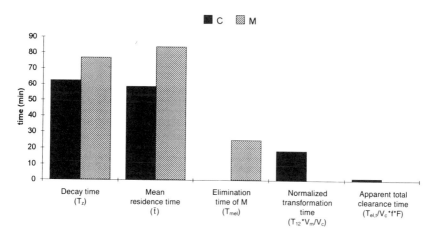

FIGURE 11.18. The time constant plot comparing the pharmacokinetics of flumazenil and its metabolite using Model 6. The hepatic elimination time $(T_{12}*V_m/V_c)$ and total elimination time of the metabolite $(T_{mel,t})$ are relatively short (within minutes), reflected also by the short decay time of the drug and the metabolite (T_zs).

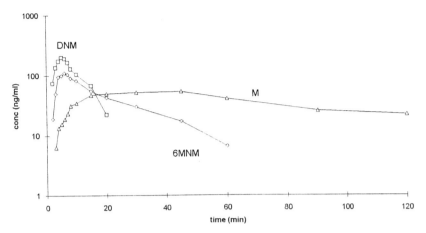

FIGURE 11.19. Mean plasma concentration profiles of nicomorphine (DNM) and its metabolites 6 MNM and M in eight patients after intramuscular injection of 20 mg nicomorphine. (Reproduced from Reference [5] with permission.) The time constant plot comparing the pharmacokinetics of the drug and its metabolite is shown in Figure 11.20.

tramuscular injection of 20 mg nicomorphine [5]. The mean plasma concentration profiles of nicomorphine (DNM) and its metabolites 6MNM and M are shown in Figure 11.19. Nicomorphine is absorbed rapidly into the bloodstream following the injection. One of the metabolites 6MNM, appears in the blood immediately after nicomorphine. However, the concentration of the other metabolite M lags consistently after nicomorphine.

It is assumed that one nicotinoyl group is removed from nicomorphine at a time along the metabolic pathway. Therefore, the two metabolites 6MNM and M appear in the pathway in series. The key time constants in this example are the elimination time of DNM, 6MNM, and M to determine the rate limiting step in the serial metabolic pathway. The pharmacokinetic parameters of nicomorphine and its metabolites are estimated using Model 2 and are listed in Table 11.7, and the estimated time constants are presented in Figure 11.20.

Now let us examine the time constant plot (Figure 11.20). The decay time of M is longer than that of 6MNM, indicating a slower elimination rate of M than of 6MNM. Similarly, the decay time of 6MNM is longer than that of the parent drug, indicating the elimination of the metabolite is slower than that of nicomorphine. The elimination time constant of M ($T_{mel,t}$) is 8.4 times longer than that of 6MNM. Therefore, the elimination of M is the rate limiting step in the pathway, and metabolite M accumulates for a longer time than do 6MNM and DNM. To summarize, the long elimination time of metabolites 6MNM and M results in the accumulation of these metabo-

TABLE 11.7. The Estimated Pharmacokinetic Parameters of
Nicomorphine Using Model 2.

Parameter*	DNM	6 MNM	M	Equation
T_z (min)	10.1	23.3	60.1	(11.4)
$\bar{t}$ (min)	12	23	115	(11.11–11.13)
$T_{mel,t}$ (min)		11.0	92.0	(11.11–11.13)
$T_{m1}*V_{m1}/V_c$ or		8.62	22.38	$AUC_{M1}/AUC_{M2}*T_{mel2,t}$ or
$T_{m2}*V_{m2}/V_{m1}$ (min)				$AUC_C/AUC_{M1}*T_{mel1,t}$
AUC (nmol·hr/L)	80	102	419	
AUC_{M1}/AUC_C or				
AUC_{M2}/AUC_{M1}		1.28	4.11	

*Parameters estimated from the mean concentration profiles or the mean reported values.

lites and may be responsible for the long-lasting pain relief after an intramuscular administration of nicomorphine [5].

Example 4: Parallel Metabolic Pathways

Pharmacokinetics of diltiazem and its metabolites were studied in twenty
healthy subjects after a single oral dose of 90 mg diltiazem [11]. The mean
plasma concentration profiles of diltiazem and its three metabolites are

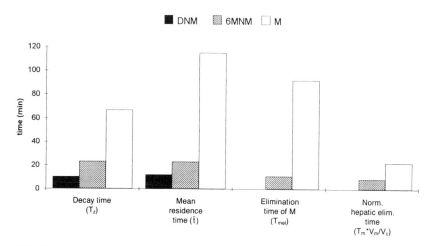

FIGURE 11.20. The time constant plot comparing the pharmacokinetics of nicomorphine
and its metabolite using Model 1. The elimination time constant of M (T_{mel}) is 8.4 times
longer than that of 6 MNM. Therefore, the elimination of M is the rate limiting step in the pathway, and metabolite M accumulates for a longer time than do 6 MNM and DNM.

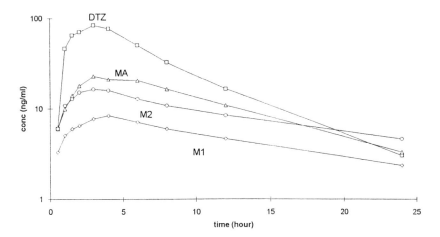

FIGURE 11.21. Mean plasma concentration profiles of diltiazem and its three metabolites M1, MA, and M2, in twenty healthy subjects following a single oral dose of 90 mg diltiazem. (Reproduced from Reference [11] with permission.) The time constant plot comparing the pharmacokinetics of the drug and its metabolites is shown in Figure 11.22.

shown in Figure 11.21. Diltiazem appears first in the blood, followed by MA, M2, and M1.

Metabolites M1 and MA are formed in parallel from diltiazem, and M2 is formed from both M1 and MA [11]. The key time constants in this example are the hepatic elimination time toward metabolites to assess the amount of each metabolite produced and the elimination time of the metabolites to evaluate possible accumulation. The pharmacokinetic parameters of diltiazem and the metabolites are estimated using Model 1 and listed in Table 11.8, and the estimated time constants are presented in Figure 11.22.

Now let us examine the time constant plot (Figure 11.22). The elimina-

TABLE 11.8. The Estimated Pharmacokinetic Parameters of Diltiazem Using Model 1.

Parameter*	DTZ	M1	MA	M2	Equation
T_z (hr)	5.98	15.38	9.62	16.13	(11.4)
$\bar{t}$ (hr)	13.5	23.9	18.7	24.2	(11.1, 11.2)
T_{mel} (hr)		10.31	5.24	10.75	(11.3)
$T_m * V_m / V_c$ (hr)		47.62	11.63		(11.6)
AUC_M / AUC_C		0.22	0.46	0.43	(11.5)
AUC (ng·hr/L)	682.5	151.8	314.7	295.8	

*Parameters estimated from the mean concentration profiles or the mean reported values.

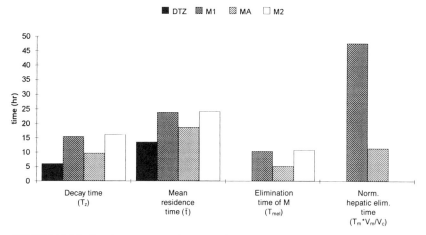

FIGURE 11.22. The time constant plot comparing the pharmacokinetics of diltiazem and its metabolites using Model 1. The hepatic elimination time ($T_m{}^* V_m / V_c$) toward MA is shorter than that of M1, which corresponds to the order of appearance of these metabolites in the blood.

tion time of M2 is estimated, assuming it is formed through a third pathway parallel to those of M1 and MA. By this assumption, the value of T_{mel} of M2 is overestimated. The decay time of all metabolites is longer than that of diltiazem, indicating that all metabolites have slower elimination rates than the parent drug. The elimination time of M1 and M2 is longer than that of MA. The hepatic elimination time toward MA is shorter than that of M1, which corresponds to the order of appearance of these metabolites in the blood. To summarize, the decay time and mean residence time of M1 and M2 are considerably longer than those of DTZ and MA; therefore, under chronic administration, M1 and M2 may accumulate more in the body than DTZ and MA, as suggested in Reference [11].

REFERENCES

1. Carrillo J. A. and Benitez J., "Caffeine metabolism in a healthy Spanish population: Nacetylator phenotype and oxidation pathways," *Clinical Pharmacology & Therapeutics,* 1994; 55(3):293–304.

2. Debruyne D., Abadie P., Barre L., Albessard F., Moulin M., Zarifian E., and Baron J. C., "Plasma pharmacokinetics and metabolism of benzodiazepine antagonist [11C] Ro 15-1788 (flumazenil) in baboon and human during positron emission tomography studies," *European Journal of Drug Metabolism and Pharmacokinetics,* 1991; 16(2):141–152.

3. Gschwind H. P., Schutz H., Wigger N., and Bentley P., "Absorption and disposition of ^{14}C-labelled oxiracetam in rat, dog and man," *European Journal of Drug Metabolism and Pharmacokinetics*, 1992; 17(1):67–82.

4. Kelloway J. S., Awni W. M., Lin C. C., Lim J., Affrime M. B., Keane W. F., Matzke G. R., and Halstenson C. E., "Pharmacokinetics of ceftibuten-*cis* and its *trans* metabolite in healthy volunteers and in patients with chronic renal insufficiency," *Antimicrobial Agents and Chemotherapy*, Nov. 1991; 2267–2274.

5. Koopman-Kimenai P. M., Vree T. B., Booij L. H. D. J., Dirksen R., and Nijhuis G. M. M., "Pharmacokinetics of intramuscular nicomorphine and its metabolites in man," *Eur. J. Clin. Pharmacol.*, 1991; 41:375–378.

6. Leroy A., Fillastre J. P., Borsa-Lebas F., Etienne I., and Humbert G., "Pharmacokinetics of meropenem (ICI 194,660) and its metabolite (ICI 213,689) in healthy subjects and in patients with renal impairment," *Antimicrobial Agents and Chemotherapy*, Dec. 1992; 2794–2798.

7. Ljungberg B. and Nilsson-Ehle I., "Pharmacokinetics of meropenem and its metabolite in young and elderly healthy man," *Antimicrobial Agents and Chemotherapy*, July 1992; 1437–1440.

8. Marquer C., Trouvin J. H., Lacolle J. Y., Dupont Ch., and Jacquot C., "Pharmacokinetics of a prodrug thymoxamine: Dose-dependence of the metabolite ratio in healthy subjects," *European Journal of Drug Metabolism and Pharmacokinetics*, 1991; 16(3):183–188.

9. Ramis J., Mis R., Forn J., Torrent J., Gorina E., and Jane F. "Pharmacokinetics of triflusal and its main metabolite HTB in healthy subjects following a single oral dose," *European Journal of Drug Metabolism and Pharmacokinetics*, 1991; 16(4):269–273.

10. Schaefer H. G., Beermann D., Horstmann R., Wargenau M., Heibel B. A., and Kuhlmann J., "Effect of food on the pharmacokinetics of the active metabolite of the prodrug repirinast," *Journal of Pharmaceutical Sciences*, 1993; 82(1):107–109.

11. Yeung P. F. K., Prescott C., Haddad C., Montague T. J., McGregor C., Quilliam M. A., Xei M., Li R., Farmer P., and Klassen G. A., "Pharmacokinetics and metabolism of diltiazem in healthy males and females following a single oral dose," *European Journal of Drug Metabolism and Pharmacokinetics*, 1993; 18(2):199–206.

12. Zylber-Katz E., Granit L., and Levy M., "Formation and excretion of dipyrone metabolism in man," *Eur. J. Clin. Pharmacol.*, 1992; 42:187–191.

13. Krause W. and Kuhne G., "Biotransformation of the antidepressant D,L-rolipram. II. Metabolite patterns in man, rat, rabbit, rhesus and cynomolgus monkey," *Xenobiotica*, 1993; 23(11):1277–1288.

14. Harvey D. J., Samara E., and Mechoulam R., "Urinary metabolites of cannabidiol in dog, rat and man and their identification by gas chromatography-mass spectrometry," *J. Chromatogr.*, 1991; 562(1–2):299–322.

15. Schroeder N. J., Trafford D. J., Cunningham J., Jones G., and Makin H. L., "In vivo dihydrotachysterol2 metabolism in normal man: 1 alpha- and 1 beta-hydroxylation of 25-hydroxydihydrotachysterol2 and effects on plasma parathyroid hormone and 1 alpha,25-dyhydroxyvitamin D3 concentrations," *J. Clin. Endocrinol Metab.*, 1994; 78(6): 1481–1487.

Relationship between Pharmacokinetics and Pharmacodynamics

INTRODUCTION

The relationship between the drug plasma concentration and the pharmacological effect can be determined in a pharmacokinetic/pharmacodynamic study. The concentration/effect correlation can be a direct or indirect relationship. In a direct relationship, the pharmacological effect is an immediate response to the appearance of the drug in the blood. In an indirect relationship, the pharmacological effect is a delayed response to the appearance of the drug in the blood [23]. The typical models for describing a direct concentration-effect relationship include linear [3,16], E_{max} [2], and sigmoid models [4]. If the pharmacokinetic/pharmacodynamic data indicate an indirect relationship between the effect and plasma concentration, a compartmental model is required to account for the lag time between the effect and concentration. There are many models and approaches used to describe a pharmacokinetic/pharmacodynamic relationship.

This chapter will be focused on the Time Constant Approach to this topic. The key time constant in a pharmacokinetics/pharmacodynamics study is the lag time between the pharmacological response and the plasma concentration. To model an indirect relationship, an effect compartment is usually assumed, where the effect concentration is synchronous with the pharmacological effect. The pharmacodynamic effect can be expressed as a linear, E_{max}, or sigmoid function of the effect concentration. The relationship between the effect and central compartments may be irreversible, reversible, or indirect. In addition, when the pharmacokinetics are complicated, the link between the pharmacodynamics and the pharmacokinetics can be simplified and described by an isolated multi-compartment model (as discussed in Chapter 3).

Some common themes in the time constant view can be observed in the pharmacokinetic/pharmacodynamic study as well as other studies. The lag time between the pharmacological effect and the plasma concentration is likely to be short for a drug with rapid distribution to the effect site. Therefore, the distribution time and redistribution time estimated from a tissue penetration study (Chapter 10) may correspond to the pharmacodynamic lag time estimated from a pharmacokinetic/pharmacodynamic study. If the pharmacological effect correlates better with a metabolite than with the parent drug, the metabolite concentration, instead of the drug concentration, should be the key consideration in all clinical studies. When time constants in pharmacokinetics are nonlinear with dose in a dose proportionality study (Chapter 7), the pharmacodynamic/dose relationship is also likely to be nonlinear even if the effect/concentration relationship is linear.

Six models are discussed in this chapter to describe the pharmacokinetics/pharmacodynamics relationship: (1) the first model describes an irreversible relationship between central and effect compartments; (2) the second model describes a reversible relationship between the central and effect compartments; (3) the third model describes a two-compartment pharmacokinetics with an irreversible relationship between pharmacokinetics and pharmacodynamics; (4) the fourth model describes a sequence of responses evoked by a drug; (5) the fifth model describes an isolated multi-compartment model with an irreversible relationship between the central and effect compartments; and (6) the sixth model describes an isolated multi-compartment model with a reversible relationship between the central and effect compartments. Five simulated case studies and three literature examples are presented in this chapter to illustrate the utilities of these models in pharmacokinetic/pharmacodynamic studies. Additional examples of pharmacokinetic/pharmacodynamic studies can be found in the literature [1–22].

PHARMACOKINETIC MODELS

This section presents six models that are useful in describing the pharmacokinetics and pharmacodynamics relationships. The goal is to establish simple relationships between time constants and measurable parameters such as (1) mean residence time, which is the sum of input and output times, and (2) area under the curves. The derivations of these relationships are straightforward and are discussed in Chapter 2.

Model 1: Irreversible Relationship between Central and Effect Compartments

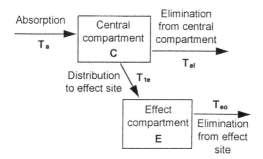

Frequently, a lag time exists between the pharmacological effect curve and the plasma concentration curve. One hypothesis is that a lag time exists between the effect site and the plasma concentration curves. In this case, the delayed pharmacological effect can be described by an effect site compartment that is connected to the central compartment.

The mean residence time of the plasma and effect concentrations in this model is simply the sum of input and output times.

$$\text{Mean residence time of C } (\bar{t}_C) = \frac{\text{AUMC}_C}{\text{AUC}_C}$$

$$= \text{Input time } (T_{c,in}) + \text{Output time } (T_{c,out}) = T_a + T_{el,t} \quad (12.1)$$

$$\text{Mean residence time in effect compartment } (\bar{t}_E) = \frac{\text{AUMC}_E}{\text{AUC}_E}$$

$$= \text{Input time } (T_{e,in}) + \text{Output time } (T_{e,out}) = T_a + T_{el,t} + T_{eo} \quad (12.2)$$

where $T_{el,t} = 1/(1/T_{el} + 1/T_{le})$. The difference in the mean residence time between the effect compartment and the central compartment gives the elimination time constant of the effect concentration:

$$\text{Elimination time of effect concentration } (T_{eo}) = \bar{t}_E - \bar{t}_C \quad (12.3)$$

This also means that T_{eo} is the only time constant responsible for the lag time between the effect concentration and the plasma concentration. The decay time of the concentration curves can be estimated from a partial area under the curve (see Appendix 2)

$$\frac{1}{\text{Decay time } (T_z)} = \lambda_z = 2\frac{(t_{ref} - t_{last}) \ln (C_{t_{ref}}) - \text{AU} \ln C_{t_{ref} - t_{last}}}{(t_{ref} - t_{last})^2} \tag{12.4}$$

The effect site concentration can be estimated by a convolution between the plasma concentration and the exponential decay function $e^{-t/T_{eo}}$.

$$C_e = C * \frac{V_c}{T_{le}V_e} e^{-t/T_{eo}} \tag{12.5}$$

However, $T_{le}V_e$ cannot be estimated since the effect concentration is not measured. An assumption [4] such as that the clearance from the central compartment to the effect compartment is equal to the clearance from the effect compartment can be made to simplify Equation (12.5) to the following:

$$T_{le}V_e = T_{eo}V_c \tag{12.6}$$

The ratio of the area under the effect curve to the area under the plasma concentration curve gives the ratio of the clearance from the central compartment to the effect compartment to the clearance from the effect compartment.

$$\frac{\text{AUC}_E}{\text{AUC}_C} = S\frac{T_{eo}V_c}{T_{le}V_e} \tag{12.7}$$

where S is a scaling factor converting the effect concentration to effect.

Model 2: Reversible Relationship between the Central and Effect Compartments

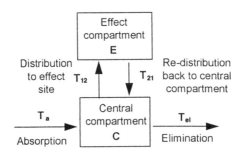

The effect concentration can have a reversible relationship with the plasma concentration as in this model. In this case, the ratio of the effect to plasma concentration versus time profile will increase initially following dosing and reach a constant after a period of time.

The mean residence times of the plasma and effect concentration in this model are the sums of input and output times (see Chapter 2):

$$\text{Mean residence time of C } (\bar{t}_C) = \frac{\text{AUMC}_C}{\text{AUC}_C}$$

$$= \text{Input time } (T_{c,in}) + \text{Output time } (T_{c,out}) = T_a + T_{el} + T_{el}\frac{T_{21}}{T_{12}} \quad (12.8)$$

$$\text{Mean residence time in effect compartment } (\bar{t}_E) = \frac{\text{AUMC}_E}{\text{AUC}_E}$$

$$= \text{Input time } (T_{e,in}) + \text{Output time } (T_{e,out}) = T_a + T_{el} + T_{el}\frac{T_{21}}{T_{12}} + T_{21}$$

$$(12.9)$$

The difference in the mean residence time between the effect and plasma concentration gives the redistribution time from the effect site:

$$\text{Redistribution time from the effect site } (T_{21}) = \bar{t}_E - \bar{t}_C \quad (12.10)$$

This indicates that T_{21} is the only time constant responsible for the lag time between the effect and the plasma concentration. The effect concentration can be estimated from the convolution of the plasma concentration with the exponential decay function $e^{-t/T_{21}}$.

$$C_e = C * \frac{V_c}{T_{12}V_e}e^{-t/T_{21}} \quad (12.11)$$

The value of T_{12} cannot be estimated from the Time Constant Approach; however, it can be eliminated from the above equation by assuming that the clearance from the central compartment to the effect compartment is equal to the clearance from the effect compartment

$$T_{12}V_e = T_{21}V_c \quad (12.12)$$

The ratio of the area under the effect curve to the area under the plasma concentration curve gives the ratio of the clearances into and from the effect compartment multiplied by a scaling factor S:

$$\frac{\text{AUC}_E}{\text{AUC}_C} = S\frac{T_{21}V_c}{T_{12}V_e} \tag{12.13}$$

Model 3: Two-Compartment Pharmacokinetics with an Irreversible Relationship between Pharmacokinetics and Pharmacodynamics

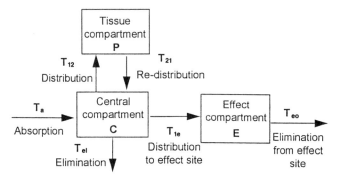

When the known pharmacokinetics of a drug follows a two-compartmental model and the pharmacodynamic effect does not follow the concentrations in either pharmacokinetic compartment, the pharmacokinetic/pharmacodynamic link may be described by Model 3.

The mean residence time is the sum of input and output times (see Chapter 2):

$$\text{Mean residence time of C } (\bar{t}_C) = \frac{\text{AUMC}_C}{\text{AUC}_C}$$

$$= \text{Input time } (T_{c,in}) + \text{Output time } (T_{c,out}) = T_a + T_{el,t} + T_{el,t}\frac{T_{21}}{T_{12}} \tag{12.14}$$

$$\text{Mean residence time in the effect compartment } (\bar{t}_E) = \frac{\text{AUMC}_E}{\text{AUC}_E}$$

$$= \text{Input time } (T_{e,in}) + \text{Output time } (T_{e,out}) = T_a + T_{el,t} + T_{el,t}\frac{T_{21}}{T_{12}} + T_{eo} \tag{12.15}$$

where $T_{el,t} = 1/(1/T_{el} + 1/T_{le})$. The mean residence time can be estimated from the ratio of the area under the first moment curve to the area under the concentration curve. The difference in the mean residence time of effect and plasma concentrations gives

$$\text{Elimination time from the effect site } (T_{eo}) = \bar{t}_E - \bar{t}_C \quad (12.16)$$

Therefore, T_{eo} is the only time constant that is responsible for the lag time between the effect and the drug concentration. The effect concentration can be estimated from the following convolution:

$$C_e = C * \frac{V_c}{T_{le}V_e}e^{-t/T_{eo}} \quad (12.17)$$

which can be simplified by assuming that the clearance from the central compartment to the effect compartment is equal to the clearance from the effect compartment:

$$T_{le}V_e = T_{eo}V_c \quad (12.18)$$

The ratio of the area under the effect curve to the area under the plasma concentration curve gives the ratio of the clearances into and from the effect compartment multiplied by a scaling factor S:

$$\frac{\text{AUC}_E}{\text{AUC}_C} = S\frac{T_{eo}V_c}{T_{le}V_e} \quad (12.19)$$

Model 4: Sequential Responses

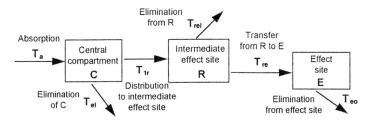

The effect site compartment may be indirectly linked to the central compartment through an intermediate compartment as described in this model. The effect curve will be delayed by two factors: the elimination time of compartment R and the elimination time of compartment E.

The mean residence time in this model is the sum of input and output times:

$$\text{Mean residence time of C } (\bar{t}_C) = \frac{\text{AUMC}_C}{\text{AUC}_C}$$

$$= \text{Input time } (T_{c,in}) + \text{Output time } (T_{c,out}) = T_a + T_{el,t} \quad (12.20)$$

$$\text{Mean residence time in effect compartment } (\bar{t}_E) = \frac{\text{AUMC}_E}{\text{AUC}_E}$$

$$= \text{Input time } (T_{e,in}) + \text{Output time } (T_{e,out}) = T_a + T_{el,t} + T_{rel,t} + T_{eo}$$

$$(12.21)$$

where $T_{el,t} = 1/(1/T_{el} + 1/T_{1r})$ and $T_{rel,t} = 1/(1/T_{rel} + 1/T_{re})$. The difference in the mean residence time of the effect and plasma concentration curve gives

$$\bar{t}_E - \bar{t}_C = T_{rel,t} + T_{eo} \quad (12.22)$$

The existence of the intermediate compartment R can be determined by comparing the time constants. The decay time of the effect concentration T_{ze} is equal to the greatest of T_{eo}, $T_{rel,t}$, $T_{el,t}$, or T_a, assuming linear kinetics for all processes involved. If the decay time of the central compartment T_{zc} (equal to the larger of $T_{el,t}$ or T_a) is smaller than the decay time of the effect compartment T_{ze}, then T_{ze} must be equal to the larger of $T_{rel,t}$ or T_{eo}. In this case (if $T_{zc} < T_{ze}$), the following relationship exists $\bar{t}_E - \bar{t}_C > t_{ze}$, which would not be true without the intermediate compartment (Model 1). Therefore, if $T_{zc} < T_{ze}$ and $\bar{t}_E - \bar{t}_C > t_{ze}$, then an intermediate compartment is likely to exist between the central and the effect compartments. However, if $T_{zc} = T_{ze}$ the existence of intermediate compartment R cannot be determined. The effect concentration can be estimated from the following convolution

$$C_e = \frac{V_c}{T_{1r}T_{re}V_e}C*e^{-t/T_{rel,t}}*e^{-t/T_{eo}} \quad (12.23)$$

which can be simplified by assuming that the clearance from the central compartment to the effect compartment is equal to the clearance from the effect compartment:

$$T_{eo}\frac{T_{rel}}{T_{rel} + T_{re}}V_c = T_{1r}V_e \quad (12.24)$$

The ratio of the area under the effect curve to the area under the plasma concentration curve gives the ratio of the clearances into and from the effect compartment multiplied by a scaling factor S:

$$\frac{\text{AUC}_E}{\text{AUC}_C} = S\frac{T_{eo}T_{rel}V_c}{T_{1r}(T_{rel} + T_{re})V_e} \qquad (12.25)$$

Model 5: Isolated Multi-Compartment Model with an Irreversible Relationship between the Central and Effect Compartments

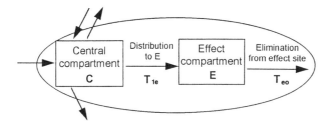

When the pharmacokinetics of a drug are complicated or the data from a study are not sufficient to characterize the pharmacokinetics, the relationship between the effect compartment and the central compartment can still be studied using an isolated multi-compartment model (Chapter 3). In Model 5, a first-order linear kinetics is assumed between the effect and the plasma concentration.

The value of T_{eo} can be estimated from the difference in the mean residence time of the effect and plasma concentration curves.

$$\text{Elimination time from the effect site } (T_{eo}) = \bar{t}_E - \bar{t}_C \qquad (12.26)$$

The effect site concentration can be estimated from the convolution of the plasma concentration curve with the exponential function $e^{-t/T_{eo}}$.

$$C_e = C * \frac{V_c}{T_{1e}V_e}e^{-t/T_{eo}} \qquad (12.27)$$

which can be simplified by assuming that the clearance from the central compartment to the effect compartment is equal to the clearance from the effect compartment

$$T_{1e}V_e = T_{eo}V_c \qquad (12.28)$$

The value of T_{eo} can also be estimated by a numerical method described as follows. (A) First, an initial guess of T_{eo} value is chosen. (B) Then the effect concentration curve is estimated using Equation (12.27). (C) The relationship between effect and effect concentration will result in a hysteresis loop. (D) Change the value of T_{eo} to obtain the minimum area within the hysteresis loop. The numerical method is especially useful when the relationship between the pharmacological effect and the effect concentration (in Step C above) is nonlinear.

The ratio of the area under the effect curve to the area under the plasma concentration curve gives the ratio of the clearances into and from the effect compartment multiplied by a scaling factor S:

$$\frac{\text{AUC}_E}{\text{AUC}_C} = S\frac{T_{eo}V_c}{T_{1e}V_e} \qquad (12.29)$$

Model 6: Isolated Multi-Compartment Model with a Reversible Relationship between the Central and Effect Compartments

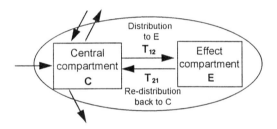

When the relationship between the effect concentration and the plasma concentration is reversible, the pharmacokinetic/pharmacodynamic link may be described by Model 6. To determine if the pharmacokinetic/pharmacodynamic relationship is reversible, the ratio of pharmacological effect to plasma concentration should be plotted against time. If the effect/concentration ratio reaches a constant with time, two models can be applied to describe the pharmacokinetic/pharmacodynamic link: a reversible model (Model 6) or an irreversible model (Model 5) with a small T_{eo}. To exclude the possibility of the irreversible model, T_{eo} should be calculated first. If the T_{eo} value is longer than the decay time of the effect curve, then reversible kinetics are likely.

The value of T_{21} can be estimated from the difference in the mean residence times of the effect and plasma concentration curves:

$$\text{Redistribution time from the effect site } (T_{21}) = \bar{t}_E - \bar{t}_C \qquad (12.30)$$

The effect site concentration can be estimated from the following convolution:

$$C_e = C * \frac{V_c}{T_{12} V_E} e^{-t/T_{21}} \qquad (12.31)$$

which can be simplified by assuming that the clearance from the central compartment to the effect compartment is equal to the clearance from the effect compartment:

$$T_{12} V_e = T_{21} V_c \qquad (12.32)$$

The value of T_{21} can be estimated numerically as described in Model 5. The ratio of the area under the effect curve to the area under the plasma concentration curve gives

$$\frac{\text{AUC}_E}{\text{AUC}_C} = S \frac{T_{21} V_c}{T_{12} V_e} \qquad (12.33)$$

CASE STUDIES

Case 1: Irreversible Relationship between Plasma and Effect Concentrations

The lag time between the pharmacological effects of a drug and the appearance of the drug in the blood can be accounted for as a delay in the distribution of the drug from the blood to an effect site (such as receptors). The required amount of the drug at the effect site to activate or inhibit the receptors is assumed to be negligible compared with the amount in the plasma. The lag time between the effect and the plasma drug concentration is a direct result of a slow elimination of the drug from the receptor sites. An irreversible distribution of the drug from the central compartment to the effect site can be described by Model 1. Simulated plasma drug concentration and pharmacological effect time profiles using the model are shown in Figure 12.1. In this example, the K_{eo} is equal to 0.25 hr^{-1}, which is reflected in the 4 to 5 hours of lag time between the maximum effect and the maximum concentration.

The key time constant in this example is the elimination time of the effect concentration, which is equal to the lag time of the effect concentration relative to the plasma concentration. The estimated pharmacokinetic pa-

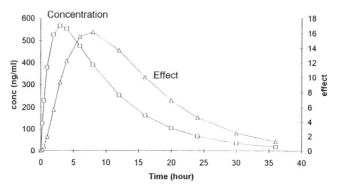

FIGURE 12.1. Simulated plasma drug concentration and pharmacological effects time profiles with an irreversible relationship between plasma and effect concentrations using Model 1. The time constant plot illustrating the pharmacokinetics and pharmacodynamics of the drug is shown in Figure 12.2. The parameters used in this simulation are $X_0 = 10$ mg, $f*F = 0.8$, $V_c = 10$ L, $K_a = 0.7$ hr^{-1}, $K_{el} = 0.1$ hr^{-1}, $K_{1e} = 0.01$ hr^{-1}, $K_{eo} = 0.25$ hr^{-1}.

rameters for the above example using the time constant analysis are listed in Table 12.1, and the estimated time constants are presented in Figure 12.2.

Now let us examine the time constant plot (Figure 12.2). The decay time of the effect compartment is equal to that of the central compartment, indicating that the elimination time of the drug at the effect site is shorter than the elimination time of the drug in the plasma. The estimated T_{eo} is 4.17 hours, which is reflected by the 4 to 5-hour lag time between the peak concentration and the peak effect. Since the value of T_{le} cannot be determined, a pseudo C_e profile that is "parallel" to the true C_e profile can be obtained assuming $T_{le}/V_c = T_{el}/V_e$ [4]. The lag time between the effect and the cen-

TABLE 12.1. Estimated Time Constants of Model 1
for the Example Shown in Figure 12.1.

Parameter	Central Cmpt. Time Constant Analysis	Central Cmpt. Model Value	Effect Cmpt. Time Constant Analysis	Effect Cmpt. Model Value	Equation
T_z (hr)	9.1	9.1 ($T_{el,t}$)	10.0	9.1 ($T_{el,t}$)	(12.4)
$\bar{t}$ (hr)	10.4	10.5	14.6	14.5	(12.1, 12.2)
T_{eo} (hr)			4.17	4.0	(12.3)
AUC (ng·hr/L)	7303	7272	291	290	

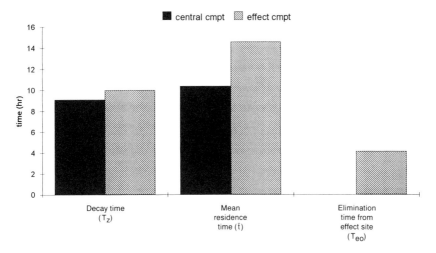

FIGURE 12.2. The time constant plot illustrating the pharmacokinetics and pharmaco-dynamics of the drug in the example shown in Figure 12.1. The estimated elimination time from the effect site (T_{eo}) is 4.17 hours, which is reflected by the difference in the mean residence time ($\bar{t}$) between the plasma concentration and the effect.

tral compartments can be illustrated by plotting the effect against the plasma concentrations (Figure 12.3). The plot of the effect versus the plasma drug concentration shows a hysteresis loop, and the loop collapses as the effect is plotted against the effect concentration.

The relationship between the effect and the effect concentration may follow an E_{max} model, as shown in the example in Figure 12.4. In this case, T_{eo} can be estimated by numerically searching for the T_{eo} value that will collapse the hysteresis loop. The numerical procedure is: first, guess a T_{eo} value; second, estimate C_e from the equation $C_e = C * [V_c/(T_{le}V_e)]e^{-t/T_{eo}}$; third, evaluate the area within the hysteresis loop; and fourth, try other values of T_{eo} until the loop collapses (i.e., the area within the loop is minimized). The criteria for collapsing the hysteresis loop is minimizing the area within the loop. Based on the above convolution calculation of C_e, the influence of the plasma concentration on the effect concentration C_e "decays retrogressively" (see the discussion of multi-compartment model in Chapter 2), where the half-life of the exponential decay is $0.693*T_{eo}$ (effect half-life). Therefore, the plasma concentration can produce the effect for a time period up to three times the effect half-life. The estimated value of T_{eo} is 4.17 hours for the example in Figure 12.4 using the numerical method. By the convolution calculation, this means that the plasma concentration will contribute to the pharmacological effect for about 9 hours (three times the

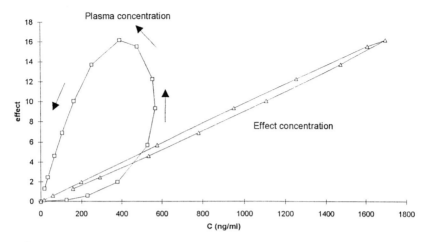

FIGURE 12.3. The relationship between the pharmacological effect and drug concentration in the central and effect compartments for the example in Figure 12.1.

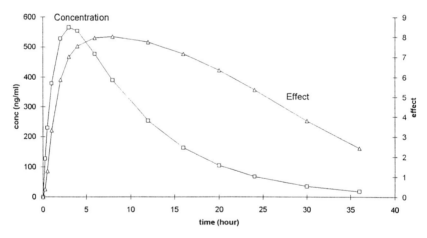

FIGURE 12.4. Simulated plasma drug concentration and pharmacological effects time profiles with nonlinear pharmacokinetics/pharmacodynamic relationship using Model 1: $X_0 = 10$ mg, $f^*F = 0.8$, $V_c = 10$ L, $K_a = 0.7$ hr^{-1}, $K_{el} = 0.1$ hr^{-1}, $K_{1e} = 0.01$ hr^{-1}, $K_{eo} = 0.25$ hr^{-1}, $E_{max} = 10$, EC$_{50} = 4$ ng/ml.

286

effect half-life). The collapsed hysteresis loop is shown in Figure 12.5, and the relationship between the effect and the effect concentration is clearly nonlinear, following an E_{max} model. Since the calculated effect concentration is "parallel" to the true effect concentration, the estimated E_{max} (≈ 10) represents the true value, but the estimated EC_{50} (≈ 450 ng/ml) is arbitrary.

Case 2: Reversible Relationship between Plasma and Effect Concentrations

The relationship between the plasma drug concentration and the effect site concentration can be reversible. This may be described by Model 2, and a simulated example using the model is shown in Figure 12.6. In this example, the value of K_{21} is 0.2 hr^{-1}, which corresponds to a 5-hour delay in pharmacological effect relative to the plasma concentration. The method for verifying the reversibility between the central and effect compartments is to plot the ratio of the effect to the plasma concentration against time. If the effect-concentration relationship is reversible, the ratio will reach an equilibrium, as shown in Figure 12.7. However, a constant ratio between the effect and the plasma concentration may also suggest an irreversible effect-concentration relationship with a fast elimination from the effect site.

In this example, the lag time between the effect and plasma concentration is determined by the redistribution time constant (T_{21}) from the effect site, which is then the key time constant. The estimated pharmacokinetic param-

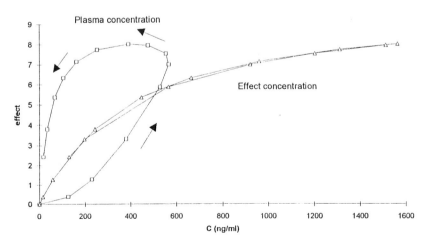

FIGURE 12.5. The relationship between the pharmacological effect and drug concentration in the central and effect compartments for the example in Figure 12.4.

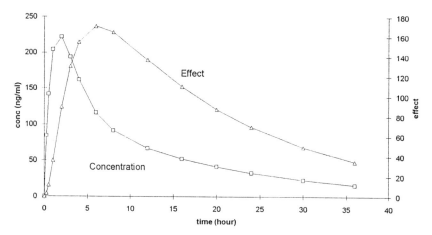

FIGURE 12.6. Simulated plasma drug concentration and pharmacological effects time profiles with reversible relationship between plasma and effect concentrations using Model 2. The time constant plot illustrating the pharmacokinetics and pharmacodynamics of the drug is shown in Figure 12.8. The parameters used in this simulation are $X_0 = 10$ mg, $f^*F = 0.8$, $V_c = 10$ L, $K_a = 0.7$ hr^{-1}, $K_{el} = 0.1$ hr^{-1}, $K_{12} = 0.6$ hr^{-1}, $K_{21} = 0.2$ hr^{-1}.

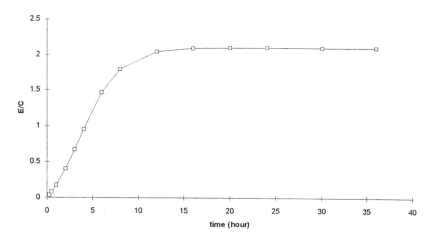

FIGURE 12.7. The ratio of effect to plasma drug concentration as a function of time for the example in Figure 12.6.

**TABLE 12.2. Estimated Time Constants of Model 2
for the Example Shown in Figure 12.6.**

| Parameter | Central Cmpt. | | Effect Cmpt. | | |
	Time Constant Analysis	Model Value	Time Constant Analysis	Model Value	Equation
T_z (hr)	17.1	17.4	17.1	17.4	(12.4)
$\bar{t}$ (hr)	15.2	15.3	20.2	20.3	(12.8, 12.9)
T_{21} (hr)			5.0	5.0	(12.10)
AUC (ng·hr/L)	2669	2666	3988	4000	

eters for the above example using the time constant analysis are listed in Table 12.2, and the estimated time constants are presented in Figure 12.8.

Now let us examine the time constant plot (Figure 12.8). The mean residence time of the effect time profile is about 5 hours longer than the mean residence time of the plasma concentration profile, which is reflected by the lag time between the maximum effect and the maximum concentration. The value of T_{21} is 5.0 hours, and thus the effect half-life is approximately 3.5 hours (= 0.693*5), suggesting that the plasma drug concentration may

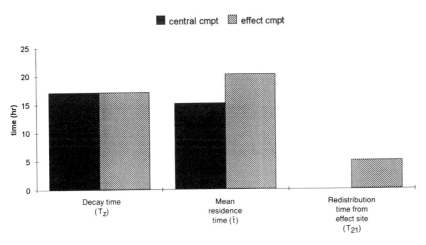

FIGURE 12.8. The time constant plot illustrating the pharmacokinetics and pharmacodynamics of the drug with a reversible relationship between plasma and effect concentrations in the example shown in Figure 12.6. The mean residence time ($\bar{t}$) of the effect time profile is about 5 hours longer than the mean residence time of the plasma concentration profile, which is equal to the redistribution time from the effect site (T_{21}).

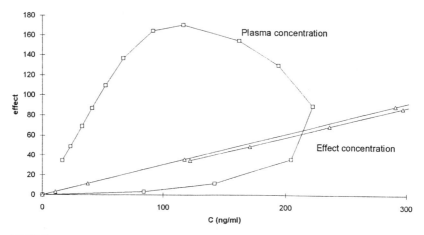

FIGURE 12.9. The relationship between the pharmacological effect and drug concentrations in the central and effect compartments for the example in Figure 12.6.

contribute to the pharmacological effect for 10.5 hours ($= 3*3.5$). A pseudo-concentration profile parallel to the true effect site concentration can be obtained using the equation $C_e = C*[V_c/(T_{12}V_e)]e^{-t/T_{21}}$. The relationships between the effect and the concentrations in the central and effect compartments are shown in Figure 12.9. The hysteresis loop collapses when the effect is plotted against the effect site concentration.

Case 3: Two-Compartment Pharmacokinetic Model

When the pharmacokinetics of a drug follows a two-compartment model and the effect does not correlate with the concentration in either compartment, the pharmacokinetic/pharmacodynamic link might be described by Model 3. Simulated time courses for plasma concentration and pharmacological effect using the model are shown in Figure 12.10. In this example, the value of K_{eo} is equal to 0.2 hr^{-1}, which is reflected by the 5-hour lag time between the maximum effect and the maximum concentration.

The distribution time between plasma and tissue does not contribute to the lag time between the effect site and plasma. The lag time is simply equal to the elimination time from the effect site [Equation (12.16)], independent of any other time constant. The estimated pharmacokinetic parameters for the above example using the time constant analysis are listed in Table 12.3, and the estimated time constants are presented in Figure 12.11. As shown in the time constant plot (Figure 12.11), the mean residence of the effect compartment is longer than that of the central compartment, and the lag time (5

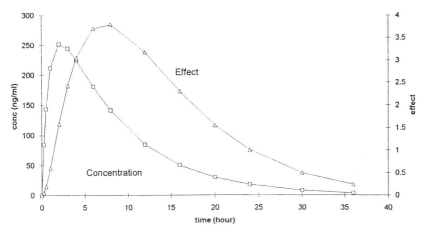

FIGURE 12.10. Simulated plasma drug concentration and pharmacological effects time profiles for a drug with biexponential decay in concentration using Model 3. The time constant plot illustrating the pharmacokinetics and pharmacodynamics of the drug is shown in Figure 12.11. The parameters used in the simulation are $X_0 = 10$ mg, $f*F = 0.8$, $V_c = 10$ L, $K_a = 0.5$ hr^{-1}, $K_{el} = 0.3$ hr^{-1}, $K_{12} = 0.6$ hr^{-1}, $K_{21} = 0.6$ hr^{-1}, $K_{1e} = 0.01$ hr^{-1}, $K_{eo} = 0.2$ hr^{-1}.

hours) is a result of a long T_{eo}. The effect half-life is 3.5 hours ($= 0.693*T_{eo}$), indicating that the plasma concentration may contribute to the pharmacological effect for 10.5 hours (3*3.5). A pseudo-concentration parallel to the effect concentration is obtained using the convolution method. The effect-concentration relationship is shown in Figure 12.12, where the hysteresis loop is collapsed as the effect is plotted against the effect site concentration.

TABLE 12.3. *Estimated Time Constants of Model 3 for the Example Shown in Figure 12.10.*

Parameter	Central Cmpt.		Effect Cmpt.		Equation
	Time Constant Analysis	Model Value	Time Constant Analysis	Model Value	
T_z (hr)	7.1	7.6	8.1	7.6	(12.4)
$\bar{t}$ (hr)	8.6	8.7	13.6	13.7	(12.14, 12.15)
T_{eo} (hr)			5.0	5.0	(12.16)
AUC (ng·hr/L)	2697	2666	67	67	

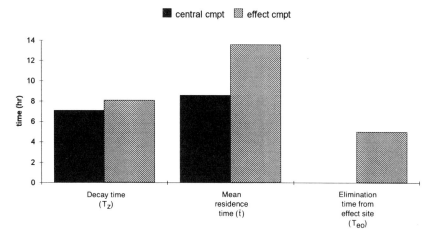

FIGURE 12.11. The time constant plot illustrating the pharmacokinetics and pharmacodynamics of the drug with biexponential decay in concentration time profile of the example shown in Figure 12.10. The mean residence time ($\bar{t}$) of the effect compartment is longer than that of the central compartment, and the lag time between the two (5 hours) is a result of a long elimination time from the effect site (T_{eo}).

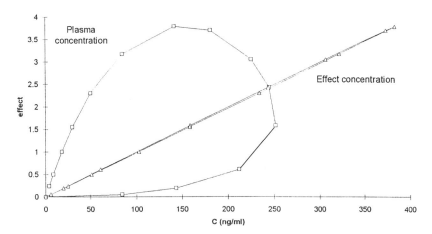

FIGURE 12.12. The relationship between the pharmacological effect and drug concentration in the central and effect compartments for the example in Figure 12.10.

Case 4: Cascade of Pharmacological Effect

The mechanism of pharmacological effects of a drug may involve a cascade, where the drug evokes a series of sequential intermediate responses prior to the clinical end result. In this case, the lag time between the pharmacological effect and the plasma drug concentration is a sum of the lag time of all processes in the cascade. This can be described using Model 4, and simulated time courses for plasma drug concentration and pharmacological effect using the model are shown in Figure 12.13. The cascade evoked by the drug in this example involves two physiological processes represented by compartments R (receptor) and E (effect). The lag time between the maximum effect and the maximum plasma drug concentration is about 8 hours.

The estimated pharmacokinetic parameters of the above example using the time constant analysis are listed in Table 12.4, and the estimated time constants are presented in Figure 12.14. If the effect compartment is directly connected to the central compartment (as in Models 1 to 3), decay time of the effect compartment should be equal to the longer one of $T_{el,t}$ and T_{eo}, depending on which one is the rate limiting step; the lag time ($\bar{t}_E - \bar{t}_C$) between the effect and the central compartments should be smaller (if T_{el} is rate limiting) or equal to (if T_{eo} is rate limiting) the decay time of the effect

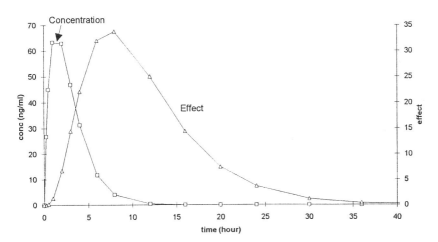

FIGURE 12.13. Simulated plasma drug concentration and pharmacological effects time profiles for a drug with a cascade of pharmacological effects using Model 4. The time constant plot illustrating the pharmacokinetics and pharmacodynamics of the drug is shown in Figure 12.14. The parameters used in this simulation are $X_0 = 10$ mg, $f^*F = 0.8$, $V_c = 40$ L, $K_a = 0.8$ hr^{-1}, $K_{el} = 0.6$ hr^{-1}, $K_{1r} = 0.01$ hr^{-1}, $K_{rel} = 0.1$ hr^{-1}, $K_{re} = 0.2$ hr^{-1}, $K_{eo} = 0.2$ hr^{-1}.

TABLE 12.4. Estimated Time Constants of Model 4
for the Example Shown in Figure 12.13.

Parameter	Central Cmpt.		Effect Cmpt.		
	Time Constant Analysis	Model Value	Time Constant Analysis	Model Value	Equation
T_z (hr)	1.64	1.64	5.26	5.0	(12.4)
$\bar{t}$ (hr)	2.9	2.9	11.2	11.2	(12.20, 12.21)
$\bar{t}_E - \bar{t}_C$ (hr)			8.3	8.3	(12.22)
T_{eo} (hr)			5.26	5.0	$T_{eo} = T_z$
$T_{rel,t}$ (hr)	3.13	3.33			(12.22)
AUC (ng·hr/L)	265	262	438	437	

profile (T_{ze}). However, as shown in the time constant plot (Figure 12.14), in this example, the lag time between the effect and central compartment is 8.3 hours, which is longer than the decay time of the effect curve T_{ze} (= 5.3 hours). This suggests that an additional compartment between the effect and central compartments exists. A pseudo-concentration parallel to the true effect concentration can be obtained using the convolution method. The

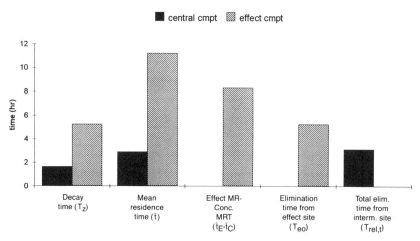

FIGURE 12.14. The time constant plot illustrating the pharmacokinetics and pharmacodynamics of the drug with a cascade of pharmacological effects in the example shown in Figure 12.13. The lag in the mean residence time ($\bar{t}$) between the effect and central compartment is 8.3 hours, which is longer than the decay time of the effect curve T_{ze} (= 5.3 hours). This suggests an additional compartment between the effect and central compartments exists.

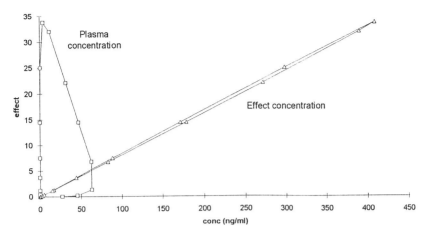

FIGURE 12.15. The relationships between the pharmacological effect and drug concentration in the central and effect compartments for the example in Figure 12.13.

hysteresis loop collapses as the effect is plotted against the effect site concentration (Figure 12.15).

Case 5: Isolated Multi-Compartment PK/PD Model

The relationship between the pharmacological effect and the plasma drug concentration can be established without the knowledge of the pharmacokinetics of the drug by using an isolated multi-compartment model as described in Models 5 and 6. This approach allows one to retrieve information from the pharmacokinetic/pharmacodynamic link when there is not enough information for a full-scale pharmacokinetic analysis. The pharmacokinetic/pharmacodynamic link can be irreversible (as in Model 1), reversible (as in Model 2), or involve cascade (as in Model 4). If the relationship between the pharmacological effect and the effect site concentration is linear, the reversibility can be identified by plotting the ratio of effect to plasma concentration versus time. If the ratio reaches an equilibrium, the relationship is likely to be reversible. The existence of cascade can be identified by examining the decay time (T_{ze}) and the lag time $(\bar{t}_E - \bar{t}_C)$, provided that the effect-concentration relationship is linear. If the lag time is longer than the decay time of the effect profile, cascade of physiological processes may be involved between the central and the effect compartments. If the effect-concentration relationship is nonlinear, the reversibility and cascade of the pharmacokinetic/pharmacodynamic link cannot be identified by the above mentioned methods, and the appropriate effect-

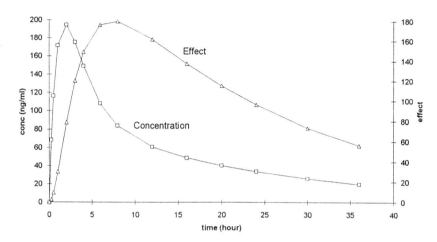

FIGURE 12.16. Simulated plasma drug concentration and pharmacological effects time profiles with reversible interaction between the plasma and effect concentrations using Model 6. The time constant plot illustrating the pharmacokinetics and pharmacodynamics of the drug is shown in Figure 12.18. The parameters used in this simulation are $K_{12} = 0.6$ hr^{-1}, $K_{21} = 0.15\ hr^{-1}$.

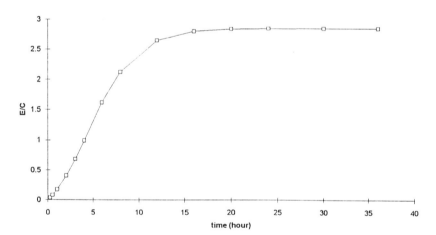

FIGURE 12.17. The ratio of effect to plasma drug concentration as a function of time for the example in Figure 12.16.

TABLE 12.5. Estimated Time Constants of Model 6
for the Example Shown in Figure 12.16.

| Parameter | Central Cmpt. | | Effect Cmpt. | | |
	Time Constant Analysis	Model Value	Time Constant Analysis	Model Value	Equation
T_z (hr)	22.2	22.2	22.2	22.2	(12.4)
$\bar{t}$ (hr)	18.9	19.2	25.7	25.8	
$\bar{t}_E - \bar{t}_C$ (hr)			6.8	6.6	(12.30)
T_{21} (hr)			6.67	6.67	(12.31)
AUC (ng·hr/L)	2667	2666	5316	5333	

concentration models can be selected by minimizing the area within the hysteresis loop (as described in Case 1).

An example illustrating a reversible interaction between the effect and central compartments is simulated by Model 6 and shown in Figure 12.16. In this example, the value of K_{eo} is the 0.15 hr^{-1}, which is reflected in the 5–6 hours of lag time between the maximum effect and the maximum concentration. The plot of E/C versus time indicates a possible reversible interaction between the effect and the central compartments (Figure 12.17).

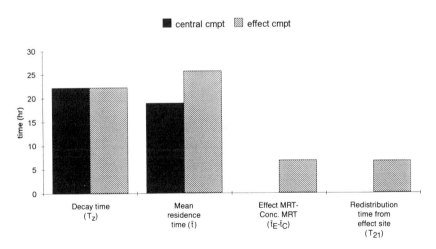

FIGURE 12.18. The time constant plot illustrating the pharmacokinetics and pharmacodynamics of the drug with a reversible relationship between plasma and effect concentrations in the example shown in Figure 12.16. The lag in the mean residence time ($\bar{t}$) between the effect and central compartments (6.8 hours) is shorter than the decay time (T_z) of the effect profile, indicating that no cascade between the two compartments is involved.

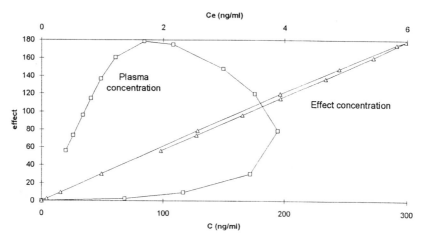

FIGURE 12.19. The relationships between the pharmacological effect and drug concentration in the central and effect compartments for the example in Figure 12.16.

The key time constant in this example is the redistribution time of the drug from the effect site to the plasma. The estimated pharmacokinetic parameters of the above example using the time constant analysis are listed in Table 12.5, and the estimated time constants are presented in Figure 12.18.

Now let us examine the time constant plot (Figure 12.18). The lag time between the effect and central compartments (6.8 hours) is shorter than the decay time of the effect profile, indicating that no cascade between the two compartments is involved. The value of T_{21} is 6.67 hours, resulting in an effect half-life of 4.6 hours (Chapter 3). Therefore, the plasma drug concentration may contribute to the pharmacological effect up to 13.8 hours. A pseudo-concentration parallel to the true effect site concentration is obtained using the convolution method. The collapse of the hysteresis loop is illustrated in Figure 12.19.

EXAMPLES

Example 1: Linear Effect-Concentration Relationship

The pharmacological effects of theophylline were studied following the oral administration of 600 mg theophylline in asthmatic patients [23]. The pharmacodynamic variable is the change in the peak expiratory flow rate (ΔPEFR). The mean plasma concentration of theophylline and the mean ΔPEFR following the oral dose are shown in Figure 12.20. There is a slight lag time between the effect and concentration profiles.

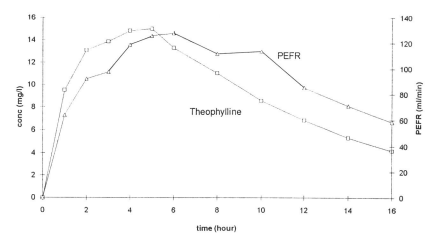

FIGURE 12.20. Mean plasma concentration of theophylline and change in peak expiratory flow rate following the oral administration of 600 mg theophylline in asthmatic patients. (Reproduced from Reference [23] with permission.) The time constant plot illustrating the pharmacokinetics and pharmacodynamics of the drug is shown in Figure 12.21.

To evaluate the lag time between the effect and the plasma concentration, the key time constant in this example is the elimination time from the effect site. The pharmacokinetic parameters of theophylline are estimated using Model 5 and listed in Table 12.6, and the estimated time constants are presented in Figure 12.21.

Now let us examine the time constant plot (Figure 12.21). The decay time of the concentration and effect profiles is similar, indicating that the elimination time of the effect is shorter than the elimination time of theophylline. This is confirmed by the small value of T_{eo} compared with the decay time. The T_{eo} value is estimated by minimizing the area within the hysteresis

TABLE 12.6. *The Estimated Pharmacokinetic Parameters of Theophylline Using Model 5.*

Parameter*	Conc.	Effect	Equation
T_z (hr)	8.55	8.26	(12.4)
$\bar{t}$ (hr)	10.2	11.8	
T_{eo} (hr)		0.55	(12.27)
$S*V_c/(V_eK_{1e})$			
(ml·L/mg/min)	10.52		(12.29)
AUC (mg·hr/L)	189.4	1993.2	

*Parameters estimated from the mean concentration profiles or the mean reported values.

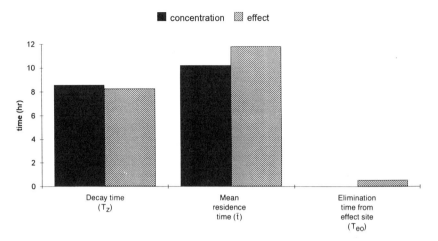

FIGURE 12.21. The time constant plot illustrating the pharmacokinetics and pharmacodynamics of theophylline using Model 5. The decay time (T_z) of the concentration and effect profiles is similar, indicating the elimination time of the effect (T_{eo}) is shorter than the elimination time of theophylline. This is confirmed by the small value of T_{eo} compared with the decay time.

loop of effect versus effect concentration curve in Figure 12.22. The effect site concentrations are estimated from the convolution of Equation (12.27). After collapsing the hysteresis loop, the resulting relationship between the effect and the effect site concentration is linear. Since the pharmacological effect has not reached a maximum at this dose, an exploration of higher dosing levels may be warranted, as suggested in Reference [16].

Example 2: Nonlinear Effect-Concentration Relationship

The pharmacodynamics of ticlopidine were studied in six normal subjects following the oral administrations of 250 mg, 500 mg, and 1000 mg of ticlopidine [2]. The pharmacodynamic variable is expressed in terms of percent inhibition of ADP-induced aggregation. The mean plasma concentration and the mean effect profiles following the three treatments are shown in Figure 12.23. There is a significant lag time between the effect and the drug concentration curves, indicating a very large T_{eo}. The lag time results in hysteresis loops between the effect and the plasma drug concentration (Figure 12.24).

The effect curves are significantly delayed relative to the plasma concentration curves; therefore, the elimination time from the effect site is the key

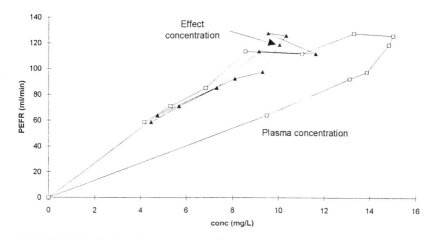

FIGURE 12.22. Relationship between the effect versus plasma concentration and effect versus effect site concentration of theophylline.

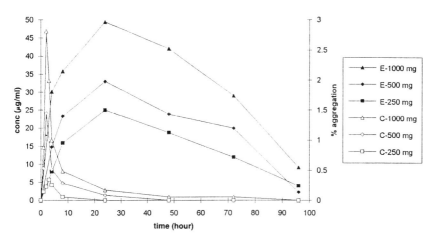

FIGURE 12.23. Mean ticlopidine plasma concentration and its pharmacological effects (percent inhibition of ADP-induced aggregation) in six normal subjects following the oral administrations of 250 mg, 500 mg, and 1000 mg of ticlopidine. (Reproduced from Reference [2] with permission.) The time constant plot illustrating the pharmacokinetics and pharmacodynamics of the drug is shown in Figure 12.25.

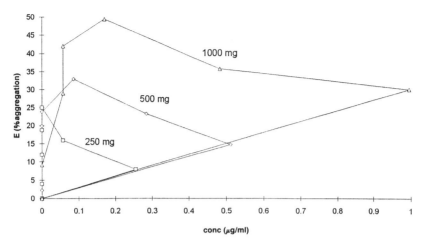

FIGURE 12.24. The relationship between the effect and the plasma concentration of ticlopidine.

time constant for collapsing the hysteresis between the effect and concentration. The pharmacokinetic/pharmacodynamic parameters of ticlopidine are estimated using Model 5 and listed in Table 12.7, and the estimated time constants are presented in Figure 12.25. The area under the concentration curves is disproportionate with the dose, indicating nonlinear kinetics. The dose normalized area under the drug concentration curve increases with dose, while the dose normalized area under the effect curve decreases, indicating a nonlinear relationship between effect and concentration.

Now let us examine the time constant plot (Figure 12.25). The mean residence time of the drug concentration increases with dose, probably due to a saturation of elimination with the high doses. The ratio of the area under the effect curve to the area under the plasma concentration curve $[\mathrm{AUC_E/AUC_C} = S*V_c/(V_eT_{le})]$ decreases with dose, indicating a nonlinear E_{max} model for the effect-concentration relationship. The values of T_{eo} are obtained by collapsing the hysteresis loops of the effect versus concentration curves. The effect versus effect site concentration relationships are shown in Figure 12.26. The slope of the effect-effect concentration curves is sharper at the low concentration range than at the high concentration range, indicating a nonlinear relationship, possibly an E_{max} model. To summarize, the pharmacological effect of ticlopidine seems to be saturable at a high dose (as indicated in Reference [2] using an E_{max} model), while the pharmacokinetics of the drug is also nonlinear.

TABLE 12.7. The Estimated Pharmacokinetic/Pharmacodynamic Parameters of Ticlopidine Using Model 5.

Parameter*	Conc.			Effect			Equation
	250 mg	500 mg	1000 mg	250 mg	500 mg	1000 mg	
$\bar{t}$ (hr)	4.5	8.5	16.0	43.6	41.7	43.7	
T_{eo} (hr)				94.6	54.8	40.8	(12.27)
$S*V_c/(V_eT_{1e})$ (ml/μg)	800	234	177				(12.29)
AUC (ng·hr/ml or %·hr)	1.9	8.8	19.1	1535	2060	3392	
AUC/D (ng·hr/ml/mg or %·hr/mg)	0.007	0.017	0.0191	6.14	4.12	3.39	
	6	6					

*Parameters estimated from the concentration profiles or the mean reported values.

303

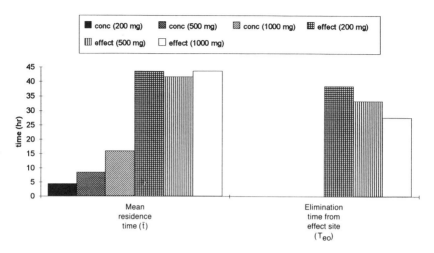

FIGURE 12.25. The time constant plot illustrating the pharmacokinetics and pharmacodynamics of ticlopidine using Model 5. The mean residence time ($\bar{t}$) of the drug concentration increases with dose, probably due to a saturation of elimination with the high doses.

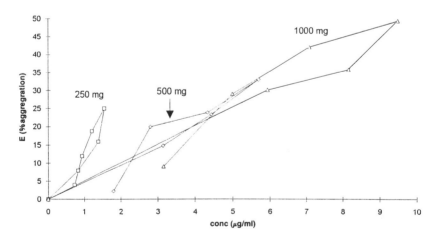

FIGURE 12.26. The effect versus effect site concentration relationship of ticlopidine.

304

Example 3: Relationship between Effect and Metabolite Concentration

The pharmacodynamics of adinazolam and its primary metabolite NDMAD were studied in sixteen healthy subjects following 30-mg oral and 15-mg intravenous doses of adinazolam [3]. The pharmacodynamic variable is expressed in terms of the Nurse-Rated Sedation Scale (NRSS) scores. The mean plasma concentration and the effect curves following the treatments are shown in Figures 12.27 and 12.28. The appearance of the metabolite NDMAD in the blood is faster following the oral dose than the intravenous dose, indicating a first pass effect. The lag time between NDMAD and effect is shorter than the lag time between adinazolam and the effect. This is expected since a metabolite always appears later in the blood than the parent drug. The relationship between the effect and adinazolam and NDMAD concentration is shown in Figure 12.29. The lag time results in hysteresis loops of the effect-concentration curves.

Earlier studies have shown that the metabolite NDMAD is twenty-five times more potent as a benzodiazepine receptor agonist than the parent drug adinazolam. Therefore, to determine whether there is a relationship between effect and NDMAD or between effect and adinazolam, both hysteresis loops of effect versus NDMAD and effect versus adinazolam must be collapsed. The pharmacokinetic/pharmacodynamic parameters of adina-

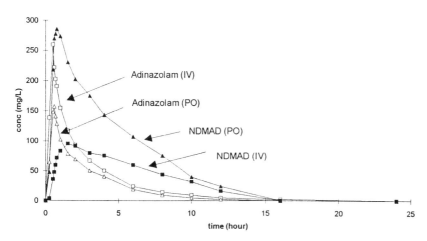

FIGURE 12.27. Mean plasma concentration profiles of adinazolam and its metabolite NDMAD in sixteen healthy subjects following 30-mg oral and 15-mg intravenous doses of adinazolam. (Reproduced from Reference [3] with permission.) The time constant plot illustrating the pharmacokinetics and pharmacodynamics of the drug is shown in Figure 12.30.

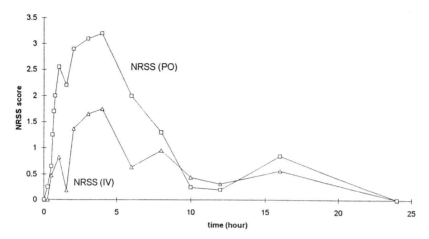

FIGURE 12.28. Mean effect (Nurse-Rated Sedation Scale scores) profiles of adinazolam and its metabolite NDMAD in sixteen healthy subjects following 30-mg oral and 15-mg intravenous doses of adinazolam. (Reproduced from Reference [3] with permission.)

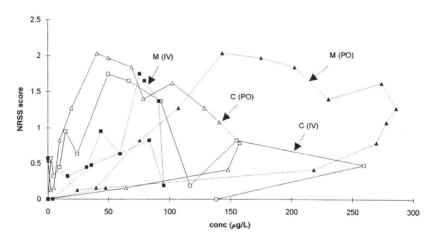

FIGURE 12.29. The relationship between the effect (E) and the plasma concentration between adinazolam (C) and NDMAD (M).

306

TABLE 12.8. *The Estimated Pharmacokinetic/Pharmacodynamic Parameters of Adinazolam Using Model 5.*

Parameter*	C-iv	C-po	M-iv	M-po	E-iv	E-po	Equation
$\bar{t}$ (hr)	3.3	3.0	5.2	4.4	6.6	6.8	
T_{eo} (hr)	3.23	3.85	1.35	2.44			
$S*V_c/(V_eK_{1e})$ (L/mg)	0.020	0.041	0.018	0.012			(12.27)
AUC (mg·hr/L)	596	400	685	1415	12.1	16.3	(12.29)

*Parameters estimated from the concentration profiles or the mean reported values.

307

zolam and NDMAD are estimated using Model 5 and listed in Table 12.8, and the estimated time constants are presented in Figure 12.30. The ratio of the area under NDMAD concentration curve to the area under adinazolam concentration curve is higher after the oral dose than the intravenous dose, indicating a first pass effect after the oral dose.

Now let us examine the time constant plot (Figure 12.30). The mean residence time of the metabolite is shorter after the oral dose than the intravenous dose because a large amount of metabolite is produced by the first pass effect immediately after the oral administration (see Chapter 5 for discussion on the first pass effect). The values of T_{eo} are estimated for both effect-adinazolam (Figure 12.31) and effect-NDMAD relationships following the oral and intravenous doses. The effect-effect concentration relationship for adinazolam and NDMAD after the oral and intravenous doses is shown in Figure 12.32. The effect versus adinazolam effect concentration relationships after the oral and intravenous doses are not consistent with each other, with a significant difference in the slopes. On the other hand, the effect versus NDMAD effect concentration relationships after the oral and intravenous doses are consistent. This suggests a better correlation between the effect and NDMAD concentration than between the effect and adinazolam concentration, as indicated in Reference [3] using a different method. The value of T_{eo} based on the effect-NDMAD model is different between the oral and intravenous dose. This may be due to a nonlinear ki-

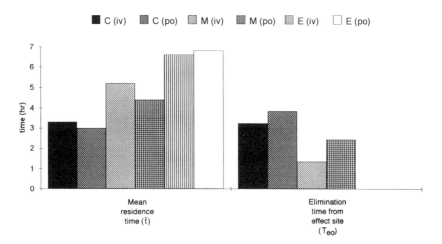

FIGURE 12.30. The time constant plot illustrating the pharmacokinetics and pharmacodynamics of adinazolam using Model 5. The mean residence time ($\bar{t}$) of the metabolite is shorter after the oral dose than the intravenous dose because a large amount of metabolite is produced by the first pass effect immediately after the oral administration.

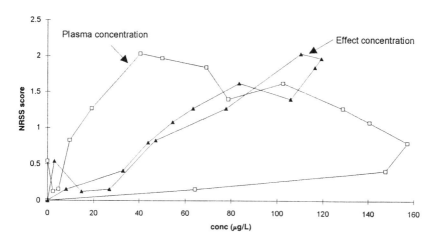

FIGURE 12.31. The relationship between effect versus plasma concentration and effect versus effect concentration of adinazolam after oral administration of adinazolam.

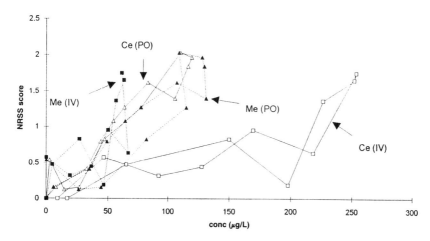

FIGURE 12.32. The effect-effect concentration plot for adinazolam and NDMAD after oral and intravenous administrations.

netics of the elimination from the effect site, where the elimination is saturable and T_{eo} is longer with higher concentrations following the oral dose.

REFERENCES

1. Derendorf H., Mollmann H., Krieg M., Tunn S., Mollmann C., Barth J., and Rothig H. J., "Pharmacodynamics of methylprednisolone phosphate after single intravenous administration to healthy volunteers," *Pharmaceutical Research,* 1991; 8(2):263–268.

2. Di Perri T., Pasini F. L., Frigerio C., Blardi P., Centini F., Messa G. L., Ghezzi A., and Volpi L., "Pharmacodynamics of ticlopidine in man in relation to plasma and blood cell concentration," *Eur. J. Clin. Pharmacol.,* 1991; 41:429–434.

3. Fleishaker J. C., Smith T. C., Friedman H. L., and Hulst L. K., "Separation of the pharmacokinetic/pharmacodynamic properties of oral and IV adinazolam mesylate and *N*-desmethyladinazolam mesylate in healthy volunteers," *Drug Invest,* 1992; 4(2):155–165.

4. Gibaldi M. and Perrier D., *Pharmacokinetics,* 1982; Marcel Dekker, Inc.

5. Girard P. Saumet J. L., Dubois F., and Boissel J. P., "Pharmacodynamic model of the haemodynamic effects of pinacidil in normotensive volunteers," *Eur. J. Clin. Pharmacol.,* 1993; 44:177–182.

6. Gumbleton M. and Benet L. Z., "Simultaneous pharmacodynamic modelling of the non-steady-state effects of three oral doses of 1,3-glyceryl dinitrate upon blood pressure in healthy volunteers," *Journal of Pharmacokinetics and Biopharmaceutics,* 1993; 21:515–532.

7. Gupta S. K., Ritchie J. C., Ellinwood E. H., Wiedemann K., and Holsboer F., "Modeling the pharmacokinetics and pharmacodynamics of dexamethasone in depressed patients," *Eur. J. Clin. Pharmacol.,* 1992; 43:51–55.

8. Hedner T., Edgar B., Edvinsson L., Hedner J., Persson B., and Pettersson A., "Yohimbine pharmacokinetics and interaction with the sympathetic nervous system in normal volunteers," *Eur. J. Clin. Pharmacol.,* 1992; 43:651–656.

9. Hochhaus G. and Mollmann H., "Pharmacokinetic/pharmacodynamic characteristics of the β-2-agonists terbutaline, salbutamol and fenoterol," *International Journal of Clinical Pharmacology, Therapy and Toxicology,* 1992; 30(9):342–362.

10. Huang M. L., Van Peer A., Woestenboughs R., De Coster R., Heykants J., Jansen A. A. I., Zylicz Z., Visscher H. W., and Jonkman J. H. G., "Pharmacokinetics of the novel antipsychotic agent risperidone and the prolactin response in healthy subjects," *Clinical Pharmacology & Therapeutics,* 1993; 54(3):257–268.

11. Le Coz F., Funck-Brentano C., Poirier J. M., Kibleur Y., Mazoit F. X., and Jaillon P., "Prediction of sotalol-induced maximum steady-state QTc prolongation from single-dose administration in healthy volunteers," *Clin. Pharmacol. Ther.,* 1992; 52(4): 417–426.

12. Mandema J. W., Tuk B., van Steveninck A. L., Breimer D. D., Cohen A. F., and Danhof M., "Pharmacokinetic-pharmacodynamic modelling of the central nervous system effects of midazolam and its main metabolite α-hydroxymidazolam in healthy volunteers," *Clin. Pharmacol. Ther.,* 1992; 51(6):715–728.

13. Ohtawa M., Morikawa H., and Shimazaki J., "Pharmacokinetics and biochemical efficacy after single and multiple oral administration of *N*-(2-methyl-2-propyl)-3-oxo-4-aza-5α-androst-1-ene-17β-carboxamide, a new type of specific competitive inhibitor of testosterone 5α-reductase, in volunteers," *European Journal of Drug Metabolism and Pharmacokinetics,* 1991, 16(1):15–21.

14. Porchet H. C., Piletta P., and Dayer P., "Pharmacokinetic-pharmacodynamic modeling of the effects of clonidine on pain threshold, blood pressure, and salivary flow," *Eur. J. Clin. Pharmacol.,* 1992; 42:655–662.

15. Provost J. C., Funck-Brentano C., Rovei V., D'Estanque J., Ego D., and Jaillon P., "Pharmacokinetic and pharmacodynamic interaction between toloxatone, a new reversible monoamine oxidase-A inhibitor, and oral tyramine in healthy subjects," *Clin. Pharmacol. Ther.,* 1992; 52(4):384–393.

16. Richer C., Mathieu M., Bah H., Thuillez C., Duroux P., Giudicelli, J., *Clin. Pharmacol. Ther.,* 1982; 31:579–586.

17. Rolan P. E., Parker J. E., Gray S. J., Weatherley B. C., Ingram J., Leavens W., Wootton R., and Posner J., "The pharmacokinetics, tolerability and pharmacodynamics of tucaresol (589C80; 4[2-formyl-3-hydroxyphenoxymethyl] benzoic acid), a potential anti-sickling agent, following oral administration to healthy subjects," *Br. J. Clin. Pharmac.,* 1993; 35:419–425.

18. Sandouk P., Serrie A., Urtizberea M., Debray M., Got P., and Scherrmann M., "Morphine pharmacokinetics and pain assessment after intracerebroventricular administration in patients with terminal cancer," *Clin. Pharmacol. Ther.,* 1991; 49(4):442–448.

19. Scheinin H., Karhuvaara S., Olkkola K. T., Kallio A., Anttila M., Vuorilehto L., and Scheinin M., "Pharmacodynamics and pharmacokinetics of intramuscular dexmedetomidine," *Clin. Pharmacol. Ther.,* 1992; 52(5):537–546.

20. Shaheen O., Zmeili, Al-Qussuois Y., Arafat T., and Mouti H., "Pharmacokinetics and pharmacodynamics of two commercial oral nifedipine products," *International Journal of Clinical Pharmacology, Therapy and Toxicology,* 1991; 29(9):337–341.

21. Sjostrom P. A., Odlind B. G., and Hammarlund-Udenaes M., "Response to furosemide during dehydration with and without naproxen pretreatment of kidney donors and renal transplant recipients," *Eur. J. Clin. Pharmacol.,* 1991; 40:209–214.

22. Uematsu T., Nagashima S., Inaba H., Mizuna A., Kosuge K., and Nakashima M., "Pharmacokinetic and pharmacodynamic profiles of CS-518, a selective, long-lasting thromboxane synthase inhibitor, after single and multiple oral administration to healthy volunteers," *J. Clin. Pharmacol.,* 1994; 34:41–47.

23. Holford N. H. G. and L. B. Sheiner, "Understanding the dose-effect relationship: Clinical application of pharmacokinetic pharmacodynamic models," *Clinical Pharmacokinetics,* 1981; 6:429–453.

INTERACTIONS

CHAPTER 13

Influence of Food on Pharmacokinetics

INTRODUCTION

In general, intake of food within 30 minutes to 2 hours before an oral dose will affect the absorption of the drug [8,19–22], but the effects are unpredictable. The effects of food on oral drug absorption can be placed into four categories: unaffected, delayed, reduced, and increased absorption [18]. Food can alter drug absorption by affecting the gastrointestinal physiology [23], for example, delaying gastric emptying, increasing gastric acid secretion, stimulating bile secretion, increasing intestinal motility, and stimulating hepatic and splanchnic blood flow. Food may also interact directly with drugs, for example, chelating with the drugs [24] or solubilizing the drugs (high-fat food) [1,7].

The following are six typical drug-food interactions. First, for well-absorbed drugs (complete and fast absorption) [16,17], food frequently reduces the maximum concentration slightly and delays the time to reach the maximum concentration, but not affect the area under the concentration curve. Second, for acid-labile drugs [8,13], bioavailability may decrease because food stimulates gastric acid secretion, delays gastric emptying, and thus promotes drug degradation in the stomach. Third, for drugs with low water solubility [1,7], the fat content in food may help the drugs solubilize, increasing the bioavailability, and the mean residence time of plasma concentration profiles frequently is prolonged possibly due to a slow release of the drug from the fat content in the food. Fourth, for lipophilic basic drugs with first pass metabolism such as hydroxylation, glucuronidation, and acetylation [2,6], food may increase the bioavailability of the drugs by stimulating hepatic blood flow and reducing the first pass effect. Fifth, for controlled release formulations [15], food may alter the gastrointestinal pH values and affect the release characteristics. Sixth, for enteric coated tablets, food may delay the absorption because the tablet will not dissolve in the stomach, and it will stay there until the fasting motility pattern resumes after all the food is digested. To summarize, the key time constants in food interaction studies include the gastric emptying time, the absorption time, and the release time of drug from the fat content of food.

Some common themes in the time constant view can be observed in the food study as well as other studies. The first pass effect is a common factor in many studies. A first pass effect may be observed in both bioequivalence (Chapter 6) and food studies. The first pass effect results in a small oral bioavailability compared with intravenous administration in a bioequivalence study, while food may reduce the first pass effect and increase the oral bioavailability in a food study. A significant first pass effect may indicate a large hepatic extraction ratio and a short hepatic elimination time; in this case, metabolism may be the predominant elimination route, and any potential factor affecting metabolism, such as hepatic impairment (Chapter 18), gender (Chapter 16), and age (Chapter 15), may influence the total elimination time. A dissolution limited absorption is also a common factor in several studies: food may improve the solubility and increase the bioavailability; dissolution limited absorption will cause nonlinearity in the absorption time, which may be identified as a dose proportionality study (Chapter 7); and a large variability in absorption time will usually be observed in a bioequivalence study (Chapter 6) for a drug with poor solubility. There is frequently a similarity between the effects of food and emulsion formulation on the mean residence time of drugs with low solubility: both factors improve the solubility and tend to prolong the mean residence time.

Four models are presented in this chapter for the estimation of pharmacokinetic parameters in food interaction studies: (1) the first model describes effects of food on gastric emptying; (2) the second model describes effects of food on drug solubility; (3) the third model describes effects of food on the first pass metabolism; and (4) the fourth model describes effects of food on both first pass metabolism and drug solubility. Four simulated case studies and four literature examples are provided in this chapter to illustrate the utility of these models in food interaction studies. Additional examples of food interaction studies can be found in the literature [1–18].

PHARMACOKINETIC MODELS

This section presents four models that are useful in describing the food effects on pharmacokinetics. The goal is to establish simple relationships between time constants and measurable parameters such as (1) mean residence time, which is the sum of input and output times, and (2) area under the curves. The derivations of these relationships are straightforward and are discussed in Chapter 2.

Model 1: Effects of Food on Gastric Emptying

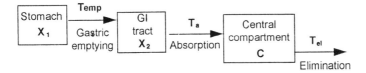

Under the fasting condition, the gastric motility consists of alternating quiescent and active phases [23]. The active phase occurs every 1 to 2 hours on the average and lasts for 5 to 20 minutes, during which time the content of the stomach is emptied into the intestine. In the fed state, the gastric motility becomes more intensive and may last continuously for several hours, depending on the size and the content of the meal. The gastric emptying of liquid (with drugs) is more rapid during the fasting state than the fed state [6,17]. Assuming gastric emptying follows first-order kinetics, then Model 1 can be used to describe the absorption process of a drug. In the model, a drug is initially in the stomach (X_1) and is constantly emptied into the intestine (X_2) with a time constant T_{emp}, where the drug is absorbed into blood (C) with a time constant T_a.

The mean residence time of the concentration profiles is simply the sum of input and output times:

$$\text{Mean residence time } (\bar{t}) = \frac{\text{AUMC}}{\text{AUC}}$$

$$= \text{ Input time } (T_{in}) + \text{ Output time } (T_{out}) = T_{emp} + T_a + T_{el} \qquad (13.1)$$

and can be estimated from the ratio of the area under the first moment curve to the area under the curve. Notice that the mean residence time is a sum of the gastric emptying time, the absorption time, and the elimination time, since the three processes are arranged in series. The difference in the mean residence time between concentration curves under the fasting and fed conditions is then

$$\bar{t}_{fed} - \bar{t}_{fast} = T_{emp,fed} - T_{emp,fast} + T_{a,fed} - T_{a,fast} \qquad (13.2)$$

Food may prolong gastric emptying and thus increase the value of T_{emp}. The absorption time constants can also be affected by food due to change in factors such as pH in the intestine, solubility of the drug in food content, improved solubility with bile salts, and degree of mixing in the intestine. The decay time of the concentration profile may be affected by food when the absorption is retarded to a degree that the absorption becomes the rate limiting step and a flip-flop occurs. The decay time constant can be estimated using a partial area under the concentration curve (see Appendix 2).

$$\frac{1}{\text{Decay time } (T_z)} = \lambda_z = 2 \frac{(t_{\text{ref}} - t_{\text{last}}) \ln (C_{t_{\text{ref}}}) - \text{AU} \ln C_{t_{\text{ref}} - t_{\text{last}}}}{(t_{\text{ref}} - t_{\text{last}})^2} \qquad (13.3)$$

The degree of absorption and renal elimination time can be estimated from the urine recovery data:

$$\text{Bioavailability } (f) = \frac{X_u}{X_0} \qquad (13.4)$$

$$\text{Renal clearance time } \left(\frac{T_{\text{el}}}{V}\right) = \frac{\text{AUC}}{X_u} \qquad (13.5)$$

Equation (13.4) applies only when the renal excretion is the predominant route of elimination.

Model 2: Effects of Food on Drug Solubility

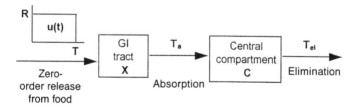

For lipophilic drugs that are poorly soluble in water, high-fat meals may improve the solubility of the drug and increase the fraction absorbed [1,7]. Frequently, as the fraction absorbed of a drug is improved by the intake of food, the peak plasma concentration of the drug is delayed substantially, the concentration profile is broadened, and the mean residence time of the concentration curve is prolonged. One possible reason for this prolonged mean residence time is that the drug is dissolved in the fat content and is slowly released into the liquid phase in the intestine for absorption. This scenario can be described by Model 2, in which the drug is released from fat at a constant rate R for a time period of T. The total amount of dose is $X_0 = R*T$. The drug is the liquid phase is subsequently absorbed by the intestine with a time constant T_a.

The mean residence time of the plasma concentration profile in the fed and fasting states is dependent only on the absorption time, the elimination time, and the releasing time.

$$\text{Mean residence time under fed condition } (\bar{t}_{fed}) = \frac{\text{AUMC}}{\text{AUC}}$$

$$= \text{Input time } (T_{fed,in}) + \text{Output time } (T_{fed,out}) = T_a + T_{el} + \frac{T}{2} \quad (13.6)$$

$$\text{Mean residence time under fast condition } (\bar{t}_{fast})$$

$$= \text{Input time } (T_{fast,in}) + \text{Output time } (T_{fast,out}) = T_a + T_{el} \quad (13.7)$$

The difference between the mean residence time of the concentration curve in the fed and fasting state is then equal to half of the releasing time:

$$\frac{\text{Release time from food } (T)}{2} = \bar{t}_{fed} - \bar{t}_{fast} \quad (13.8)$$

Model 3: Effects of Food on the First Pass Metabolism

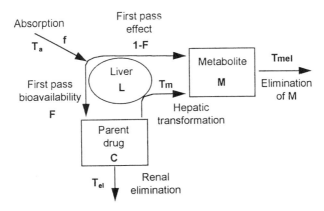

If a drug is subjected to the first pass effect, intake of food may improve the bioavailability of the drug by reducing the portion of the drug that is metabolized in the liver immediately after the absorption [3]. The pharmacokinetics of such drugs can be described by Model 3.

When the first pass effect is reduced by food, the fraction (F) that is not metabolized (by the first pass) increases; thus, the area under the drug concentration curve increases, and the area under the metabolite concentration curve decreases. As a result, the ratio of the area under the metabolite con-

centration curve to the area under the drug concentration curve decreases if
food reduces the first pass effect.

$$\frac{AUC_M}{AUC_C} = \frac{V_c T_{mel}}{V_m T_m} + \frac{V_c}{V_m}\frac{1 - FT_{mel}(T_m + T_{el})}{F}\frac{(T_m + T_{el})}{T_m T_{el}} = \frac{V_c}{V_m}\frac{1}{F}\frac{T_{mel}(T_m + T_{el})}{T_m T_{el}} - \frac{V_c T_{mel}}{V_m T_{el}}$$

$$(13.9)$$

By rearrangement of Equation (13.9), the fraction of the absorbed drug
that is not metabolized by the first pass effect can be estimated from the area
under the curve (AUC_C and AUC_M), renal clearance time of the drug
(T_{el}/V_c) and the metabolite (T_m/V_m), and total clearance time of the drug
($T_{el,t}/V_c$):

$$\frac{1}{\text{First pass bioavailability } (F)} = \left(\frac{AUC_M}{AUC_C} + \frac{T_m V_c}{T_C V_m}\right)\frac{T_{el,t} V_m}{T_{mel} V_c} \quad (13.10)$$

The mean residence of the concentration curve is the sum of input and output times (see Chapter 2):

$$\text{Mean residence time of C } (\bar{t}_C) = \frac{AUMC_C}{AUC_C}$$

$$= \text{Input time } (T_{c,in}) + \text{Output time } (T_{c,out}) = T_a + T_{el,t} \quad (13.11)$$

$$\text{Mean residence time of M } (\bar{t}_M) = \frac{AUMC_M}{AUC_M}$$

$$= \text{Input time } (T_{m,in}) + \text{Output time } (T_{m,out})$$

$$= \frac{FT_m T_{el}^2}{(T_m + T_{el})(T_{el} + T_m - FT_m)} + T_a + T_{mel} \quad (13.12)$$

where $T_{el,t} = 1/(1/T_m + 1/T_{el})$. The mean residence time of the parent
drug is not affected by a change in the first pass effect, while the mean residence time of the metabolite increases with a decrease in the first pass
effect. In the extreme case, if there is no first pass effect, the mean residence
time of the metabolite concentration curve is reduced to a sum of all time
constants involved in the model:

$$\bar{t}_M = T_{el,t} + T_a + T_{mel} \quad \text{if } F \to 1 \quad (13.13)$$

Model 4: Effects of Food on Both First Pass Metabolism and Drug Solubility

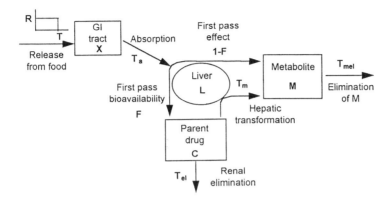

The bioavailability of lipophilic basic drugs may increase following a meal by both improved solubility and reduced first pass effect. This case can be described by Model 4, in which the drug is dissolved in the fat content of food and slowly released to the liquid phase in the intestine at a constant rate R for a time period of T. Then, the drug is absorbed by the intestine with an absorption time constant T_a. Immediately after the absorption, the drug is subjected to the first pass effect with a fraction $(1 - F)$ being metabolized. Once the drug enters the systemic circulation, it can be eliminated through renal or hepatic routes.

After a meal, the drug concentration increases, while the metabolite concentration decreases with a decrease in the first pass effect. As a result, the ratio of the area under the metabolite concentration curve to the area under the drug concentration curve decreases with a decrease in the first pass effect:

$$\frac{AUC_M}{AUC_C} = \frac{V_c T_{mel}}{V_m T_m} + \frac{V_c}{V_m} \frac{1-F}{F} \frac{T_{mel}(T_m + T_{el})}{T_m T_{el}} = \frac{V_c}{V_m} \frac{1}{F} \frac{T_{mel}(T_m + T_{el})}{T_m T_{el}} - \frac{V_c}{V_m} \frac{T_{mel}}{T_{el}}$$

$$(13.14)$$

By rearrangement of Equation (13.14), the first pass effect can be evaluated as follows:

$$\frac{1}{\text{First pass bioavailability }(F)} = \left(\frac{AUC_M}{AUC_C} + \frac{T_m V_c}{T_c V_m}\right) \frac{T_{el,t} V_m}{T_{mel} V_c} \quad (13.15)$$

The mean residence time is the sum of input and output times (see Chapter 2):

$$\text{Mean residence time of C } (\bar{t}_C) = \frac{\text{AUMC}_C}{\text{AUC}_C}$$

$$= \text{Input time } (T_{c,in}) + \text{Output time } (T_{c,out}) = T_a + T_{el,t} + \frac{T}{2} \quad (13.16)$$

$$\text{Mean residence time of M } (\bar{t}_M) = \frac{\text{AUMC}_M}{\text{AUC}_M}$$

$$= \text{Input time } (T_{m,in}) + \text{Output time } (T_{m,out})$$

$$= \frac{FT_m T_{el}^2}{(T_m + T_{el})(T_{el} + T_m - FT_m)} + T_a + T_{mel} + \frac{T}{2} \quad (13.17)$$

where $T_{el,t} = 1/(1/T_m + 1/T_{el})$. Therefore, the slow release of the drug from fat content will prolong the mean residence times of both the drug and the metabolite. A reduction in the first pass effect will not affect the mean residence time of the parent drug but will increase the mean residence time of the metabolite.

CASE STUDIES

Case 1: Food Delays Gastric Emptying

Most of the completely and rapidly absorbed drugs exhibit high dissolution, solubility, and permeability and are absorbed by the intestine immediately after gastric emptying [16,17]. Because of the short absorption time, the extent of absorption is almost complete in the first few hours after dosing. Therefore, the rate limiting step for the absorption process is the gastrc emptying. In this case, delaying gastric emptying by giving food will delay the absorption, but the extent of absorption will not increase since a complete absorption is achieved under the fasting condition. The food effects on gastric emptying can be described by Model 1, and a simulated example of plasma concentration profiles for a drug given under fasting and fed conditions is shown in Figure 13.1. It is assumed that no metabolism is involved, and the bioavailability is 100%. Only one pharmacokinetic parameter is different between the fasting and fed conditions: the gastric emptying rate constant (K_{emp}) is smaller in the fed condition. The only

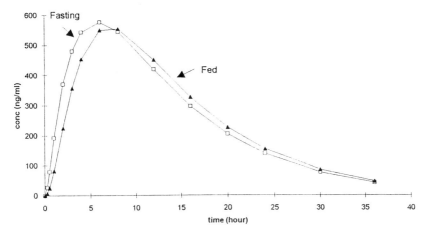

FIGURE 13.1. Simulated plasma drug concentration profiles under fasting and fed conditions using Model 1, with food delaying the gastric emptying. The time constant plot comparing the two treatments is shown in Figure 13.2. The parameters used in this simulation are fasting: $X_0 = 10$ mg, $f = 1$, $F = 1$, $V = 10$ L, $K_{emp} = 4$ hr^{-1}, $K_a = 0.3$ hr^{-1}, $K_{el} = 0.1$ hr^{-1}; fed: $X_0 = 10$ mg, $f = 1$, $F = 1$, $V = 10$ L, $K_{emp} = 0.8$ hr^{-1}, $K_a = 0.3$ hr^{-1}, $K_{el} = 0.1$ hr^{-1}.

difference in the concentration profiles between the fasting and fed conditions is that the maximum concentration is slightly decreased and the time to reach the maximum concentration is delayed by 1–2 hours under the fed condition.

The plasma drug concentration profiles under the fasting and fed conditions do not show much difference, except a slight delay of maximum concentration after a meal. Therefore, food may affect only the gastric emptying rate but not bioavailability, and the key time constant is the absorption time or the mean residence time. The estimated pharmacokinetic parameters for the above example using the time constant analysis are listed in Table 13.1, and the estimated time constants are presented in Figure 13.2. The results show little difference in the extent of absorption, indicated by the area under the plasma concentration curve. As shown in the time constant plot (Figure 13.2), the mean residence time is delayed under the fed condition, and the difference in mean residence time between the fasting and fed conditions should be equal to the difference in the emptying time $(\bar{t}_{fed} - \bar{t}_{fast} = T_{emp,fed} - T_{emp,fast})$. The normal delay in gastric emptying after a standard breakfast is about 1 hour. Therefore, if food prolongs the mean residence time of the plasma drug concentration profile by more than 2 hours, a mechanism other than the delayed gastric emptying may be responsible for the delayed absorption.

TABLE 13.1. The Estimated Time Constants of Model 1
for the Example in Figure 13.1.

Parameter	Fasting		Fed		
	Time Constant Analysis	Model Value	Time Constant Analysis	Model Value	Equation
$\bar{t}$ (hr)	14.0	13.6	14.6	14.6	(13.1)
T_z (hr)	11.1	10.0	10.5	10.0	(13.3)
AUC_C (ng·hr/L)	10,121	10,000	10,010	10,000	

Case 2: Food Improves Solubility

For lipophilic drugs with low water solubility [1,7], the dissolution or solubilization of the drugs can be the rate limiting step. Often, in these cases, the absorption is incomplete because the drug is not readily dissolved in the intestine. The fat content of food and the bile secretion stimulated after the meal may enhance the solubility of the drugs and increase the bioavailability. The delay in absorption (T_{max}) is often longer than 2 hours when the extent of absorption is enhanced by food. There are several possible mechanisms for this long delay other than an inhibited gastric empty-

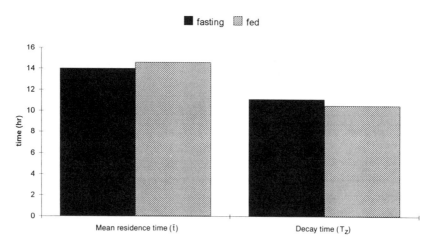

FIGURE 13.2. The time constant plot comparing the fasting and fed treatments in the example shown in Figure 13.1. The mean residence time ($\bar{t}$) is delayed under the fed condition, and the difference in mean residence time between the fasting and fed conditions should be equal to the difference in the emptying time ($\bar{t}_{fed} - \bar{t}_{fast} = T_{emp,fed} - T_{emp,fast}$).

ing: the drug is physically blocked by food in the intestine, or the drug is slowly released from the fat content (delayed absorption is also seen in the emulsion formulation [1,3]). The improved but slow absorption after a meal can be described by Model 2, assuming the drug is slowly released from the fat content in the food. Simulated plasma drug concentration profiles are shown in Figure 13.3. In this example, the difference in parameters between the fed and fasting conditions is that the releasing time of the drug in the intestine in 4 hours under the fed condition compared to a bolus under the fasting condition, and the extent of absorption is improved under the fed condition. As a result, there are significant increases in the maximum concentration and the time to reach the maximum concentration under the fed condition. The concentration profile is broader under the fed condition, which is typical for drugs with improved absorption with food.

Since there is a delay in the time to reach the maximum concentration under the fed condition compared with the fasting condition, the mean residence time is a key time constant to determine the magnitude of delay. The estimated pharmacokinetic parameters for the above example using the time constant analysis are listed in Table 13.2, and the estimated time constants are presented in Figure 13.4. The area under the concentration curve significantly increases by 60% under the fed condition, compared with the fasting condition. As shown in the time constant plot, the mean residence

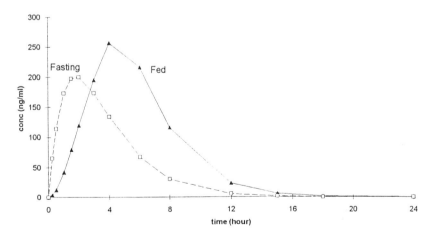

FIGURE 13.3. Simulated plasma drug concentration profiles under fasting and fed conditions using Model 2, with food improving the solubility of the drug. The time constant plot comparing the two treatments is shown in Figure 13.4. The parameters used in this simulation are fasting: $X_0 = 10$ mg, $f = 0.5$, $F = 1$, $V = 10$ L, $K_a = 0.6$ hr^{-1}, $K_{el} = 0.5$ hr^{-1}; fed: $X_0 = 10$ mg, $R = 2.5$ mg/hr, $f = 0.8$, $F = 1$, $T = 4$, $V = 10$ L, $K_a = 0.6$ hr^{-1}, $K_{el} = 0.5$ hr^{-1}.

TABLE 13.2. The Estimated Time Constants of Model 2
for the Example in Figure 13.3.

| Parameter | Fasting | | Fed | | |
	Time Constant Analysis	Model Value	Time Constant Analysis	Model Value	Equation
$\bar{t}$ (hr)	3.7	3.7	5.6	5.7	(13.6, 13.17)
T_z (hr)	2.0	2.0	2.0	2.0	(13.3)
AUC_C (ng·hr/L)	1017	1000	1620	1600	

time is delayed by 2 hours with food, and the increase in the mean residence time after the meal is equal to half the releasing time (Equation 13.8). Because of the broad peak under the fed condition and prolonged mean residence time (Figure 13.3), the delayed absorption is more likely caused by a slow release process than an inhibited gastric emptying, which should preserve the sharpness of the concentration profile (as in Figure 13.1).

Case 3: Food Reduces First Pass Metabolism

Food may increase the bioavailability of a drug by reducing the first pass effect [3]. High-protein content meals are known to increase the hepatic

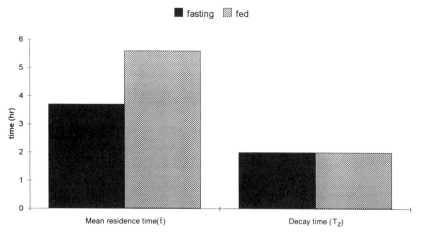

FIGURE 13.4. The time constant plot comparing the fasting and fed conditions in the example shown in Figure 13.3. The mean residence time ($\bar{t}$) is delayed by 2 hours with food, and the increase in the mean residence after the meal is equal to half the releasing time (T).

blood flow so that the absorbed drug will rapidly exit the hepatic vein and have a short exposure time to the hepatic enzymes. Lipophilic basic drugs with extensive first pass metabolism by hydroxylation, glucuronidation, and acetylation are candidates subjected to food effects [2,6]. In these cases, metabolites, as well as the parent drug concentrations, must be assayed for a meaningful pharmacokinetic analysis. The food effects on first pass metabolism can be described by Model 3, and simulated plasma concentration profiles using the model are shown in Figure 13.5. In this example, the only change in parameter after the meal is the percentage of first pass effect (from 50% to 20% metabolized). The time to reach the maximum concentration and the shape of the concentration profile for both parent and metabolite are not affected by the meal. The maximum concentration for the parent drug increases, while that of the metabolite decreases. This indicates that less of the absorbed drug is converted to the metabolite by the first pass effects after the meal.

Since the drug is metabolized quite extensively, it is reasonable to assume that the drug may be subjected to a first pass metabolism and food may reduce the first pass effect. Therefore, they key pharmacokinetic parameter in this example in the ratio of the area under the metabolite concentration curve to the area under the drug concentration curve for the evaluation of the extent of the first pass effect. The estimated pharmacokinetic parame-

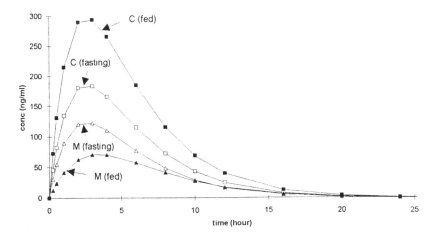

FIGURE 13.5. Simulated plasma drug concentration profiles under fasting and fed conditions using Model 3, with food reducing the first pass effect. The time constant plot comparing the two treatments is shown in Figure 13.6. The parameters used in this simulation are fasting: $X_0 = 10$ mg, $f = 0.8$, $F = 0.5$, $V = 10$ L, $V_m = 15$ L, $K_a = 0.5$ hr^{-1}, $K_{el} = 0.2$ hr^{-1}, $K_m = 0.1$ hr^{-1}, $K_{mel} = .4$ hr^{-1}; fed $X_0 = 10$ mg, $f = 0.8$, $F = 0.8$, $V = 10$ L, $V_m = 15$ L, $K_a = 0.5$ hr^{-1}, $K_{el} = 0.2$ hr^{-1}, $K_m = 0.1$ hr^{-1}, $K_{mel} = 0.4$ hr^{-1}.

*TABLE 13.3. The Estimated Time Constants of Model 2
for the Example in Figure 13.5.*

Parameter	Fasting		Fed		
	Time Constant Analysis	Model Value	Time Constant Analysis	Model Value	Equation
$\bar{t}_C$ (hr)	5.3	5.3	5.3	5.3	(13.11)
$\bar{t}_M$ (hr)	5.3	5.3	6.4	6.4	(13.12)
$T_{z,c}$ (hr)	3.45	3.33 $(T_{el,t})$	3.33	3.33 $(T_{el,t})$	(13.3)
$T_{z,m}$ (hr)	3.45	3.33 $(T_{el,t})$	3.57	3.33 $(T_{el,t})$	(13.3)
AUC_C (ng·hr/ml)	1338	1333	2141	2133	
AUC_M (ng·hr/ml)	892	888	624	622	
AUC_M/AUC_C	0.67	0.67	0.29	0.29	(13.9)

ters using the time constant analysis are listed in Table 13.3, and the estimated time constants are presented in Figure 13.6. The area under the concentration curve for the parent drug increases from 1338 to 2141 ng·hr/ml and the area under the concentration curve for the metabolite decreases from 892 to 624 ng·hr/ml under the fed condition. This indicates less

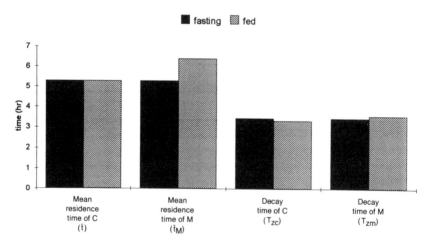

FIGURE 13.6. The time constant plot comparing the fasting and fed conditions in the example shown in Figure 13.5. The mean residence time for the parent drug ($\bar{t}_C$) does not change, while that of the metabolite ($\bar{t}_M$) increases by 1 hour because of the reduced first pass effects.

metabolite is produced by the first pass effects after a meal. The reduction in the first pass effect is confirmed by comparing the ratio of area under the curve of the metabolite to the parent drug AUC_M/AUC_C, which decreases dramatically by more than twofold from 0.67 (fasting) to 0.29 (fed).

Now let us examine the time constant plot (Figure 13.6). The mean residence time for the parent drug does not change, while that of the metabolite increases by 1 hour because of the reduced first pass effects (Equation 13.12). The delay time of the metabolite $T_{z,m}$ is dominated by $T_{el,t}$ because $T_{mel} < T_{el,t}$.

Case 4: Food Improves Solubility and Reduces First Pass Effect

The bioavailability of a lipophilic drug with the first pass effects can be enhanced after a meal by a combination of increased solubility and reduced first pass effect. This type of food effect can be described by Model 4, which is a combination of Models 2 and 3. Simulated plasma drug concentration profiles using the model are shown in Figure 13.7. The difference in parameters between the fasting and the fed conditions includes a greater fraction absorbed, a smaller first pass effect, and an additional release time from the food under the fed condition. The time to reach the maximum

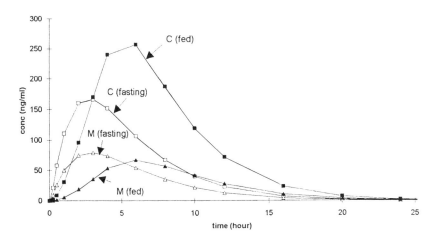

FIGURE 13.7. Simulated plasma drug concentration profiles under fasting and fed conditions using Model 4, with food improving solubility and reducing first pass effect. The time constant plot comparing the two treatments is shown in Figure 13.8. The parameters used in this simulation are fasting: $X_0 = 10$ mg, $f = 0.6$, $F = 0.6$, $R = 40$ mg/hr, $T = 0.25$ hr, $V = 10$ L, $V_m = 15$ L, $K_a = 0.5$ hr^{-1}, $K_{el} = 0.2$ hr^{-1}, $K_m = 0.1$ hr^{-1}, $K_{mel} = 0.4$ hr^{-1}; fed: $X_0 = 10$ mg, $f = 0.8$, $F = 0.8$, $R = 2.5$ mg/hr, $T = 4$ hr, $V = 10$ L, $V_m = 15$ L, $K_a = 0.5$ hr^{-1}, $K_{el} = 0.2$ hr^{-1}, $K_m = 0.1$ hr^{-1}, $K_{mel} = 0.4$ hr^{-1}.

concentrations for both parent drug and metabolite is delayed by 3 hours, which is longer than the normal food effect on gastric emptying. The area under the concentration curve for the parent drug and the maximum concentration significantly increases, while that for the metabolite remains about the same. The concentration profiles for both parent and metabolite are broader under the fed condition, suggesting a slow release process of the drug from food.

Since the time to reach the maximum concentration is significantly prolonged by food, the mean residence time is a key time constant to determine the cause of the delay (retarded gastric emptying, slow release from food, or other mechanism). In addition, the drug is likely to be subjected to a first pass effect; therefore, the ratio of the area under the metabolite concentration curve to the area under the drug concentration curve must be estimated to evaluate the food effect on the first pass metabolism. The estimated pharmacokinetic parameters for the above example using the time constant analysis are shown in Table 13.4, and the estimated time constants are presented in Figure 13.8.

The area under the concentration curve for the parent drug increases by 77% from 1204 to 2133 ng·hr/ml, while that of the metabolite only slightly changes from 602 to 623 ng·hr/ml. From this observation of the areas under the curves, one might erroneously conclude that the improved bioavailability of the parent drug after food is not due to a reduction in first pass effect since the bioavailability of the metabolite does not decrease concurrently. However, the change in the first pass effects by food can only be revealed by examining the ratio of the area under the curve for the metabo-

TABLE 13.4. The Estimated Time Constants of Model 2
for the Example in Figure 13.7.

Parameter	Fasting		Fed		Equation
	Time Constant Analysis	Model Value	Time Constant Analysis	Model Value	
$\bar{t}_C$ (hr)	5.5	5.5	7.4	7.3	(13.16)
$\bar{t}_M$ (hr)	5.7	5.7	8.4	8.4	(13.17)
$T_{z,c}$ (hr)	3.33	3.33 $(T_{el,t})$	3.33	3.33 $(T_{el,t})$	(13.3)
$T_{z,m}$ (hr)	3.33	3.33 $(T_{el,t})$	3.57	3.33 $(T_{el,t})$	(13.3)
AUC_C (ng·hr/ml)	1204	1200	2133	2133	
AUC_M (ng·hr/ml)	602	600	623	622	
AUC_M/AUC_C	0.5	0.5	0.29	0.29	(13.14)

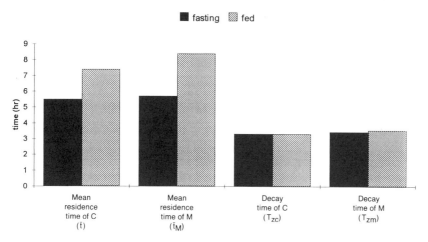

FIGURE 13.8. The time constant plot comparing the fasting and fed treatments in the example shown in Figure 13.7. The mean residence time of both parent ($\bar{t}_C$) and metabolite ($\bar{t}_M$) are delayed by food, due to the slow release of the drug from the food. The delay in mean residence time of the metabolite is longer than the delay in the parent drug because of the reduced first pass effects.

lite to the parent drug AUC_M/AUC_C [Equation (13.14)]. This ratio actually decreases by 42% after the meal, indicating a significant reduction in the first pass effects.

Now let us examine the time constant plot (Figure 13.8). The mean residence time of both parent and metabolite is delayed by food, due to the slow release of the drug from the food. The delay in mean residence time of the metabolite is longer than the delay in the parent drug because of the reduced first pass effects [Equation (13.17)].

EXAMPLES

Example 1: Food Slightly Delays Gastric Emptying

The effects of food on the absorption of moxonidine were studied in eighteen healthy male subjects [16]. Single doses of 0.2 mg moxonidine were administered under fasting and fed conditions. The mean plasma moxonidine concentration profiles following the two treatments are shown in Figure 13.9. The concentration profiles under the fasting and the fed conditions are similar. Moxonidine has a high absolute bioavailability (88%), and as typical with completely absorbed drugs, foods slightly delay and reduce its absorption.

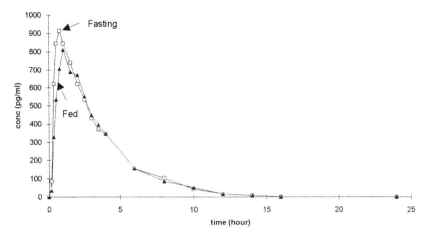

FIGURE 13.9. Mean plasma moxonidine concentration profiles following the oral administration of 0.2 mg moxonidine to eighteen healthy male subjects under fasting and fed conditions. (Reproduced with permission from Reference [16].) The time constant plot comparing the two treatments is shown in Figure 13.10.

Moxonidine is known to be completely absorbed and excreted predominantly via the renal route; therefore, the most likely food effect on the drug is a delayed gastric emptying. This is consistent with the concentration profiles in Figure 13.9. To evaluate the gastric emptying rate, the key time constant is the mean residence time. The concentration profiles of moxonidine exhibit a monoexponential terminal phase; therefore, Model 1 is used to estimate the pharmacokinetic parameters. The estimated pharmacokinetic parameters are listed in Table 13.5, and the estimated constants are pre-

TABLE 13.5. Estimated Pharmacokinetic
Parameters of Moxonidine Using Model 1.

Parameter*	Fasting	Fed	Equation
T_z (hr)	2.94	3.03	(13.3)
T_0 (hr)	0.20	0.23	(13.3)
			stripping
$\bar{t}$ (hr)	3.21	3.35	(13.1)
T_{el}/V (hr/L)	0.0375	0.0356	(13.5)
AUC (pg·hr/ml)	3452	3234	
X_u (μg)	92	91	
f	0.46	0.46	(13.4)

*Parameters estimated from the mean concentration curves or the reported mean values.

sented in Figure 13.10. There is no significant difference in all the estimated parameters. This example illustrates the typical food effects on drugs with complete absorption. The maximum concentration is slightly reduced, and the mean residence time is slightly prolonged under the fed condition, as shown in the time constant plot (Figure 13.10). However, the difference in these parameters between the fasting and fed conditions is too small to be detected statistically [16].

Example 2: Food Reduces Bioavailability

The effect of the time of food administration on the absorption of didanosine, administered as a 300-mg chewable tablet, was evaluated in ten men with positive HIV [8] Didanosine was administered (1) under fasting conditions, Didanosine was administered (1) under fasting conditions, (2) 30 minutes before a meal, (3) 1 hour before a meal, (4) 1 hour after a meal, and (5) 2 hours after a meal. The mean plasma concentration profiles of didanosine in the ten subjects following the five treatments are shown in Figure 13.11. The concentration profiles can be divided into two groups. The concentration profiles following the administration of the drug (1) under the fasting condition, (2) 30 minutes before a meal, and (3) 1 hour before a meal are similar, while the concentration profiles following the administration of the drug (4) 1 hour after a meal and (5) 2 hours after a meal are similar. The concentrations under the fasting condition and before a meal are

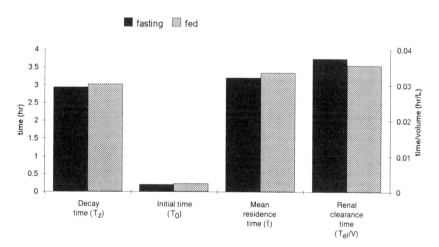

FIGURE 13.10. The time constant plot comparing the pharmacokinetics of moxonidine under fasting and fed conditions using Model 1. The mean residence time ($\bar{t}$) is slightly prolonged under the fed condition.

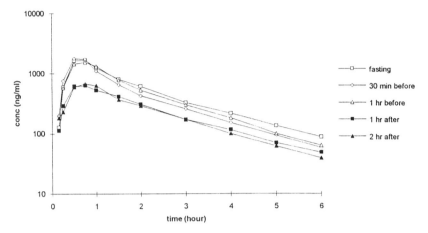

FIGURE 13.11. Mean plasma didanosine concentration profiles following the oral administration of 300 mg didanosine to ten subjects with positive HIV under fasting conditions and at various times relative to a meal. (Reproduced from Reference [8] with permission.) The time constant plot comparing the five treatments is shown in Figure 13.12.

higher than those after a meal. Therefore, food reduces the bioavailability of didanosine, and the food effects may last at least 2 hours after a meal.

Based on the concentration profiles in Figure 13.11, it is clear that food reduces the bioavailability of the drug. However, there is no shift of the concentration profile by food. Therefore, the key pharmacokinetic parameter in this example is the area under the curve to assess the change in bioavailability after a meal. The pharmacokinetic parameters of didanosine are estimated using Model 1, since the concentration profiles follow a monoexponential terminal phase. The estimated parameters are listed in Table 13.6, and the estimated time constants are presented in Figure 13.12.

TABLE 13.6. Estimated Pharmacokinetic Parameters
of Didanosine Using Model 1.

Parameter*	Fasting	30 min Before	1 hr Before	1 hr After	2 hr After	Equation
T_z (hr)	1.92	1.96	1.85	2.0	1.92	(13.3)
$\bar{t}$ (hr)	2.11	1.85	1.94	2.31	2.15	(13.1)
T_{el}/V (min/ml)	0.00272	0.00281	0.00299	0.00282	0.00278	(13.5)
AUC (ng·hr/ml)	3141	2690	2824	1414	1400	
X_u (mg)	65.1	57.3	57.9	28.8	28.8	
f	0.22	0.19	0.19	0.096	0.096	(13.4)

*Parameters estimated from the mean concentration curves or the reported mean values.

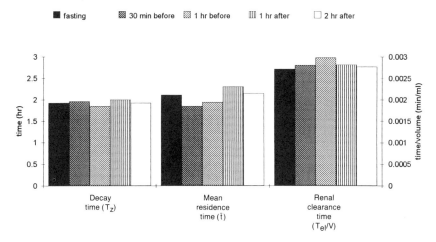

FIGURE 13.12. The time constant plot of didanosine comparing the fasting and fed conditions using Model 1. The renal elimination time (T_{el}/V) and decay time (T_z) are similar after the five treatments, indicating that in this case the elimination is not affected by the food.

The area under the concentration curve is reduced when the drug is dosed 1 hour and 2 hours after a meal, compared to the fasting condition. In general, a decrease in area under the curve may be due to reduced fraction absorbed, increased first pass effect, increased volume of distribution, or decreased elimination time. However, food in most cases affect only the fraction absorbed and the first pass effect. As shown in the time constant plot (Figure 13.12), the renal elimination time and decay time are similar after the five treatments, indicating that in this case the elimination is not affected by the food. The cumulative urine recovery of the drug under the fed conditions decreases proportionally with the decrease in the area under the curve, indicating a reduction in the fraction absorbed by food. Didanosine is acid-labile and may be hydrolyzed by the stomach acid, which is increased by food [8]. This may be responsible for the reduced bioavailability under the fed conditions. Other possible mechanisms of the reduced bioavailability after a meal include competition of food constituents with didanosine for transport carrier system in the intestine or interaction of the drug with the food components. To summarize, to avoid any reduction in bioavailability, the drug should not be given with 2 hours after a meal, as suggested in Reference [8].

Example 3: Food Improves Solubility

The bioavailability of a single dose of 100 mg danazol delivered from a capsule and an emulsion formulation was studied in eleven healthy female subjects under both fasting and fed conditions [1]. The mean plasma concentration profiles of danazol after the four treatments are shown in Figure 13.13. Danazol is poorly soluble in water, and clearly, the emulsion formulation improves the absorption over the capsule under the fasting condition. Food increases the bioavailability of danazol in capsule to almost the same degree as the emulsion formulation. There seems to be a shift of the concentration profiles to the right as the bioavailability increases. However, food does not have much effect on the concentration profile of the emulsion formulation, and this is similar to the typical food effect on well-absorbed drugs.

The time to reach the maximum concentration is significantly delayed by food; therefore, the mean residence time is a key time constant to assess the magnitude of the delay. Since danazol is a poorly soluble drug, its pharmacokinetic parameters under the fed and fasting conditions can be estimated using Model 2. The estimated pharmacokinetic parameters are listed in Table 13.7, and the estimated time constants are presented in Figure 13.14. The intake of food improves the bioavailability of both capsule and emulsion formulations. The emulsion formulation improves the bioavailability 3.8-fold over the capsule, and food further increases the absorption of the emulsion formulation by a small margin.

Now let us examine the time constant plot (Figure 13.14). The mean residence time of the concentration profile under the fed conditions is sig-

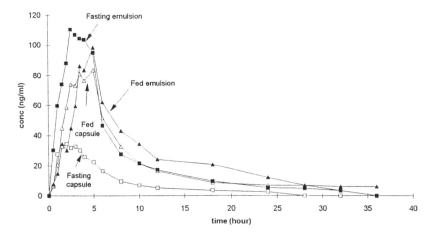

FIGURE 13.13. Mean plasma danazol concentration profiles following the oral administration of 100 mg danazol (capsule and emulsion) to eleven healthy subjects under fed and fasting conditions. (Reproduced from Reference [1] with permission.) The time constant plot comparing the four treatments is shown in Figure 13.14.

TABLE 13.7. Estimated Pharmacokinetic
Parameters of Danazol Using Model 2.

Parameter*	Fasting Capsule	Fed Capsule	Fasting Emulsion	Fed Emulsion	Equation
T_z (hr)	6.25	7.14	5.88	10.0	(13.3)
$\bar{t}$ (hr)	7.06	8.96	7.63	11.05	(13.6, 13.7)
AUC (ng·hr/ml)	204	639	779	844	

*Parameters estimated from the mean concentration curves or the reported mean values.

nificantly longer than that under the fasting condition, especially for the emulsion formulation. This is probably due to a slow gastric emptying under the fed condition and a slow release of the drug from fat content in the food. The prolongation of the mean residence time under the fed condition in this example is more significant than that in Examples 1 and 2. Therefore, mechanisms (specific to danazol) other than a slow gastric emptying must be responsible for the delayed absorption of danazol by food.

The decay times of the concentration profile following the administration of emulsion formulation under the fed conditions are longer than the decay time in other treatments. This is probably due to (1) a slow release of the

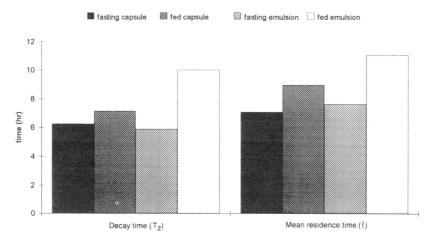

FIGURE 13.14. The time constant plot of danazol comparing capsule and emulsion formulations under the fasting and fed treatments using Model 2. The mean residence time ($\bar{t}$) of the concentration profile under the fed conditions is significantly longer than that under the fasting condition, especially for the emulsion formulation. The decay times (T_z) of the concentration profile following the administration of emulsion formulation under the fed conditions are longer than the decay times in other treatments.

drug in the intestine becoming the rate limiting step or (2) a large estimation error of the decay time resulting from the erratic terminal phase. To summarize, food significantly increases the bioavailability and delays the absorption of danazol administered as a capsule formulation. However, the food effect on the bioavailability of emulsion formulation seems minimal.

Example 4: Food Reduces First Pass Effect

The effects of food on the bioavailability of fenretinide and its metabolite were examined in two separate studies [3]. In study A, thirteen healthy subjects received three treatments: (1) 300-mg capsule under fasting conditions, (2) a 300-mg capsule after a high-fat breakfast, and (3) a 300-mg neutral suspension under fasting conditions. In study B, fifteen subjects received 300 mg fenretinide after three different test meals: high-fat, high-protein, and high-carbohydrate. The mean plasma concentration of fenretinide and its metabolite MPR after the six treatments is shown in Figures 13.15–13.18. In study A, the suspension formulation improves the bioavailability of fenretinide over the capsule, and food further increases the absorption. There is a shift in the peak concentration to the right after the administration of the suspension formulation compared with the concentration profile after the administration of the capsule, indicating a delayed absorption with the suspension formulation. In study B, the ab-

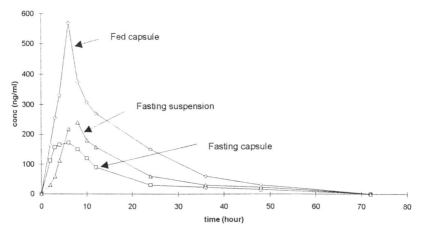

FIGURE 13.15. Mean plasma fenretinide concentration profiles following the oral administration of 300 mg fenretinide to thirteen healthy subjects in three treatments: (1) a 300-mg capsule under fasting condition, (2) a 300-mg capsule after a high-fat breakfast, and (3) 300-mg neutral oil suspension under fasting condition. (Reproduced from Reference [3] with permission.) The time constant plot comparing the three treatments is shown in Figure 13.19.

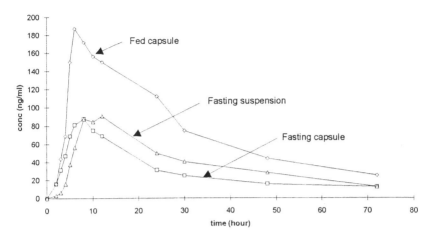

FIGURE 13.16. Mean plasma MPR concentration profiles following the oral administration of 300 mg fenretinide to 13 healthy subjects in three treatments: (1) a 300 mg capsule under fasting condition, (2) a 300 mg capsule after a high-fat breakfast, and (3) 300 mg neutral oil suspension under fasting condition. (Reproduced from Reference [3] with permission.)

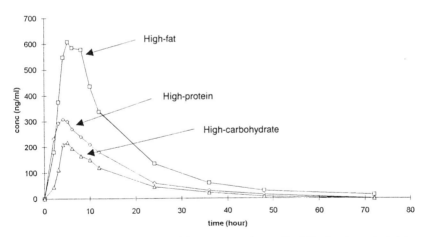

FIGURE 13.17. Mean plasma fenretinide concentration profiles following the oral administration of a 300-mg fenretinide capsule to fifteen healthy subjects after three test meals: (1) high-fat, (2) high-protein, and (3) high-carbohydrate. (Reproduced from Reference [3] with permission.)

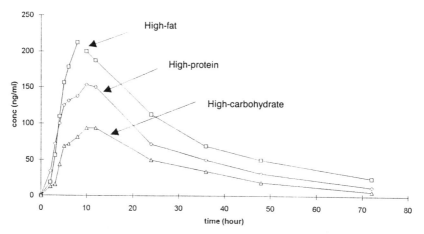

FIGURE 13.18. Mean plasma MPR concentration profiles following the oral administration of a 300-mg fenretinide capsule to fifteen healthy subjects after three test meals: (1) high-fat, (2) high-protein, and (3) high-carbohydrate. (Reproduced from Reference [3] with permission.)

sorption after the high-fat meal is much greater than that after the high-protein or the high-carbohydrate meals, while the bioavailability after the high-protein meal is better than that after the high-carbohydrate meal.

Since (1) the first pass effect of fenretinide may be affected by the intake of food and (2) the plasma concentration profiles show a broad profile after a high-fat meal compared with the low-fat meal and fasting conditions, Model 4 is used for the estimation of the pharmacokinetic parameters of fenretinide. The estimated pharmacokinetic parameters are listed in Table 13.8, and the estimated time constants are presented in Figure 13.19. In study A, the suspension formulation increase the area under the curve by 40% over the capsule, while food improves the bioavailability of capsule formulation by 188%. The first pass effect is slightly reduced by the high-fat breakfast in study A, according to the ratio of area under the metabolite concentration curve to the area under the parent drug concentration curve.

Now let us examine the time constant plot (Figure 13.19). The mean residence time increases with suspension formulation or food, suggesting the possibility of a slow release of the drug from the suspension solution and food in the intestine. In study B, the area under the curve after the high-fat meal is the greatest, and that after the high-carbohydrate meal is the lowest among all three treatments. The mean residence time after the high-fat meal is also prolonged as in study A. The ratio of AUC_M/AUC_C decreases after the high-fat meal compared with the other two treatments, indicating a possible reduction in the first pass effect after the high-fat meal. Notice that the

TABLE 13.8. Estimated Pharmacokinetic Parameters of Fenretinide Using Model 2.

Parameter*	Study A			Study B			Equation
	Fasting (capsule)	High-Fat Breakfast (capsule)	Fasting (suspension)	High-Fat Meal (capsule)	High-Protein Meal (capsule)	High-Carbohydrate Meal (capsule)	
T_{zc} (hr)	13.3	15.6	13.5	12.9	12.9	12.7	(13.3)
T_{zm} (hr)	24.4	32.3	34.5	27.8	23.8	23.8	(13.3)
$\bar{t}_C$ (hr)	15.9	16.5	17.8	16.0	14.2	14.8	(13.11)
$\bar{t}_M$ (hr)	24.6	25.9	27.4	25.0	23.1	23.5	(13.12)
AUC_C (ng·hr/ml)	2908	8396	4102	9382	4920	3230	
AUC_M (ng·hr/ml)	2284	5673	2848	5076	3664	2251	
AUC_M/AUC_C	0.79	0.68	0.69	0.54	0.75	0.70	(13.9)

*Parameters estimated from the mean concentration curves or the reported mean values.

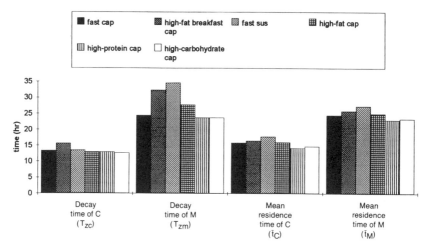

FIGURE 13.19. The time constant plot of fenretinide comparing the capsule and suspension formulations under six treatments using Model 2. The mean residence time ($\bar{t}_C$) increases with suspension formulation or food, suggesting the possibility of a slow release of the drug from the suspension solution and food in the intestine.

ratio AUC_M/AUC_C after the high-protein and high-carbohydrate meals in study B are similar to the ratio AUC_M/AUC_C under the fasting condition in study A. To summarize, fenretinide can be administered with a meal combining protein, fat, and carbohydrate to improve the bioavailability of the drug, as suggested in Reference [3].

REFERENCES

1. Charman W. N., Rogge M. C., Boddy A. W., and Berger B. M., "Effect of food and a monoglyceride emulsion formulation on danazol bioavailability," *J. Clin. Pharmacol.*, 1993, 33:381–386.

2. Degen P. H., Cardot J. M., Czendlik C., and Dieterle W., "Influence of food on the disposition of the monoamine oxidase-a inhibitor brofaromin in healthy volunteers," *Biopharmaceutics & Drug Disposition*, 1993; 14:209–215.

3. Doose, D. R., Minn F. L., Stellar S., and Nayak R. K., "Effects of meals and meal composition on the bioavailability of fenretinide," *J. Clin. Pharmacol.*, 1992; 32:1089–1095.

4. Granneman G. R. and Mukherjee D., "The effect of food on the bioavailability of temafloxacin," *Clin. Pharmacokinet.*, 1992; 22(suppl. 1):48–56.

5. Hilleman D. E., Mohiuddin S. M., Destache C. J., Stoysich A. M., Nipper H. C., and Malesker M. A., "Impact of food on the bioavailability of encainide," *J. Clin. Pharmacol.*, 1992; 32:833–837.

6. Ingwersen S. H., Matt T. G. K., and Larsen J. J., "Food intake increases the relative oral bioavailability of vanoxerine," *Br. J. Clin. Pharmac.*, 1993; 35:308–310.

7. Kaniwa N., Ogata H., Aoyagi N., Ejima A., Takahashi T., Uezono Y., and Imazato Y., "Effect of food on the bioavailability of cyclandelate from commercial capsules," *Clin. Pharmacol. Ther.*, June 1991; 641–647.

8. Knupp, C. A., Milbrath R., and Barbhaiya R. H., "Effect of time of food administration on the bioavailability of didanosine from a chewable tablet formulation," *J. Clin. Pharmacol.*, 1993; 33:568–573.

9. Kopitar Z., Vrhovac B., Povsic L., Plavsic F., and Francetic I., "The effect of food and metoclopramide on the pharmacokinetics and side effects on bromocriptine," *European Journal of Drug Metabolism and Pharmacokinetics*, 1991; 16(3):177–181.

10. Levine M. A. H., Walker S. H., and Paton T. W., "The effect of food or sucralfate on the bioavailability of S(+) and R(−) enantiomers of ibuprofen," *J. Clin. Pharmacol.*, 1992; 32:1110–1114.

11. Ohdo S., Nakano S., and Ogawa N., "Circadian change of valproate kinetics depending on meal condition in human," *J. Clin. Pharmacol.*, 1992; 32:822–826.

12. Pieniaszek, H. J., Jr., Rakestraw D. C., Schary W. L., and Williams R. L., "Influence of food on the oral absorption and bioavailability of moricizine," *J. Clin. Pharmacol.*, 1991; 31:792–795.

13. Shyu W. C., Knupp C. A., Pittman K. A., Dunkle L., and Barbhaiya R. N., "Food-induced reduction in bioavailability of didanosine," *Clin. Pharmacol. Ther.*, November 1991; 503–507.

14. Tay L. K., Sciacca M. A., Sostrin M. B., Farmen R. H., and Pittman K. A., "Effect of food on the bioavailability of gepirone in humans," *J. Clin. Pharmacol.*, 1993; 33:631–635.

15. Thakker K. M., Mangat S., Wagner W., Castellana J., and Kochak M., "Effect of food and relative bioavailability following single doses of diclofenac 150 mg hydrogel bead (HGB) capsules in healthy humans," *Biopharmaceutics & Drug Disposition*, 1992; 13:327–335.

16. Theodor R. A., Weimann H. J., Weber W., Muller M., and Michaelis K., "Influence of food on the oral bioavailability of moxonidine," *European Journal of Drug Metabolism and Pharmacokinetics*, 1992; 17(1):61–66.

17. Van Harten J., Van Bemmel P., Dobrinska M. R., Ferguson R. K., and Raghoebar M., "Bioavailability of fluvoxamine given with and without food," *Biopharmaceutics & Drug Disposition*, 1991; 12:571–576.

18. Welling P. G., "Interactions affecting drug absorption," *Clin. Pharmacokin.*, 1984; 9:404.

19. Birkett D. J., Lines D. R., Kneebone G. M., Green B., and Hughes H. M., "Effects of time of dose in relation to food on the bioavailability of theo-dur sprinkle at steady state in asthmatic children," *Clin. Pharmacol. Ther.*, 1989; 45(3):305–311.

20. Baruzzi A., Contin M., Riva R., Proaccianti G., Albani F., Tonello C., Zoni E., and Martinelli P., "Influence of meal ingestion time on pharmacokinetics of orally administered levodopa in parkinsonian patients," *Clin. Neuropharmacol.*, 1987; 10(6):527–537.

21. Lohmann A., Dingler E., Sommer W., Schaffler K., Wober W., and Schmidt W., "Bioavailability of vinpocetine and interference of the time of application with food intake," *Arznemittelforschung*, 1992; 42(7):914–917.

22. Washington N., Greaves J. L., and Wilson C. G., "Effect of time of dosing relative to a meal on the raft formation on an anti-reflux agent," *J. Pharm. Pharmacol.*, 1990; 42(1):50–53.

23. Anderson K. E., "Influences of diet and nutrition on clinical pharmacokinetics," *Clin. Pharmacokinet.*, 1988; 14:325–346.

24. Banker G. S. and Rhodes C. T., *Modern Pharmaceutics,* Marcel Dekker, Inc., 1979.

Effects of Drug Interactions on Pharmacokinetics

INTRODUCTION

Coadministration of one drug may influence potentially every aspect of the pharmacokinetics of another drug, including absorption, distribution, metabolism, and excretion. Absorption may be affected by binding or chelating of drugs in the gastrointestinal tract or inhibition or increase of gastrointestinal motility as a result of drug interaction [5]. The extent of protein binding may be affected by competition between different drugs for binding sites [3,12]. Drug interaction affecting the renal excretion of a drug may involve change in tubular reabsorption, tubular secretion, glomerular filtration, or renal blood flow [9]. Metabolism of a drug may be induced or inhibited by the coadministration of another drug [1].

Some common themes in the time constant view can be observed in the drug interaction study as well as other studies. The predominant route of elimination is a common factor among many studies. The predominant route of elimination can be determined in a drug interaction study, when the hepatic time or the renal elimination time is affected. If the hepatic elimination time is affected by the drug interaction while the total elimination time does not change accordingly, the hepatic elimination is not significant compared with other routes. On the other hand, if the total elimination time changes to a similar degree as the change in the hepatic elimination time in a drug interaction study, the hepatic elimination is the predominant elimination route. The role of renal elimination can be determined similarly. If metabolism is the predominant elimination route, total elimination time and decay time will be influenced by factors affecting metabolism, such as those in hepatic impairment (Chapter 18), dose proportionality (Chapter 7), gender (Chapter 16), and age (Chapter 15) studies. Similarly, if renal excretion is the predominant elimination route, total elimination time and decay time should be the key time constants when renal function may be altered, such as in renal impairment (Chapter 17) and age (Chapter 15) studies. Protein binding is another common factor. Altered protein binding usually coexists with additional change in pharmacokinetic processes, such as prolonged renal elimination time in renal impairment study (Chapter 17), increased hepatic elimination time in hepatic disease study (Chapter 18), and altered absorption in Crohn's disease (Chapter 19). However, a drug interaction study involving a protein binding displacer is frequently without other change in pharmacokinetic process; therefore, it can be a good opportunity to examine the effect of protein binding alone on pharmacokinetics of the drug. The key questions to be answered include the following: (1) Does the altered protein binding affect volume of distribution? (2) Does it affect renal elimination or hepatic elimination? (3) In the case of drugs with biexponential decay, does the altered protein binding affect the distribution time (affecting the first decay time) or the redistribution time (affecting the second decay time)? The answers to these questions will also be common themes in other studies where protein binding is altered.

Three models are discussed in this chapter: (1) the first one describes the drug interaction affecting absorption and renal excretion; (2) the second model describes the drug interaction affecting protein binding; and (3) the third model describes the drug interaction involving metabolism. Three simulated case studies and four literature examples are discussed in this chapter to illustrate the utility of these models. Additional examples of drug interaction studies can be found in the literature [1–12].

PHARMACOKINETIC MODELS

This section presents three models that are useful in describing drug interactions affecting pharmacokinetics. The goal is to establish simple relationships between time constants and measurable parameters such as (1) mean residence time, which is the sum of input and output times, and (2) area under the curves. The derivations of these relationships are straightforward and are discussed in Chapter 2.

Model 1: Drug Interaction Affecting Absorption and Renal Excretion

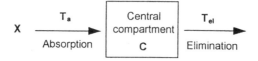

When the absorption or elimination of a drug is affected by the presence of another drug and the elimination of the affected drug exhibits a monoexponential phase, then Model 1 can be used to estimate the pharmacokinetic parameters in the drug interaction study. In this model, metabolism and distribution are not involved. The key pharmacokinetic parameters estimated from this model following the oral administration of a drug are listed below. The mean residence time is simply the sum of input and output times:

$$\text{Mean residence time } (\bar{t}) = \frac{\text{AUMC}}{\text{AUC}}$$

$$= \text{Input time } (T_{in}) + \text{Output time } (T_{out}) = T_a + T_{el} \quad (14.1)$$

The decay time can be estimated from the following equation:

$$\frac{1}{\text{Decay time } (T_z)} = \lambda_z = 2 \frac{(t_{ref} - t_{last}) \ln (C_{t_{ref}}) - \text{AU} \ln C_{t_{ref} - t_{last}}}{(t_{ref} - t_{last})^2} \quad (14.2)$$

The estimation of the decay time T_z is described in detail in Appendix 2. The mean residence time of a drug may be affected by another drug, if the absorption time or the elimination time changes after the coadministration.

Model 2: Drug Interaction Affecting Protein Binding

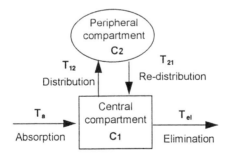

Drug interactions may involve competition between drugs for protein binding sites or inhibition of protein binding of a drug by another [3,12]. The results of altered protein binding include change in the following parameters: volume of distribution, free fraction of the drug in the plasma, elimination time constant, and distribution time constants. Drug interactions involving altered protein binding can be described by a two-compartment model, if the drugs show a biexponential terminal phase. The mean residence time estimated from the model for an oral administration is the sum of input and output times (see Chapter 2):

$$\text{Mean residence time in the central compartment } (\bar{t}_{Cl}) = \frac{\text{AUMC}_{Cl}}{\text{AUC}_{Cl}}$$

$$= \text{Input time } (T_{cl,in}) + \text{Output time } (T_{cl,out}) = T_a + T_{el} + T_{el}\frac{T_{21}}{T_{12}} \quad (14.3)$$

The mean residence time may be affected by an altered protein binding, if the distribution time constant or the elimination time constant changes.

Model 3: Drug Interaction Involving Metabolism

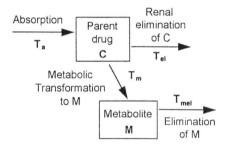

Drug interaction may involve metabolism, where the hepatic enzymes may be inhibited or induced [1]. When the metabolism of a drug is suspected to be affected by the coadministration of another drug, metabolites, as well as the parent drug, should be assayed, and urine samples should also be collected and assayed. The importance of the urine data is illustrated by Example 2 of this chapter.

The mean residence time of the parent drug and the metabolite is the sum of input and output times:

$$\text{Mean residence time of C } (\bar{t}_C) = \frac{\text{AUMC}_C}{\text{AUC}_C}$$

$$= \text{Input time } (T_{c,in}) + \text{Output time } (T_{c,out}) = T_a + T_{el,t} \quad (14.4)$$

$$\text{Mean residence time of M } (\bar{t}_M) = \frac{\text{AUMC}_M}{\text{AUC}_M}$$

$$= \text{Input time } (T_{m,in}) + \text{Output time } (T_{m,out}) = T_a + T_{el,t} + T_{mel} \quad (14.5)$$

where $T_{el,t} = 1/(1/T_{el} + 1/T_m)$. The elimination time constant of the metabolite can be obtained from the difference between the mean residence time of the metabolite and the parent drug:

$$\text{Elimination time of metabolite } (T_{mel}) = \bar{t}_M - \bar{t}_C \qquad (14.6)$$

The accuracy of estimation of T_{mel} from Equation (14.6) depends on the difference between the mean residence of the metabolite and the parent drug. The error involved in the estimated T_{mel} increases with decreasing difference in the mean residence time between the parent and the metabolite.

The ratio of the area under the metabolite concentration curve to the area under the parent drug curve gives the ratio of elimination time of the metabolite to the formation time of the metabolite.

$$\frac{AUC_M}{AUC_C} = \frac{V_c T_{mel}}{V_m T_m} = \frac{\text{Elimination clearance time of metabolite}}{\text{Formation clearance time toward metabolite}}$$

$$(14.7)$$

The above equation is useful when only one of T_m or T_{mel} is affected by the drug interaction. If both formation and elimination time of the metabolite are affected by the drug interaction, the renal elimination time of the metabolite and the hepatic elimination time of the parent drug should be calculated separately by the following equations:

$$\text{Renal clearance time } \left(\frac{T_{el}}{V}\right) = \frac{AUC}{X_u} \qquad (14.8)$$

$$\text{Hepatic clearance time } \left(\frac{T_m}{V_c}\right) = \frac{AUC_C}{X_{um}} \qquad (14.9)$$

Therefore, it is important to have urine data in a drug interaction study when the metabolism is affected. The hepatic elimination time can also be estimated from the following equation [obtained by combining Equations (14.6) and (14.7)]:

$$\begin{array}{l}\text{Normalized hepatic} \\ \text{elimination time}\end{array} \left(\frac{T_m V_m}{V_c}\right) = T_{mel}\frac{AUC_C}{AUC_M} = (\bar{t}_M - \bar{t}_C)\frac{AUC_C}{AUC_M} \quad (14.10)$$

CASE STUDIES

Case 1: Drug Interaction Affecting Absorption

The rate and extent of absorption of a drug may be affected by the presence of another drug [5]. The interaction may be due to chelating or binding between the two drugs, change in gastrointestinal pH, or change in gastric emptying and gastrointestinal motility. The simplest model to describe this phenomena is a one-compartment model (Model 1). Simulated plasma concentration profiles using the model are shown in Figure 14.1. The key pharmacokinetic parameters in this example, the fraction absorbed and the absorption time constant, decrease when the affected drug A is coadministered with drug B.

Clearly, the coadministration of drug B reduces the area under the concentration curve of drug A. However, since the time to reach the maximum concentration and the terminal phase of drug A are not changed by drug B, the elimination of drug A may not be affected by the coadministration. Therefore, the potential interaction, which affects the area under the curve, may exist at the level of the extent of absorption or the volume of distribution. The pharmacokinetic parameters are estimated using the time constant analysis, assuming it is known that the absorption time is shorter than

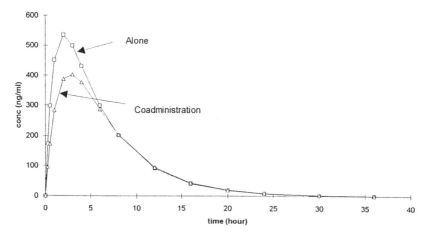

FIGURE 14.1. The simulated plasma drug concentration profiles using Model 1 for a drug administered alone or with another drug, illustrating drug interaction affecting absorption. The time constant plot comparing the two treatments is shown in Figure 14.2. The parameters used in the simulation are administered alone: $X_0 = 10$ mg, $f = 0.8$, $F = 1$, $V = 10$ L, $K_a = 1$ hr^{-1}, $K_{el} = 0.2$ hr^{-1}; coadministration: $X_0 = 10$ mg, $f = 0.7$, $F = 1$, $V = 10$ L, $K_a = 0.6$ hr^{-1}, $K_{el} = 0.2$ hr^{-1}.

TABLE 14.1. *The Estimated Pharmacokinetic Parameters of Model 1 for the Example in Figure 14.1.*

| Parameter | Administered Alone | | Coadministration | | |
	Time Constant Analysis	Model Value	Time Constant Analysis	Model Value	Equation
T_a (hr)	1.06	1.0	1.75	1.67	(14.1)
T_{el} (hr)	5.0	5.0	5.0	5.0	(14.2)
$\bar{t}$ (hr)	5.9	6	6.6	6.7	(14.1)
AUC (ng·hr/L)	4037	4000	3532	3500	

the elimination time and the elimination time dominates the decay time of the terminal phase (no flip-flop). The estimated pharmacokinetic parameters are listed in Table 14.1, and the estimated time constants are presented in Figure 14.2. The area under the curve decreases from 4037 to 3532 due to a decrease in the extent of absorption. The decrease in the area under the concentration curve is not likely caused by a reduction in protein binding due to drug interaction because the renal elimination time does not change (Figure 14.2). (A reduction in protein binding frequently results in a decrease in the renal elimination time.)

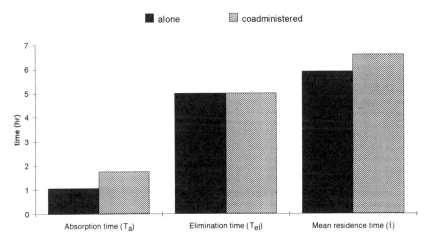

FIGURE 14.2. The time constant plot comparing the pharmacokinetics of a drug administered alone or with another drug in the example shown in Figure 14.1. The absorption time (T_a) increases when the drug is coadministered with the other drug, indicating drug interaction affecting absorption.

Case 2: Drug Interaction Affecting Protein Binding

One drug may affect the protein binding of another drug by competitive displacement [3,12]. As a result, the apparent volume of distribution of the affected drug may drop significantly, and the central compartment volume may also decrease. The unbound fraction of the drug in the plasma increases due to the displacement, and consequently, both distribution and elimination time constants decrease. Model 2 is used to describe the drug interaction affecting protein binding. Simulated plasma concentration profiles of a drug administered alone and with a protein binding displacer are shown in Figure 14.3. In this example, as a result of reduced protein binding, the renal elimination rate constant and the distribution rate constant of drug A increase when the drug is coadministered with drug B. Consequently, the plasma concentration of drug A decreases due to an increase in the peripheral distribution.

The lowering of the concentration of drug A after the coadministration with drug B implies a possibility of increased volume of distribution of A as a result of interaction. The estimated pharmacokinetic parameters are listed in Table 14.2, and the estimated time constants are presented in Figure 14.4.

Now let us examine the time constant plot (Figure 14.4). The decrease in

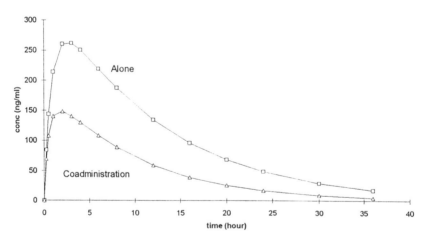

FIGURE 14.3. The simulated plasma drug concentration profiles using Model 2 for a drug administered alone or with another drug, illustrating drug interaction affecting protein binding. The time constant plot comparing the two treatments is shown in Figure 14.4. The parameters used in this simulation are administered alone: $X_0 = 10$ mg, $f = 0.8$, $F = 1$, $V_1 = 10$ L, $V_2 = 20$ L, $K_a = 0.5$ hr^{-1}, $K_{el} = 0.2$ hr^{-1}, $K_{12} = 0.7$ hr^{-1}, $K_{21} = 0.6$ hr^{-1}; coadministration: $X_0 = 10$ mg, $f = 0.8$, $F = 1$, $V_1 = 10$ L, $V_2 = 20$ L, $K_a = 0.5$ hr^{-1}, $K_{el} = 0.4$ hr^{-1}, $K_{12} = 1.4$ hr^{-1}, $K_{21} = 0.6$ hr^{-1}.

TABLE 14.2. *The Estimated Pharmacokinetic Parameters of Model 2 for the Example in Figure 14.2.*

| Parameter | Administered Alone | | Coadministration | | Equation |
	Time Constant Analysis	Model Value	Time Constant Analysis	Model Value	
T_z (hr)	11.4	11.8	9.1	9.6	(14.2)
$\bar{t}$ (hr)	12.7	12.8	10.2	10.3	(14.3)
AUC (ng·hr/L)	4003	4000	1824	1818	

the area under the curve when the drug is coadministered with the displacer is due to a decrease in T_{el}, secondary to the decrease in protein binding. The ratio of the areas under the curves between the two treatments gives the ratio of the elimination times, assuming the bioavailability of the drug is not affected by the protein displacer. However, the ratio of the decay time ($= 1.25$) is not equal to the ratio of elimination time ($= 2.19$) between the two treatments, because the decay time is a function of distribution as well as elimination. The possibility that the decrease in AUC is a result of decreased absorption can be excluded by taking urine samples and comparing the cumulated amount of drug in the urine after the two treatments.

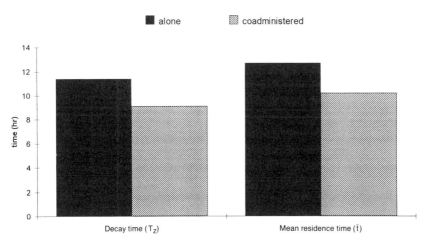

FIGURE 14.4. The time constant plot comparing the pharmacokinetics of a drug administered alone or with another drug in the example shown in Figure 14.3. A decrease in T_z occurs, secondary to the decrease in protein binding.

Case 3: Drug Interaction Affecting Metabolism

Drug interaction may also involve metabolism [1], which can be either induced or inhibited. In this example, a drug has two metabolites, M1 and M2, and the metabolic pathway to M1 is affected by coadministration of a metabolic inhibitor, while the other metabolic pathway (to M2) is not affected. The elimination time is shorter than the absorption time due to a fast metabolism, and a flip-flop of the concentration profile occurs. The simulated plasma drug concentration profiles of the drug and metabolites M1 and M2 using Model 3 are shown in Figure 14.5. The concentrations of the parent drug and metabolite M2 increase after the drug interaction, while the concentration of metabolite M1 decreases.

To identify and quantify an interaction involving metabolism, the key time constant is the hepatic elimination time. Therefore, the metabolite concentrations must be measured, since they are needed to determine the hepatic elimination time. The estimated pharmacokinetic parameters using the time constant analysis are listed in Table 14.3; the estimated time constants are presented in Figure 14.6.

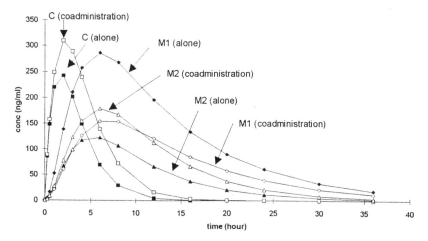

FIGURE 14.5. The simulated plasma drug concentration profiles using Model 3 for a drug administered alone or with another drug, illustrating drug interaction affecting metabolism. The time constant plot comparing the two treatments is shown in Figure 14.6. The parameters used in the simulation are dose alone: $X_0 = 10$ mg, $f^*F = 0.8$, $V_c = 10$ L, $V_m = 10$ L, $K_a = 0.5$ hr^{-1}, $K_{el} = 0.1$ hr^{-1}, $K_{m1} = 0.4$ hr^{-1}, $K_{m2} = 0.2$ hr^{-1}, $K_{mel1} = 0.1$ hr^{-1}, $K_{mel2} = 0.15$ hr^{-1}; coadministration: $X_0 = 10$ mg, $f^*F = 0.8$, $V_c = 10$ L, $V_m = 10$ L, $K_a = 0.5$ hr^{-1}, $K_{el} = 0.1$ hr^{-1}, $K_{m1} = 0.15$ hr^{-1}, $K_{m2} = 0.2$ hr^{-1}, $K_{mel1} = 0.1$ hr^{-1}, $K_{mel2} = 0.15$ hr^{-1}.

TABLE 14.3. The Estimated Pharmacokinetic Parameters of Model 3 for the Example in Figure 14.5.

| Parameter | Administered Alone | | Coadministration | | |
	Time Constant Analysis	Model Value	Time Constant Analysis	Model Value	Equation
T_z (hr)	2.04	2.0 (T_a)	2.44	2.22	(14.2)
$\bar{t}_C$ (hr)	3.4	3.4	4.2	4.2	(14.4)
$\bar{t}_{M1}$ (hr)	13.3	13.4	14.2	14.2	(14.5)
$\bar{t}_{M2}$ (hr)	10	10.1	10.8	10.9	(14.5)
T_{mel1} (hr)	9.9	10.0	10.0	10.0	(14.6)
T_{mel2} (hr)	6.6	6.7	6.6	6.7	(14.6)
$T_{m1}*V_{m1}/V_c$ (hr)	2.51	2.5	6.8	6.67	(14.10)
$T_{m2}*V_{m2}/V_c$ (hr)	5.0	5.04	5.04	5.04	(14.10)
AUC_C (ng·hr/L)	1157	1142	1802	1777	
AUC_{M1} (ng·hr/L)	4573	4571	2666	2666	
AUC_{M2} (ng·hr/L)	1529	1523	2375	2370	
AUC_{M1}/AUC_C	3.95	4.0	1.47	1.5	(14.7)
AUC_{M2}/AUC_C	1.32	1.33	1.31	1.33	(14.7)

Now let us examine the time constant plot (Figure 14.6). First, one notices that the decay time does not change much after coadministration with the inhibitor, in contrast to the significant change in the area under the curve. This is because, when the drug is administered alone, there is a flip-flop of the concentration profile and the decay time is equal to the absorption time T_a ($= 2.0$ hour), which is longer than the total elimination time $T_{el,t}$ ($= 1.43$ hour); after coadministered with the inhibitor, $T_{el,t}$ increases to 2.22 hours, which dominates the decay time. As a result, the decay time changes slightly from 2.0 hours ($= T_a$) when administered alone to 2.22 hours ($= T_{el,t}$) after the drug interaction.

The area under the curve of metabolite M1 decreases while that of metabolite M2 increases after the drug interaction. Based on the change in area under the curve, an incorrect conclusion may be drawn that the metabolism toward M2 is induced by the coadministration of the second drug. The correct analysis on the metabolism inhibition or induction is based on the ratio of area under the curve of each metabolite to that of the parent drug. From the values of AUC_{M1}/AUC_C and AUC_{M2}/AUC_C, it is concluded that the metabolism to M1 is inhibited and the metabolism to M2 is not affected by the second drug. In addition, the metabolic elimination time toward M1 ($T_{m1}*V_{m1}/V_c$) increases after the coadministration, while the metabolic elimination time toward M2 ($T_{m2}*V_{m2}/V_c$) is not affected (Figure 14.6).

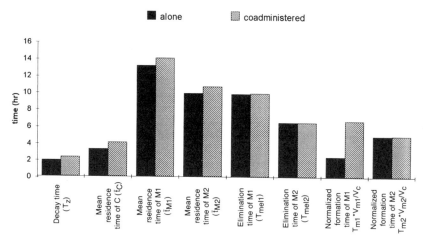

FIGURE 14.6. The time constant plot of a drug administered alone or with another drug in the example shown in Figure 14.5. The metabolic elimination time toward M1 ($T_{m1} * V_{m1}/V_c$) increases after the coadministration, while the metabolic elimination time toward M2 ($T_{m2} * V_{m2}/V_c$) is not affected.

EXAMPLES

Example 1: Drug Interaction Affecting the Extent of Absorption

Studies were conducted to investigate the interaction between ranitidine and an excipient, SAPP (sodium acid pyrophosphate), by dosing 150 mg ranitidine solution and tablet with and without SAPP to healthy subjects [5]. The mean concentration profiles following the four different treatments are shown in Figure 14.7. The plasma concentrations following the administration of ranitidine with SAPP is much lower than those following the administration of ranitidine alone. The excipient SAPP has the same effect on the solution as on the tablet.

Sodium pyrophosphate salts are known to affect the intestinal motility, which may be a reason for the reduction in the fraction absorbed and, consequently, the area under the curve of a drug. In addition, any change in elimination time or volume of distribution may also affect the area under the curve. However, urine data are not available in this example for the estimation of renal elimination time; therefore, the decay time will be used to determine the effect of SAPP on the elimination time of ranitidine. The concentration profiles of ranitidine show a monoexponential terminal phase, and thus the pharmacokinetic parameters are estimated using Model 1. The estimated pharmacokinetic parameters are listed in Table 14.4, and the esti-

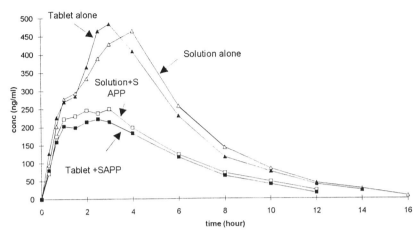

FIGURE 14.7. Mean plasma concentration profiles of ranitidine following the oral administration of 150 mg ranitidine in solution with 1132 mg SAPP, 150 mg ranitidine in solution,
150-mg ranitidine tablet, and 150-mg ranitidine tablet containing 1132 mg SAPP, to healthy
subjects. (Reproduced from Refernce [5] with permission.) The time constant plot comparing the four treatments is shown in Figure 14.8.

mated time constants are presented in Figure 14.8. The area under the
ranitidine concentration curve is much smaller when the drug is dosed with
SAPP than when it is dosed alone. The possible factors that can reduce the
area under the curve include a decreased extent of absorption, a decreased
elimination time, and an increased volume of distribution.

Now let us examine the time constant plot (Figure 14.8). The mean residence time, the decay time T_z, and the initial time constant T_0' are similar
between the four treatments, which excludes the possibility of change in the
elimination time. If the volume of distribution of ranitidine were increased

TABLE 14.4. *The Pharmacokinetic Parameters of Ranitidine Estimated for
the Example in Figure 14.7 by the Time Constant Analysis Using Model 1.*

Parameter*	Soln. Alone	Soln. + SAPP	Tablet Alone	Tablet + SAPP	Equation
AUC (ng·hr/ml)	2891	1586	2757	1449	
$\bar{t}$ (hr)	4.9	4.2	4.5	4.2	(14.1)
T_z (hr)	3.3	4.0	3.3	3.7	(14.2)
T_0 (hr)	1.1	0.9	1.0	1.1	(14.2) stripping

*Parameters estimated from the mean concentration curves or the reported mean values.

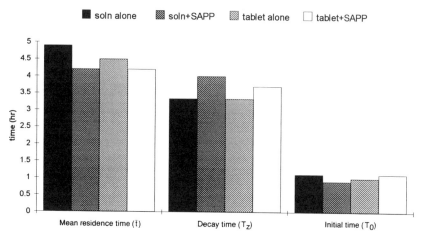

FIGURE 14.8. The time constant plot of ranitidine using Model 1, comparing four treatments: 150 mg ranitidine in solution with 1132 mg SAPP, 150 mg ranitidine in solution, 150-mg ranitidine tablet, and 150-mg ranitidine tablet containing 1132 mg SAPP. The mean residence time ($\bar{t}$), the decay time (T_z), and the initial time constant (T_0) are similar between the four treatments, which exclude the possibility of change in the elimination time (T_{el}).

by SAPP, the decay time would likely have changed due to a decreased renal elimination time or a decreased tissue distribution time secondary to the increase in the free fraction in the plasma. Therefore, the most likely cause for the decreased area under the concentration curve when ranitidine is dosed with SAPP is a reduced extent of absorption. This is confirmed by the observation (by scintigraphic imaging) that the gastric emptying is not affected, but the intestinal transit time is reduced by 56% in the presence of SAPP. To summarize, SAPP reduces the plasma concentration of ranitidine probably due to a decrease in the fraction absorbed; therefore, SAPP should not be used as an excipient in the ranitidine tablet, as suggested in Reference [5].

Example 2: Drug Interaction Affecting Renal Excretion

The pharmacokinetics of zidovudine were studied following a 1-hour constant intravenous infusion of 3 mg/kg in nine HIV patients without and with trimethoprim (150 mg) and trimethoprim-sulphamethoxazole (160 and 800 mg) [1]. The mean concentration profiles of zidovudine and its glucuronide metabolite are shown in Figure 14.9. The concentrations of zidovudine and its glucuronide metabolite during the infusion phase (0–1 hour) are higher when dosed alone than with trimethoprim or trimethoprim-sulphamethoxazole; however, after the completion of infusion, the concentration profiles become similar.

The main route of elimination of zidovudine is by metabolism to glucuronide, and the glucuronide is mainly excreted by the kidney. On the other hand, trimethoprim and sulphamethoxazole are also eliminated by the liver, as well as the kidney. Therefore, the potential interaction between zidovudine and trimethoprim or sulphamethoxazole may involve metabolism and renal secretion. The key time constants in this example are then the hepatic and renal elimination times. The pharmacokinetic parameters of zidovudine are estimated using Model 3, since the metabolite concentration is measured. The estimated pharmacokinetic parameters are listed in Table 14.5, and the estimated time constants are presented in Figure 14.10.

The area under the concentration curves of zidovudine and its metabolite increases when zidovudine is dosed with trimethoprim or trimethoprim-sulphamethoxazole. The ratios of the area under the glucuronide concentration curve to the area under the zidovudine concentration curve are similar between the three treatments. However, the renal elimination time $T_{el}V$ and the hepatic elimination time T_m/V of zidovudine increase substantially when zidovudine is dosed with trimethoprim or trimethoprim-sulphamethoxazole (from the time constant plot, Figure 14.10), which may contribute to the increase in the area under the curve. The renal elimination

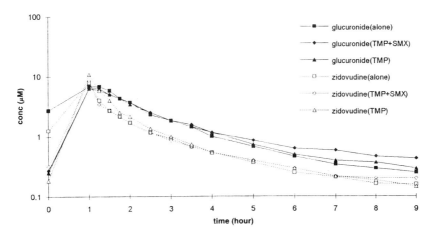

FIGURE 14.9. Mean plasma concentration profiles of zidovudine and its glucuronide metabolite following the 1-hour constant intravenous infusion of 3 mg/kg zidovudine, 3 mg/kg zidovudine with 150 mg trimethoprim, and 3 mg/kg zidovudine with 160 mg trimethoprim and 800 mg sulphamethoxazole to nine HIV patients. (Reproduced from Reference [1] with permission from Blackwell Science Ltd.) The time constant plot comparing the three treatments is shown in Figure 14.10.

TABLE 14.5. The Pharmacokinetic Parameters of Zidovudine Estimated for the Example in Figure 14.9 by the Time Constant Analysis Using Model 3.

Parameter*	Alone Z	Alone ZG	+TMP +SMX Z	+TMP +SMX ZG	+TMP Z	+TMP ZG	Equation
T_z (hr)	2.56		2.5	1.96	2.78	1.79	(14.2)
T_{el}/V (hr·kg/L)	2.94	1.43	7.14	5.0	5.88	4.76	(14.8)
T_m/V_c (hr·kg/L)		2.04					(14.9)
$\bar{t}$ (hr)	2		1.8		1.9		(14.4)
AUC (μM·hr)	9.5	13.6	11.2	16.3	12.4	15	
AUC_M/AUC_C		1.43		1.46		1.21	

*Parameters estimated from the mean concentration curves or the reported mean values.

Z: zidovudine, ZG: zidovudine glucuronide.

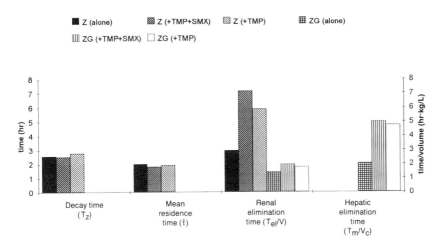

FIGURE 14.10. The time constant plot of zidovudine using Model 3, comparing three treatments: 3 mg/kg zidovudine, 3 mg/kg zidovudine with 150 mg trimethoprim, and 3 mg/kg zidovudine with 160 mg trimethoprim and 800 mg sulphamethoxazole. The renal elimination time (T_{el}/V) and the hepatic elimination time (T_m/V) of zidovudine increases substantially when zidovudine is dosed with trimethoprim or trimethoprim-sulphamethoxazole, which may contribute to the increase in the area under the curve.

time of the glucuronide metabolite also increases when zidovudine is dosed with trimethoprim or trimethoprim-sulphamethoxazole, which may be partly responsible for the increase in the area under the glucuronide concentration curve. If the urine data were not available, the altered renal and hepatic elimination time would not have been identified. To summarize, the hepatic elimination time and the renal elimination time of zidovudine are prolonged when the drug is coadministered with trimethoprim or sulphamethoxazole. The increased elimination time results in a slight increase in the area under the zidovudine concentration curve. However, the decay time is not affected by the drug interaction, suggesting a possible increase in zidovudine elimination in a nonrenal, nonhepatic route, probably biliary excretion.

Example 3: Drug Interaction Affecting Protein Binding

The interaction between warfarin and etodolac was studied in eighteen healthy subjects following a multiple oral dose of warfarin with and without etodolac [3]. The mean plasma concentration profiles of warfarin after the last dose (the third day) are shown in Figure 14.11. The plasma concentration of warfarin is reduced by the coadministration of etodolac. Warfarin is

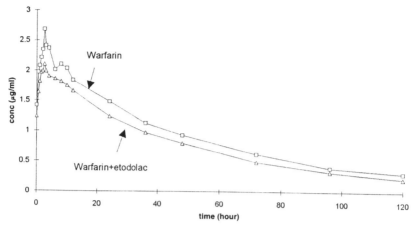

FIGURE 14.11. Mean plasma concentration profiles of warfarin following the oral administration of 10 mg warfarin without and with 200 mg b.i.d. etodolac. (Reproduced from Reference [3] with permission.) The time constant plot comparing the two treatments is shown in
Figure 14.12.

known to be completely absorbed orally, highly bound to plasma albumin,
and almost entirely eliminated by hepatic metabolism. Mechanisms frequently associated with the interaction of warfarin with other drugs include
inhibited metabolism and competition for protein binding.

Etodolac is also highly bound to plasma protein; therefore, a competition
between etodolac and warfarin for the plasma protein binding sites may be
the potential cause for the decrease in the warfarin concentration. The pharmacokinetic parameters of warfarin are estimated using Model 2, since the
drug interaction may involve a change in protein binding and distribution.
The estimated pharmacokinetic parameters are listed in Table 14.6, and the
estimated time constants are presented in Figure 14.12. The area under the

TABLE 14.6. *The Pharmacokinetic Parameters of Warfarin Estimated for
the Example in Figure 14.11 by the Time Constant Analysis Using Model 2.*

Parameter*	Warfarin	Warfarin + Etodolac	Equation
T_z (hr)	50.0	50.0	(14.2)
$\bar{t}$ (hr)	62.6	64.2	(14.3)
$T_{el,t}*f*F/V$ (hr·kg/ml)	0.357	0.313	(14.a3)
$(T_{el,t})_u*F/V$ (hr·kg/ml)	0.00346	0.00351	(14.a3)
AUC (μg·hr/ml)	128	106	
F_u (%)	1.05%	1.25%	measured

*Parameters estimated from the mean concentration curves or the reported mean values.

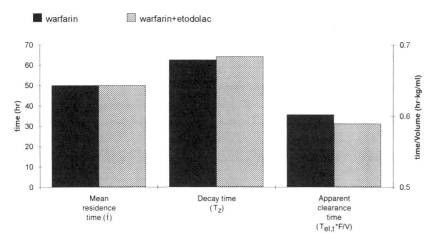

FIGURE 14.12. The time constant plot of warfarin using Model 2, comparing two treatments: 10 mg warfarin without and with 200 mg b.i.d. etodolac. The total clearance time ($T_{el,t}*F/V$) decreases with the coadministration of etodolac, implicating a possible increase in the volume of distribution of warfarin when dosed with etodolac.

warfarin concentration curve decreases with the coadministration of etodolac.

Now let us examine the time constant plot (Figure 14.12). The decay time and mean residence time of the concentration curve for both treatments are similar, indicating that the elimination and the absorption of warfarin are probably not affected by etodolac. However, the total clearance time characterized by $T_{el}*F/V$ decreases with the coadministration of etodolac, implicating a possible increase in the volume of distribution of warfarin when dosed with etodolac. The total clearance time of the unbound fraction characterized by $(T_{el,t})_u*F/V$ is similar between treatments, indicating that the intrinsic (unbound) hepatic and renal clearances of warfarin are not affected by etodolac. It is also shown that the unbound fraction of warfarin in plasma increases with the coadministration of etodolac, indicating that etodolac displaces warfarin from the plasma protein binding sites. To summarize, the total clearance time of warfarin increases, but the unbound clearance time of the drug is not affected by the coadministration of etodolac. However, the drug interaction does not affect the pharmacological effect of warfarin, which is determined by the prothrombin time [3].

Example 4: Drug Interaction Affecting Elimination

The pharmacokinetics of phenytoin were studied in nine healthy male subjects following the oral administration of 250 mg phenytoin suspension

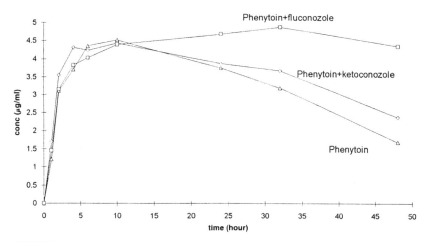

FIGURE 14.13. Mean plasma concentration profiles of phenytoin following the oral administration of 250 mg phenytoin, 250 mg phenytoin with 200 mg ketoconazole b.i.d., and 250 mg phenytoin with 400 mg fluconazole q.d. in nine healthy male subjects. (Reproduced from Reference [11] with permission from Blackwell Science Ltd.)

without and with ketoconazole 200 mg b.i.d. or 400 mg fluconazole q.d. [11]. The mean plasma concentration profiles of phenytoin following the three treatments are shown in Figure 14.13. The concentration of phenytoin increases with the coadministration of ketoconazole and fluconazole, especially the latter. The decay time of the plasma phenytoin concentration curve drastically increases with the coadministration of fluconazole, indicating an interaction involving the elimination of phenytoin.

Fluconazole and ketoconazole are known to inhibit oxidative metabolism. However, metabolite concentrations are not available in this example for the estimation of the hepatic elimination time. Therefore, the decay time will be used to assess the potential interaction affecting the metabolism. The area under the plasma phenytoin concentration curve and the decay time of the concentration profiles of both treatments are listed in Table 14.7.

TABLE 14.7. The Pharmacokinetic Parameters of Phenytoin Estimated for the Example in Figure 14.13 by the Time Constant Analysis.

Parameter*	Alone	+ Ketoconazole	+ Fluconazole	Equation
T_z (hr)	3.45	6.25	5000	(14.2)
AUC_{0-48} ($\mu g \cdot hr/ml$)	146	156	195	

*Parameters estimated from the mean concentration curves or the reported mean values.

The effect of fluconazole on the area under the phenytoin concentration curve is more significant than the effect of ketoconazole. The increase in the decay time of phenytoin concentration curve with the coadministration of ketoconazole and fluconazole indicates a reduced elimination rate of phenytoin by the other two drugs. To summarize, the plasma concentration of phenytoin increases with the coadministration of fluconazole probably due to an inhibition of phenytoin metabolism.

REFERENCES

1. Chatton J. Y., Munafo A., Chave J. P., Steinhauslin F., Roch-Ramel F., Glauser M. P., and Biollaz J., "Trimethoprim, alone or in combination with sulphamethoxazole, decreases the renal excretion of zidovudine and its glucuronide," *Br. J. Clin. Pharmac.*, 1992; 34:551–554.

2. Edner M., Jogestrand T., and Dahlqvist R., "Effect of salbutamol on digoxin pharmacokinetics," *Eur. J. Clin. Pharmacol.*, 1992; 42:197–201.

3. Ermer J. C., Hicks D. R., Wheeler S. C., Kraml M., Jusko W. J., "Concomitant etodolac affects neither the unbound clearance nor the pharmacologic effect of warfarin," *Clinical Pharmacology & Therapeutics*, 1994; 55(3):305–316.

4. Honig P. K., Wortham C. W., Hull R., Zamani K., Smith J. E., and Cantilena L. R., "Itraconazole affects single-dose terfenadine pharmacokinetics and cardiac repolarization pharmacodynamics," *J. Clin. Pharmacol.*, 1993; 33:1201–1206.

5. Koch K. M., Parr A. F., Tomlinson J. J., Sandefer E. P., Digenis G. A., Donn K. H., and Powell J. R., "Effect of sodium acid pyrophosphate on ranitidine bioavailability and gastrointestinal transit time," *Pharmaceutical Research*, 1993; 10(7):1027–1030.

6. Ohashi K., Sakamoto K., Sudo T., Tateishi T., Fujimura A., Shiga T., and Ebihara A., "Effects of diltiazem and cimetidine on theophylline oxidative metabolism," *J. Clin. Pharmacol.*, 1993; 33:1233–1237.

7. Ohashi K., Sudo T., Sakamoto K., Tateishi T., Fujimura A., Kumagai Y., and Ebihara A., "The influence of pretreatment period with diltiazem on nifedipine kinetics," *J. Clin. Pharmacol.*, 1993; 33:222–225.

8. Sommers K., van Wyk M., Snyman J. R., and Moncrieff J., "The effects of omeprazole-induced hypochlorhydria on absorption of theophylline from a sustained release formulation," *Eur. J. Clin. Pharmacol.*, 1992; 43:141–143.

9. Sudoh T., Fujimura A., Shiga T., Tateishi T., Sunaga K. I., Ohashi K. I., and Ebihara A., "Influence of lisinopril on urinary electrolytes excretion after furosemide in healthy subjects," *J. Clin. Pharmacol.*, 1993; 33:640–643.

10. Stringer K. A., Lebsack M. E., Cetnarowski-Cropp A. B., Chang T., and Sedman J., "Effect of cimetidine administration on the pharmacokinetics of primenol," *J. Clin. Pharmacol.*, 1992; 32:91–94.

11. Touchette M. A., Chandrasekar P. H., Milad M. A., and Edwards D. J., "Contrasting effects of fluconazole and ketoconazole on phenytoin and testosterone disposition in man," *Br. J. Clin. Pharmac.*, 1992; 34:75–78.

12. Wade J. R., Meredith P. A., Hughes D. M., and Elliott H. L., "The effect of saturation of ACE binding sites on the pharmacokinetics of enalaprilat in man," *Br. J. Clin. Pharmac.*, 1992; 33:155–160.

SPECIAL POPULATIONS

CHAPTER 15

Influence of Age on Pharmacokinetics

INTRODUCTION

The difference in the pharmacokinetics of a drug between different age groups can be assessed in a young versus elderly study. The absorption of drugs may be affected by age because the gastric acid secretion, gastrointestinal blood flow, number of absorbing cells in the gastrointestinal tract, and gastrointestinal motility are reduced in the elderly [3]. The body mass compositions, as well as the body size of different age groups, are varied significantly [25]. The total body water decreases with age, while the fat to lean ratio of body mass increases. This change in body mass composition with increasing age may result in a slight decrease in the volume of distribution of a hydrophilic drug or a pronounced increase in the volume of distribution of a lipophilic drug [19]. Serum albumin concentration decreases with age [22,23], while serum α-acid glycoprotein increases in the elderly [20,21]. Due to the change in plasma protein concentration, the free fraction, and apparent volume of distribution of highly bound acidic drug may increase with age, and those of highly bound basic drugs may decrease with age. Renal clearance of drug may decline with age [6], which results in an increase in renal elimination time constant. Hepatic blood flow [18] and liver volume [16] decline with age, which may increase the hepatic elimination time of drugs with high extraction ratios. Liver microsomal enzyme activity may diminish with age [25,26], which also increases hepatic elimination time constants. To summarize, the key time constants in the young versus elderly study are the distribution time constants, the renal elimination time constant, the hepatic elimination time constant, and the volume of distribution. All these time constants affect the decay time of a

369

drug; therefore, care must be taken to identify the cause for a change in half-life between different age groups.

Some common themes in the time constant view can be observed in the age study as well as other studies. The distribution characteristic is a common factor among different clinical studies. The distribution characteristics of drugs may be different between age groups for several reasons. If a drug does not distribute to tissue very well, as is typical with hydrophilic drugs, the volume of distribution may decrease with age without a considerable change in the distribution time and the redistribution time [19]. For the same hydrophilic drug, a change in the volume of distribution, but not in the distribution and redistribution time, may also be observed in a male versus female study (Chapter 16), where women may have, on average, a smaller body size but larger fat to lean ratio than the men.

If a drug distributes extensively into tissue, as is typical with lipophilic drugs, the volume of distribution, as well as the redistribution time, may increase with age. A similar increase in both volume of distribution and redistribution time may also be observed for the same lipophilic drug in (1) a male versus female study and (2) a drug interaction study (Chapter 14) involving protein binding displacer. The hepatic elimination time is also a common factor. A decrease in hepatic blood flow may or may not have a significant effect on the hepatic elimination time, depending on the magnitude of the hepatic extraction ratio [24]. If the first pass effect, determined by the bioavailability study (Chapter 5), is extensive, the extraction ratio is high, and it is likely that the hepatic elimination time will be prolonged with age. On the other hand, if the first pass effect is insignificant, the extraction ratio is low, and the hepatic elimination time may not increase much with age. Whether a drug is a base or acid is another common factor between the age study and other studies. The dissolution time and the absorption time of acidic and basic drugs may change with age, since the decrease in gastric acid secretion results in a high pH in the gastrointestinal tract of elderly subjects [19]. The acidic drugs tend to bind with albumin, while the basic drugs tend to bind with α_1-acid glycoprotein. Therefore, the dissociation constant pK of a drug may play an important role in studies where the protein binding may be affected, such as in the age study, the renal impairment study (Chapter 17), the inflammatory disease study (Chapter 19), and the drug interaction study (Chapter 14) involving protein binding displacers. In addition, the pK of a drug also dertemines the effect of urine pH on the renal elimination time.

Three models are discussed in this chapter: (1) the first model describes effects of age on absorption and elimination; (2) the second model describes effects of age on absorption, elimination, and distribution; and (3) the third model describes effects of age on absorption, distribution, and metabolism. Three simulated case studies and three literature examples are presented in this chapter to illustrate the utility of these models in young versus elderly studies. Additional examples of young versus elderly studies can be found in the literature [1–18].

PHARMACOKINETIC MODELS

This section presents three models that are useful in describing the effects of age on pharmacokinetics. The goal is to establish simple relationships between time constants and measurable parameters such as (1) mean residence time, which is the sum of input and output times, and (2) area under the curves. The derivations of these relationships are straightforward and are discussed in Chapter 2.

Model 1: Effects of Age on Absorption and Elimination

The absorption and elimination of drugs may be different in young and elderly subjects. Model 1 describes the pharmacokinetics of drugs with a monoexponential terminal phase.

The mean residence time of the drug concentration curve may be different in young and elderly groups due to a change in absorption or elimination time constants. The mean residence time is simply the sum of input and output times:

$$\text{Mean residence time } (\bar{t}) = \text{Input time } (T_{in}) + \text{Output time } (T_{out}) = T_a + T_{el}$$

(15.1)

The decay time of the concentration curve can be estimated from a partial area under the curve (see Appendix 2):

$$\frac{1}{\text{Decay time } (T_z)} = \lambda_z = 2\frac{(t_{ref} - t_{last})\ln(C_{t_{ref}}) - \text{AU}\ln C_{t_{ref}-t_{last}}}{(t_{ref} - t_{last})^2}$$ (15.2)

The renal clearance time can be estimated from the ratio of the area under the concentration curve to the cumulative urine recovery:

$$\text{Renal clearance time } \left(\frac{T_{el}}{V}\right) = \frac{\text{AUC}}{X_u} \qquad (15.3)$$

The bioavailability can be estimated from the total urine recovery, assuming the renal excretion is the predominant route of elimination:

$$\text{Fraction absorbed } (f) = \frac{X_{uc}}{X_0} \qquad (15.4)$$

If the renal excretion is the predominant route of elimination, the first pass effect can be determined:

$$\text{First pass bioavailability } (F) = \frac{\text{AUC} \cdot V}{f \cdot X_0 \cdot T_{el}} \qquad (15.5)$$

The total clearance time is defined as

$$\text{Apparent total clearance time } \left(\frac{T_{el,t}}{V} fF\right) = \frac{\text{AUC}}{X_0} \qquad (15.6)$$

Following an intravenous administration, the volume of the central compartment can be estimated from the extrapolated initial concentration (C_0) at time 0:

$$\text{Volume of central compartment } (V_c) = \frac{X_0}{C_0} \qquad (15.7)$$

The apparent volume of distribution can be estimated from the following two ways:

$$\text{Steady-state volume of distribution } \left(\frac{V_{ss}}{fF}\right) = \bar{t}\,\frac{X_0}{\text{AUC}} \qquad (15.8)$$

$$\text{Apparent volume of distribution } \left(\frac{V_z}{fF}\right) = T_z\,\frac{X_0}{\text{AUC}} \qquad (15.9)$$

The initial time constant T_0 of the concentration profile is equal to either T_a or T_{el}, whichever is shorter. Therefore, it is uncertain whether the initial time constant represents the absorption time. An unambiguous parameter for characterizing the absorption is T_a*V. With known values of the initial slope λ_0, the terminal slope λ_z, and the bioavailability $f*F$, the value of T_a*V can be expressed as follows:

$$\frac{1}{\text{Absorption time} \times \text{volume } (T_a \cdot V)} = \frac{A(\lambda_0 - \lambda_z)}{fFX_0} \quad (15.10)$$

where A is the intercept of the monoexponential curve fitted to the terminal portion of the concentration profile. From this equation, the value of T_a*V can be estimated whether a flip-flop occurs or not. Therefore, T_a*V is a more direct and unambiguous parameter for characterizing the absorption time than is T_0.

Model 2: Effects of Age on Absorption, Elimination, and Distribution

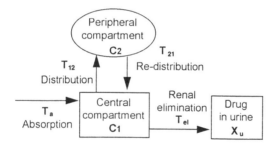

When the drug concentration profiles exhibit a biexponential terminal phase, the two-compartmental model can be used in a young versus elderly study. When the drug plasma protein binding changes with age, volume of distribution, distribution time constant, and elimination time constant may be affected.

The mean residence time in this model is dependent on the absorption, elimination, and distribution time constants (see Chapter 2):

$$\text{Mean residence time } (\bar{t}) = \text{Input time } (T_{in})$$

$$+ \text{Output time } (T_{out}) = T_a + T_{el} + T_{el}\frac{T_{21}}{T_{12}} \quad (15.11)$$

The slopes of the three exponential phases can be estimated from the curve-stripping technique. Let λ_0, λ_{z1}, and λ_{z2} represent the three exponentials, where $\lambda_0 > \lambda_{z1} > \lambda_{z2}$. Thus, λ_{z1} and λ_{z2} represent the first and second decay exponents terminal portion of the concentration curve, respectively, and λ_0 represents the initial slope of the concentration curve. Because of the possibility of flip-flop, the initial time constant T_0 ($= 1/\lambda_0$) does not always represent the absorption time constant. A less ambiguous parameter than T_0 for characterizing the absorption time is $T_a * V_1$.

The value of $T_a * V_1$ can be obtained from the following expression (see Chapter 6):

$$\frac{1}{\text{Absorption time} \times \text{volume } (T_a V_1)} = \frac{A + B}{fFX_0} \frac{(\lambda_{z1} - \lambda_0)(\lambda_{z2} - \lambda_0)}{\lambda_0 - K_{21}}$$

(15.12)

where A and B are the intercepts of the first and second terminal phases, according to the following equation:

$$C = Ae^{-\lambda_{z1}} + Be^{-\lambda_{z2}}$$

(15.13)

Under the following condition (1), only two of the three exponential phases can be identified using the curve-stripping method because the first decay phase lasts for a very short period of time. Therefore, in this case, the two-compartmental model collapses to a one-compartmental model. Under condition (2), the second decay phase lasts very long, and the variability involved in estimating λ_{z2} can be large. Two special cases of condition (2) are discussed below (conditions 3 and 5):

(1)   if $K_{21} \to \lambda_1$ and $\lambda_1 = \lambda_{z1}$ then $A \to 0$ (15.14)

(2)   if $K_{21} \to \lambda_2$ and $\lambda_2 = \lambda_{z2}$ then $B \to 0$ (15.15)

where λ_1 and λ_2 are derived from the elimination and distribution rate constants (see Appendix 3). In conditions (3) to (5), the concentration profiles typically show long tails, and the error involved in the estimation of λ_{z2} ($\lambda_{z2} = \lambda_2$ unless $K_a < \lambda_2$) can be large. Fortunately, under conditions (3) and (5), the denominator in Equation (15.12) cancels out with one term in the numerator (when $\lambda_{z2} = \lambda_2$). In addition, under conditions (3) to (5), exponent λ_{z2} in the numerator of Equation (15.12) is very small and can be ignored compared with λ_0. Thus, the estimation of $T_a \cdot V_1$ is not strongly affected by the large variability of λ_{z2} under conditions (3) to (5).

(3)   if $K_{el}, K_{21} \gg K_{12}$ then $\lambda_1 \to K_{el}, \lambda_2 \to K_{21}$ (15.16)

(4)   if $K_{12}, K_{21} \gg K_{el}$ then $\lambda_1 \to K_{12} + K_{21}, \lambda_2 \to K_{el}$ (15.17)

(5)   if $K_{el}, K_{12} \gg K_{21}$ then $\lambda_1 \to K_{el} + K_{12}, \lambda_2 \to K_{21}$ (15.18)

Therefore, under the above five conditions, Equation (15.12) collapses and contains only one of the two decay exponents. In other conditions ($\lambda_{z2} = K_a$), when the second decay time is much longer than the first decay time, λ_{z2} in the numerator of Equation (15.12) is very small and can be ignored compared with λ_0.

Another equation for estimating T_a*V_1 is shown below:

$$\frac{\text{Absorption time} \times \text{volume } (T_aV_1)}{\text{Bioavailability } (fF)} = \frac{X_0}{A(\lambda_0 - \lambda_{z1}) + B(\lambda_0 - \lambda_{z2})}$$

(15.19)

When the second decay time is much longer than the first decay time, the value of B becomes very small and can be dropped out from Equation (15.19). As a result, Equation (15.19) collapses to Equation (15.10) when the second decay time is long. Therefore, the large variability (or error) involved in estimating λ_{z2} does not affect the accuracy of $T_a*V_1/f/F$.

Model 3: Effects of Age on Absorption, Distribution, and Metabolism

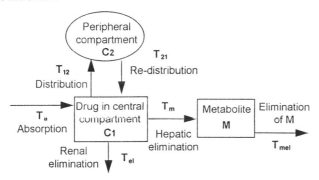

The metabolism of drugs may be affected by age. Hepatic blood flow declines with age [18], which may affect the hepatic clearance of drugs with high extraction ratios. Liver microsomal enzyme activity may diminish with age [25,26], which also affects hepatic elimination time constants. The pharmacokinetic parameters of the parent drug can be estimated as in the previous model (Model 2).

The mean residence time of the metabolite concentration curve in this model is the sum of input and output times (see Chapter 2):

$$\text{Mean residence time of metabolite } (\overline{t}_M)$$

$$= \text{Input time } (T_{m,in}) + \text{Output time } (T_{m,out}) = T_a + T_{el,t} + T_{el,t}\frac{T_{21}}{T_{12}} + T_{mel}$$

(15.20)

The ratio of the area under the metabolite concentration to the area under the drug concentration results in the ratio of the renal clearance time of the metabolite to the hepatic clearance time of the drug:

$$\frac{\text{AUC}_M}{\text{AUC}_C} = \frac{T_{mel}V_1}{T_m V_m} = \frac{\text{Renal clearance time of metabolite}}{\text{Hepatic clearance time of the drug}} \quad (15.21)$$

The hepatic clearance time can be obtained as follows:

$$\text{Hepatic clearance time} \left(\frac{T_m}{V_1}\right) = \frac{X_{um}}{\text{AUC}_C} \quad (15.22)$$

CASE STUDIES

Case 1: Renal Excretion and Volume of Distribution Change with Age

The area under the plasma concentration curve may change with age due to a number of reasons: the volume of distribution may increase as a result of an increase in fat tissue [25] or a decrease in protein binding [20–23]; the elimination rate may decrease because of reduced renal [6] or hepatic functions [16,18]; and the extent of absorption may change due to increased gastrointestinal pH, decreased gastrointestinal motility, or decreased number of absorbing cells [3]. Because of the complexity of the pharmacokinetics, identifying the cause for a change in area under the curve with age becomes a mixture of art and science. An example is illustrated by Model 1, and simulated plasma concentration profiles of a young and an elderly subject are shown in Figure 15.1. In this example, the renal elimination is slower, and the volume of distribution is greater in the elderly than the young subject. The maximum plasma concentration of the elderly subject appears later than that of the young subject, reflecting the reduced elimination rate with age. The decreased renal function in the elderly may result in a greater area under the curve, while the increased volume of distribution may reduce the area under the curve. The overall result of the change in renal function and volume of distribution in this example is an increase in the area under the curve, indicating that the effect of the reduced renal function is more significant than that of the increased volume of distribution.

Urine data are especially important in young versus elderly studies since renal function decreases with age. The key time constant for the assessment of renal excretion is the renal elimination time. The estimated pharmacokinetic parameters of the above example using the time constant analysis

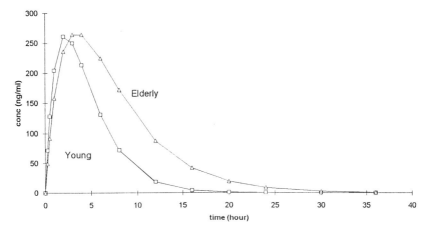

FIGURE 15.1. Simulated plasma concentration profiles of young and elderly subjects using Model 1, with age affecting renal excretion and volume of distribution. The time constant plot comparing the two age populations is shown in Figure 15.2. The parameters used in this simulation are young: $X_0 = 10$ mg, $f^*F = 0.8$, $V = 10$ L, $K_a = 0.4$ hr^{-1}, $K_{el} = 0.5$ hr^{-1}; elderly: $X_0 = 10$ mg, $f^*F = 0.8$, $V = 15$ L, $K_a = 0.4$ hr^{-1}, $K_{el} = 0.2$ hr^{-1}.

are listed in Table 15.1, and the estimated time constants are presented in Figure 15.2. The area under the curve is greater in the elderly than the young, indicating possible change in absorption, renal elimination, or volume of distribution.

Now let us examine the time constant plot (Figure 15.2). The mean residence time increases in the elderly, indicating a possible increase in either

TABLE 15.1. Estimated Time Constants of Model 1 for the Example Shown in Figure 15.1.

Parameter	Young Time Constant Analysis	Young Model Value	Elderly Time Constant Analysis	Elderly Model Value	Equation
$\bar{t}$ (hr)	4.5	4.5	7.4	7.5	(15.1)
T_0 (hr)	1.85	2.0 (T_{el})	2.5	2.5 (T_a)	(15.2)
T_z (hr)	2.5	2.5 (T_a)	5.0	5.0 (T_{el})	(15.2)
T_{el}/V (hr/L)	0.20	0.20	0.33	0.33	(15.3)
T_a^*V (hr/L)	25.0	25.0	35.7	37.0	(15.10)
AUC (ng·hr/L)	1621	1600	2686	2666	
X_u (μg)	8108	8000	8060	8000	
f^*F	0.81	0.8	0.81	0.8	(15.5)

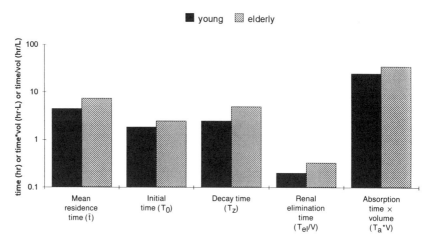

FIGURE 15.2. The time constant plot comparing the two age populations in the example shown in Figure 15.1. The time constant T_a*V_c increases with age, which may likely be a result of an increased volume of distribution in the elderly.

absorption or elimination time. Because of the possibility of flip-flop, the interpretation of T_{z0} and T_{z1} must be made with caution. On the contrary, T_a*V_c and T_{el}/V_c are better indicators for the absorption and elimination times for an obvious reason. The extent of absorption $f*F$, estimated from the cumulative urine drug recovery, is the same between the two subjects; therefore, it is not likely that the absorption is affected by age. Assuming the absorption is not affected by age, the fact that T_a*V_c increases with age may likely be a result of an increased volume of distribution in the elderly. The fact that only one of T_0 and T_z is different between the two subjects suggests that only one of the two time constants, T_{el} and T_a, changes with age. The exact difference in the volume of distribution between the young and elderly can be determined by giving an intravenous dose to the subjects.

Case 2: Protein Binding Changes with Age

The decay time of a drug may change with age due to several reasons, for example, an increase in volume of distribution or a decrease in renal elimination. If a drug is extensively bound to the plasma protein and the amount of plasma protein decreases with age, the volume of distribution and the distribution rate constant K_{12} may increase in the elderly. An example is described by Model 2, where the volume of distribution and the distribution rate constant K_{12} increase and the renal elimination decreases with age. Simulated plasma concentration profiles of young and elderly subjects are shown in Figure 15.3. There is an increase in the decay time of the concentration profile of the elderly subject, indicating a decreased elimination rate with age; however, the maximum concentration in the elderly is lower than that in the young subject in spite of the decreased elimination in the elderly, reflecting an increase in the volume of distribution with age.

The concentration profiles of the drug in the elderly show a typical result reflecting decreased protein binding: the maximum concentration drops while the decay time prolongs. The estimated pharmacokinetic parameters of the above example using the time constant analysis are listed in Table 15.2, and the estimated time constants are presented in Figure 15.4. The area under the curve increases only slightly (16%) in the elderly compared with the young subject, despite a drastic increase in the mean residence time (82%) and a significant increase in the second decay time T_{z2} (90%). This indicates that other factors (bioavailability or volume of distribution), in addition to the elimination time, may have changed with age to compensate the effect of the increased elimination time on the area under the curve. However, the urine data shows that the bioavailability is the same between the subjects.

Now let us examine the time constant plot (Figure 15.4). The ratio of renal clearance time of the young to the elderly is equal to the ratio of the area under the curve of the young to the elderly, indicating that the renal

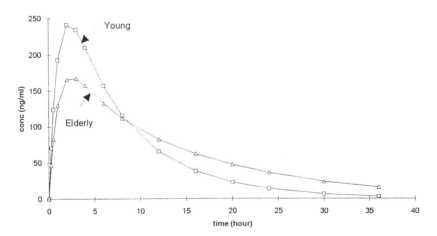

FIGURE 15.3. Simulated plasma concentration profile of young and elderly subjects using Model 2, with age affecting protein binding. The time constant plot comparing the two age groups is shown in Figure 15.4. The parameters used in this simulation are young: $X_0 = 10$ mg, $f^*F = 0.8$, $V_1 = 10$ L, $V_2 = 20$ L, $K_a = 0.4$ hr^{-1}, $K_{12} = 0.3$ hr^{-1}, $K_{21} = 0.3$ hr^{-1}, $K_{el} = 0.35$ hr^{-1}; elderly: $X_0 = 10$ mg, $f^*F = 0.8$, $V_1 = 15$ L, $V_2 = 20$ L, $K_a = 0.4$ hr^{-1}, $K_{12} = 0.45$ hr^{-1}, $K_{21} = 0.3$ hr^{-1}, $K_{el} = 0.2$ hr^{-1}.

TABLE 15.2. Estimated Time Constants of Model 2
for the Example Shown in Figure 15.3.

Parameter	Young Time Constant Analysis	Young Model Value	Elderly Time Constant Analysis	Elderly Model Value	Equation
$\bar{t}$ (hr)	8.1	8.2	14.8	15	(15.11)
T_0 (hr)	1.19	1.22	1.14	1.12	(15.2)
T_{z1} (hr)	2.22	2.5 (T_a)	2.22	2.5 (T_a)	(15.2)
T_{z2} (hr)	7.69	7.69	14.71	14.71	(15.2)
T_{el}/V_1 (hr/L)	0.29	0.29	0.33	0.33	(15.3)
T_a*V_1 (hr/L)	25.0	25.0	35.7	37.0	(15.12)
AUC (ng·hr/L)	2299	2285	2667	2666	
X_u (µg)	8048	8000	8002	8000	
$f*F$	0.8	0.8	0.8	0.8	(15.5)

clearance time alone is responsible for the change in the area under the curve. Only one of T_0, T_{z1}, and T_{z2} changes with age, indicating that only one of T_{el}, T_a, and T_{12} changes with age. Since the extent of absorption is the same between the two subjects and the renal clearance time decreases in the elderly, T_a is likely to be the same between the two subjects, and T_{el} is likely to increase in the elderly since renal function decreases with age. The

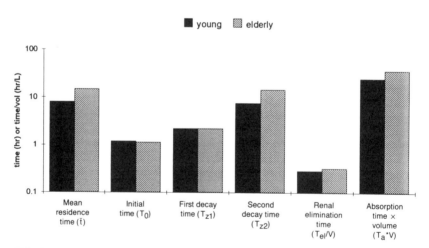

FIGURE 15.4. The time constant plot comparing the two age groups in the example shown in Figure 15.3. Only one of T_0, T_{z1}, and T_{z2} changes with age, indicating that only one of T_{el}, T_a, and T_{12} changes with age.

volume of distribution is likely to increase in the elderly based on two facts: (1) the maximum concentration decreases while the area under the curve increases with age, and (2) T_a*V_1 increases in the elderly while the value of T_a is likely to be the same between the two subjects. However, the exact volume of distribution can only be determined by giving intravenous doses to the subjects.

Case 3: Distribution and Metabolism Changes with Age

The metabolic rate in the elderly may decrease due to reduced hepatic blood flow [18], decreased liver mass size [16], or decreased hepatic enzyme activity [25,26]. As a result of a change in the metabolic rate, the decay time may vary with age. Additional factors, such as volume of distribution and protein binding, may also affect the decay time of a drug in the elderly. This can be described by Model 3, and simulated plasma concentration profiles in young and elderly subjects are shown in Figure 15.5. In this example, the elderly subject has a slower metabolic rate, a greater volume of distribution, and a faster distribution rate (K_{12}) than does the young subject. Tha parent drug concentration, as well as the metabolite concentration, is reduced in the elderly. The lag time between the maxi-

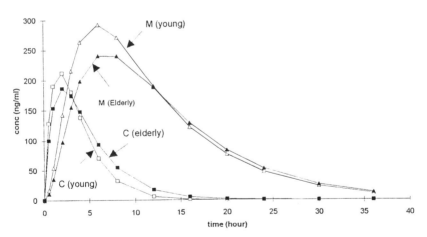

FIGURE 15.5. Simulated plasma concentration profiles of young and elderly subjects using Model 3, with age affecting distribution and metabolism. The time constant plot comparing the two age populations is shown in Figure 15.6. The parameters used in this simulation are young: $X_0 = 10$ mg, $f*F = 0.7$, $V_1 = 12$ L, $V_2 = 18$ L, $V_m = 10$ L, $K_a = 0.6$ hr^{-1}, $K_{12} = 0.1$ hr^{-1}, $K_{21} = 1$ hr^{-1}, $K_{el} = 0.15$ hr^{-1}, $K_m = 0.4$ hr^{-1}, $K_{mel} = 0.12$ hr^{-1}; elderly: $X_0 = 10$ mg, $f*F = 0.7$, $V_1 = 16$ L, $V_2 = 18$ L, $V_m = 10$ L, $K_a = 0.6$ hr^{-1}, $K_{12} = 0.15$ hr^{-1}, $K_{21} = 1$ hr^{-1}, $K_{el} = 0.12$ hr^{-1}, $K_m = 0.25$ hr^{-1}, $K_{mel} = 0.12$ hr^{-1}.

mum metabolite concentration and the maximum parent drug concentration is 4 hours, reflecting a slow elimination of the metabolite.

The key time constant in this example is the hepatic elimination time, which cannot be estimated without measuring the metabolite concentration. If the metabolite concentration is not available, the next useful time constant is the decay time for the assessment of the elimination rate. However, a change with age in renal or hepatic elimination cannot be distinguished without metabolite concentration and urine data. Therefore, if a drug is extensively metabolized, the metabolite concentration, in addition to the drug concentration, is critical for evaluating the age effect on the metabolism. The estimated pharmacokinetic parameters of the above example using the time constant analysis are listed in Table 15.3, and the estimated time constants are presented in Figure 15.6. The ratio of area under the parent drug concentration (AUC_C) between the two subjects is equal to the ratio of the total clearance time between the two subjects. In addition, the bioavailability ($f*F$), estimated from the culumative urine drug amount, is the same for the two subjects. Therefore, the total clearance time alone is responsible for the difference in the area under the parent drug concentration curve between the young and elderly subjects. The maximum concentration of the parent drug decreases in spite of an increase in the area under the curve in the elderly, indicating an increased volume of distribu-

TABLE 15.3. Estimated Time Constants of Model 3
for the Example Shown in Figure 15.5.

| Parameter | Young | | Elderly | | |
	Time Constant Analysis	Model Value	Time Constant Analysis	Model Value	Equation
$\bar{t}_C$ (hr)	3.7	3.7	4.8	4.8	(15.11)
$\bar{t}_M$ (hr)	12	12	13.1	13.1	(15.20)
T_0 (hr)	1.49	1.67	1.49	1.67	(15.2) stripping
T_{zl} (hr)	2.17	2.17	3.33	3.33	(15.2)
T_{el}/V_c (hr/L)	0.56	0.56	0.52	0.52	(15.3)
T_{mel}/V_m (hr/L)	0.83	0.83	0.83	0.83	(15.3)
T_m/V_c (hr/L)	0.21	0.21	0.25	0.25	(15.22)
T_a*V_c (hr/L)	20.0	20.0	28.6	27.0	(15.12)
AUC_C (ng·hr/L)	1071	1060	1194	1182	
AUC_M (ng·hr/L)	4254	4242	3953	3941	
X_{uc} (μg)	1929	1909	2294	2270	
X_{um} (μg)	5105	5090	4744	4729	
$f*F$	0.7	0.7	0.7	0.7	(15.5)
V_z (L)	14.5	14.2	19.5	19.5	(15.9)

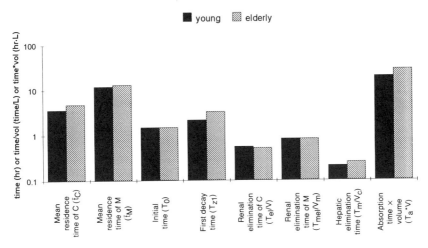

FIGURE 15.6. The time constant plot comparing the two age populations in the example shown in Figure 15.5. Only one of T_0 and T_{z1} is different between the two subjects; therefore, it is likely that only one of the time constants T_{el} and T_a changes with age.

tion of the central compartment in the subject. This is consistent with the fact that the apparent volume of distribution V_z increases in the elderly.

Now let us examine the time constant plot (Figure 15.6). In this example, only one of the two time constants, T_{z1} and T_{z2}, is determinable using the stripping method, indicating that the concentration curve may have collapsed to a two-compartment model [one of the scenarios in Equations (15.14) and (15.15)]. Only one of T_0 and T_{z1} is different between the two subjects; therefore, it is likely that only one of the time constants T_{el} and T_a changes with age.

EXAMPLES

Example 1: Volume of Distribution or First Pass Metabolism Changes with Age

The pharmacokinetics of nisoldipine were studied in nine young and twelve elderly subjects following the oral administration of 10 mg nisoldipine [1]. The mean plasma concentration profiles of nisoldipine in the young and elderly subjects are shown in Figure 15.7. The plasma nisoldipine concentrations are very low due to an extensive first pass effect (less than 1% excreted unchanged in the urine). The plasma nisoldipine concentration is higher in the elderly than in the young subjects. The drug is rapidly ab-

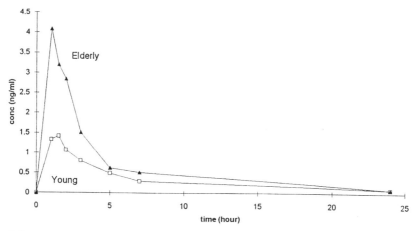

FIGURE 15.7. Mean plasma concentration profiles of nisoldipine in nine young and twelve elderly subjects following the oral administration of 10 mg nisoldipine. (Reproduced from Reference [1] with permission from Blackwell Science Ltd.) The time constant plot comparing the two age groups is shown in Figure 15.8.

sorbed in both population groups, with fast alpha phases and prolonged beta phases.

Nisoldipine is subjected to an extensive first pass effect and is highly bound to plasma protein. Bioavailability and volume of distribution are the potential parameters that may vary with age since metabolic rate and amount of plasma protein tend to change with age. The pharmacokinetic parameters of nisoldipine are estimated using Model 2 since the concentration profiles show biexponential terminal phases. The estimated pharmacokinetic parameters are listed in Table 15.4, and the estimated time constants are presented in Figure 15.8. The area under the nisoldipine concentration curve is twice as high in the elderly as in the young subjects.

TABLE 15.4. *The Estimated Pharmacokinetic Parameters of Nisoldipine Using Model 2.*

Parameter*	Young	Elderly	Equation
T_{z2} (hr)	6.21	6.21	(15.2)
$\bar{t}$ (hr)	7.57	5.57	(15.11)
$T_{el,t}*f*/V$ (hr/L)	0.00070	0.00150	(15.6)
AUC (ng·hr/ml)	7.0	15.0	
$V_{ss}/f/F$ (L)	10,809	3706	(15.8)

*Parameters estimated from the mean concentration curves or the reported mean values.

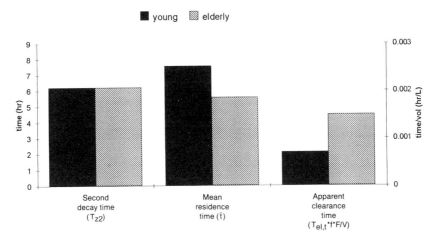

FIGURE 15.8. The time constant plot of nisoldipine comparing two age populations using Model 2. The total clearance time $(T_{el,t}*f*F/V)$ is much shorter in the young subjects, resulting in a smaller area under the concentration curve in this group.

Now let us examine the time constant plot (Figure 15.8). The second decay time constants T_{z2} are similar between the two groups, but the mean residence time is longer in the young subjects, indicating that the first decay time constant T_{z1} may be longer in the young subjects. The total clearance time is much shorter in the young subjects, resulting in a smaller area under the concentration curve in this group. The value of $V_{ss}/f/F$ is very large, probably due to an extremely small F value (extensive first pass effect).

Nisoldipine is highly bound to the plasma protein (99.73 %), and a change in protein concentration in different age groups may affect the volume of distribution. The larger area under the concentration curve in the elderly subjects can be caused by a decreased volume of distribution or a decreased first pass effect. To summarize, nisoldipine has little cardiovascular effect on young subjects while it significantly reduces the blood pressure in the elderly [1], probably due to the much higher plasma concentration in the elderly than the young subjects.

Example 2: Elimination and Volume of Distribution Change with Age

The pharmacokinetics of ofloxacin were studied in twelve young and twelve elderly subjects following the oral administration of 300 mg of ofloxacin [12]. The mean plasma concentration profiles of ofloxacin in the two groups are shown in Figure 15.9. The ofloxacin plasma concentration is

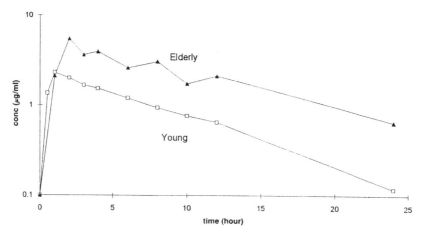

FIGURE 15.9. Mean plasma ofloxacin concentration profiles in twelve young and twelve elderly subjects following the oral administration of 300 mg of ofloxacin. (Reproduced from Reference [12] with permission.) The time constant plot comparing the two age populations is shown in Figure 15.10.

higher in the elderly subjects than the young subjects. The absorption is rapid in both groups, followed by a relatively slow elimination phase.

Ofloxacin is rapidly absorbed after oral administration, its bioavailability is very high, and it is eliminated almost entirely by renal excretion [12]. Therefore, the potential parameter that may vary with age is the renal elimination time since renal function decreases with age. However, urine data are not available in this example for the assessment of the renal elimination-time. The next useful key time constant is the decay time, which may well represent the renal elimination time since the drug is predominantly excreted through the renal route. The concentration profiles of ofloxacin exhibit a monoexponential terminal phase, and Model 1 is used to estimate

TABLE 15.5. The Estimated Pharmacokinetic
Parameters of Ofloxacin Using Model 1.

Parameter*	Young	Elderly	Equation
T_z (hr)	9.0	12.2	(15.2)
$\bar{t}$ (hr)	8.35	12.35	(15.1)
$T_{el,t}*f*F/V$ (min/ml)	0.0043	0.012	(15.6)
AUC (ng·hr/ml)	21.5	60.4	
$V_{ss}/f/F$ (L)	116.6	61.7	(15.8)

*Parameters estimated from the mean concentration curves or the
reported mean values.

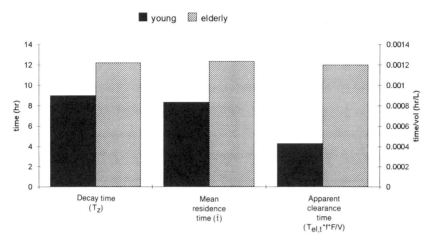

FIGURE 15.10. The time constant plot of ofloxacin comparing two age populations using Model 1. The decay time (T_z) of the concentration profile is longer in the elderly, suggesting that the elimination is probably responsible for part of the increase in the area under the curve in the elderly.

the pharmacokinetic parameters. The estimated pharmacokinetic parameters are listed in Table 15.5, and the estimated time constants are presented in Figure 15.10. The area under the plasma concentration curve in the elderly subjects is almost three times higher than in the young subjects. Ofloxacin is well absorbed in young adults (more than 95%); therefore, the increased area under the curve in the elderly cannot be due to an increase in the extent of absorption.

Now let us examine the time constant plot (Figure 15.10). The decay time of the concentration profile is longer in the elderly, suggesting that the elimination is probably responsible for part of the increase in the area under the curve in the elderly. The total clearance time is three times longer in the elderly. The steady-state volume of distribution in the elderly is half of that in the young subjects, indicating that a smaller volume of distribution may cause the greater area under the concentration curve in the older subjects. To summarize, ofloxacin concentration is higher in the elderly subjects, probably due to reduced renal excretion or decreased volume of distribution. Therefore, a reduction in the dosing level may be necessary in the elderly patients, as suggested in Reference [12].

Example 3: Elimination Changes with Age

Doxacurium pharmacokinetics were evaluated in nine young and nine

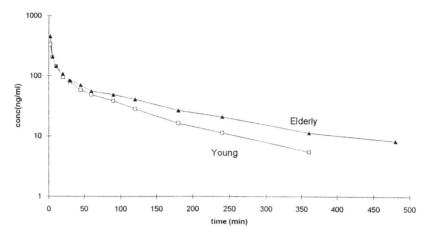

FIGURE 15.11. Mean plasma concentration profiles of doxacurium in nine young and nine elderly patients under nitrous oxide–isoflurane anesthesia, following the intravenous administration of 30 μg/kg doxacurium. (Reproduced from Reference [7] with permission.) The time constant plot comparing the two age groups is shown in Figure 15.12.

elderly patients under nitrous oxide–isoflurane anesthesia, following the intravenous administration of 30 μg/kg doxacurium [7]. The mean plasma concentration profiles of doxacurium in the young and elderly subjects are shown in Figure 15.11. The concentration profiles in both groups show biexponential terminal phases. The doxacurium plasma concentration is higher in the elderly subjects than in the young subjects.

Preliminary studies indicate that doxacurium could be excreted by both renal and biliary routes, and it is not extensively bound to the plasma protein (30%) [7]. Therefore, a key time constant that may potentially change

TABLE 15.6. The Estimated Pharmacokinetic
Parameters of Ofloxacin Using Model 1.

Parameter*	Young	Elderly	Equation
T_z (min)	109.5	172.7	(15.2)
$\bar{t}$ (min)	91.9	151.5	(15.1)
$T_{el,t}*f*F/V$ (min·kg/ml)	0.394	0.571	(15.6)
AUC (ng·min/ml)	11,602	16,966	
V_c (L/kg)	0.08	0.08	(15.7)
V_z (L/kg)	0.28	0.28	(15.9)
V_{ss} (L/kg)	0.23	0.25	(15.8)

*Parameters estimated from the mean concentration curves or the reported mean values.

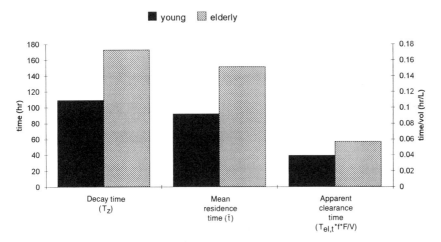

FIGURE 15.12. The time constant plot of doxacurium comparing two age groups using Model 1. The decay time (T_z) and the mean residence time ($\bar{t}$) of the concentration curve are longer in the elderly subjects, indicating that a slower elimination may be responsible for the greater area under the concentration curve in the elderly group.

with age is the renal elimination time. Since urine data are not available in this example, the next useful key time constant is the decay time. The pharmacokinetic parameters of doxacurium are estimated using Model 2. The estimated parameters are listed in Table 15.6, and the estimated time constants are presented in Figure 15.12. As shown in the time constant plot (Figure 15.12), the decay time and the mean residence time of the concentration curve are longer in the elderly subjects, indicating that a slower elimination may be responsible for the greater area under the concentration curve in the elderly group. The volumes of distribution, V_c, V_z, and V_{ss}, are similar between the two groups; therefore, they are not responsible for the difference in the area under the curve. The similarity in the volumes of distribution between age groups is probably because the large, positively charged molecule of doxacurium is confined to the extracellular water [7], the volume of which does not vary with total body water or body fat. To summarize, the concentration of doxacurium increases with age, probably due to a decreased renal function.

REFERENCES

1. Baksi A. K., Edwards J. S., and Ahr G., "A comparison of the pharmacokinetics of nisoldipine in elderly and young subjects," *Br. J. Clin. Pharmac.*, 1991; 31:367–370.
2. Barbhaiya R. H., Knupp C. A., and Pittmann K. A., "Effects of age and gender on

pharmacokinetics of cefepime," *Antimicrobial Agents and Chemotherapy,* 1992; 36(6):1181–1185.

3. Benet L. Z., Massoud N., and Gambertoglio J. G., *Pharmacokinetic Basis for Drug Treatment,* Raven Press, New York, 1984.

4. Chu S. Y., Wilson D. S., Guay D. R. P., and Craft C., "Clarithromycin pharmacokinetics in healthy young and elderly volunteers," *J. Clin. Pharmacol.,* 1992; 32:1045–1049.

5. Davis D. F. and Shock N. W., "Age changes in glomerular filtration rate, effective renal plasma flow, and the tubular excretory capacity in adult males," *J. Clin. Invest.,* 1950; 29:496.

6. Ferry D. G., Campbell A. J., Bland R., Beasley M., Gazeley L., and Edwards I. R., "Pharmacokinetics of primenol in young and elderly subjects," *Eur. J. Clin. Pharmacol.,* 1992; 43:437–439.

7. Gariepy L. P., Varin F., Donati F., Salib Y., and Bevan D. R., "Influence of aging on the pharmacokinetics and pharmacodynamics of doxacurium," *Clinical Pharmacology & Therapeutics,* 1993; 53(3):340–347.

8. Holmes D., Nuesch E., Houle J. M., and Rosenthaler J., "Steady state pharmacokinetics of hydrolysed bopindolol in young and elderly men," *Eur. J. Clin. Pharmacol.,* 1991; 41:175–178.

9. Jeandel C., Lapicque F., Netter P., Bannwarth B., Monot C., Gillet P., Payan E., Guillaume M., and Cuny G., "Effect of age on the disposition of sodium fluoride," *Eur. J. Clin. Pharmacol.,* 1992; 43:295–297.

10. McElnay J. C., Passmore A. P., Crawford V. L. S., McConnel J. G., Taylor I. C., and Walker F. S., "Steady state pharmacokinetic profile of indomethacin in elderly patients and young volunteers," *Eur. J. Clin. Pharmacol.,* 1992; 43:77–80.

11. Meyers B. R., Wilkinson P., Mendelson M. H., Bournazos C., Tejero C., and Hirschman S. Z., "Pharmacokinetics of aztreonam in healthy elderly and young adult volunteers," *J. Clin. Pharmacol.,* 1993; 33:470–474.

12. Molinaro M., Villani P., Regazzi M. B., Rondanelli R., and Doveri G., "Pharmacokinetics of ofloxacin in elderly patients and in healthy young subjects," *Eur. J. Clin. Pharmacol.,* 1992; 43:105–107.

13. Schwinghammer T. L., Antal E. J., Kubacka R. T., Hackimer M. E., and Johnston J. M., "Pharmacokinetics and pharmacodynamics of glyburide in young and elderly nondiabetic adults," *Clinical Pharmacy,* 1991; 10:532–538.

14. Shah J., Teitelbaum P., Molony B., Gabuzda T., and Massey I., "Single and multiple dose pharmacokinetics of ticlopidine in young and elderly subjects," *Br. J. Clin. Pharmac.,* 1991; 32:761–764.

15. Sitar D. S., Warren C. P., and Aoki F. Y., "Pharmacokinetics and pharmacodynamics of bambuterol, a long-acting bronchodilator pro-drug of terbutaline, in young and elderly patients with asthma," *Clin. Pharmacol. Ther.,* 1992; 52(3):297–306.

16. Swift C. G. et al. "Antipyrine disposition and liver size in the elderly," *Eur. J. Clin. Pharmacol.,* 1978; 12:149.

17. Tan A. C. I. T. L., Jansen T. L. Th. A ., Termond E. F. S., Russel F. G. M., Thien Th., Kloppenborg P. W. C., and Benraad Th. J., "Kinetics of atrial natriuretic peptide in young and elderly subjects," *Eur. J. Clin. Pharmacol.,* 1992; 42:449–452.

18. Vestal R. E. et al., "Effects of age and cigarette smoking on propranolol disposition," *Clin. Pharmacol. Ther.,* 1979; 26:8.

19. Evans W. E., Schentag J. J., and Jusko W. J., *Applied Pharmacokinetics,* Applied Therapeutics, Inc., 1992.

20. Cammarata P. J. et al., "Serum anti-γ globulin and anti-nuclear factors in the aged," *JAMA,* 1967; 199:445–458.

21. Greenblatt D. J., "Reduced serum albumin concentration in the elderly: A report from the Boston Collaborative Drug Surveillance Program," *J. Am. Geriatr. Soc.,* 1979; 27:20–22.

22. David D. et al., "Age related changes in the plasma protein binding of lidocaine and diazepam," *Clin. Res.,* 1980; 28:234A.

23. Lalonde R. L. et al., "Effects of age on the protein binding and disposition of propanolol stereoisomers," *Clin. Pharmacol. Ther.,* 1990; 47:447–455.

24. Rowland M. and Tozer T. N., *Clinical Pharmacokinetics, Concepts and Applications,* Lea & Febiger, 1980.

25. Crook J., O'Malley K., and Stevenson I. H., "Pharmacokinetics in the elderly," *Clin. Pharmacokinet.,* 1976; 1:280–296.

26. Ouslander J. G., "Drug therapy in the elderly," *Ann. Intern. Med.,* 1981; 95:711–722.

CHAPTER 16

Difference in Pharmacokinetics between Genders

INTRODUCTION

Gender differences in the pharmacokinetics of a drug can be determined in a male versus female clinical study. Among the most common differences in the pharmacokinetics between men and women are the volume of distribution [11] and rate of metabolism [4]. The difference in body weight and body mass composition between males and females [21] may result in a difference in the volume of distribution of drugs. The average body weight and lean to fat ratio is greater in males than in females; therefore, the volume of the central compartment is larger in males, but the peripheral compartment of lipophilic drugs may be disproportionally larger in females due to favorable distribution of the drugs to the fat tissue. The metabolism of some drugs (e.g., oxazepam [7] and metoprolol [8]) is slower in female than in male subjects. The coadministration of oral contraceptives inhibits the oxidative metabolism of many drugs [1,10,13]. Pregnancy also influences many aspects of drug pharmacokinetics. Late pregnancy is associated with delayed gastric emptying and decreased gastrointestinal motility, which may result in a decrease in absorption rate but an increase in the extent of absorption [20]. The apparent volume of distribution increases during pregnancy due to weight gain and decrease in protein binding. The glomerular filtration increases and nonrenal clearance of some drugs decreases with pregnancy [12]. Therefore, the key pharmacokinetic parameters in a male versus female study are volume of distribution (due to body size, composition, or plasma protein binding), absorption time constant (due to gastric emptying), bioavailability (due to gastrointestinal motility), distribution time constants (due to protein binding or body mass composition), hepatic elimination time constant (due to generic difference or drug interaction), and renal elimination time constant (due to glomerular filtration or protein binding).

Some common themes in the time constant view can be observed in the male versus female study as well as in other studies. One of the common factors among various pharmacokinetic studies is the importance of pre-dominant elimination route. If the predominant elimination route is af-fected by a clinical condition, the concentration of the drug will be greatly affected. On the other hand, if a less important elimination route is affected by a clinical condition, the plasma drug concentration will only be slightly affected. Hepatic elimination time is affected by factors such as gender, age (Chapter 15), and hepatic impairment (Chapter 18). Therefore, if the hepatic elimination time is very different but the drug concentration changes only slightly between genders, one can expect the same theme to occur in age and hepatic impairment studies. Examples of factors that may affect renal elimination time are renal impairment (Chapter 17), age (Chap-ter 15) and gender. If drug plasma concentrations change corresponding to a change in renal elimination time between genders, a similar theme should also be observed in renal impairment and age studies. Another common factor between studies is the lipophilicity of drugs. Lipophilic drugs may have a larger peripheral volume of distribution in women than in men, due to a more extensive distribution to the tissue in women. Lipophilic drugs, in general, have large volumes of distribution compared with hydrophilic drugs. Lipophilic drugs also tend to show slow dissolution time but fast absorption time. However, food may improve the dissolution of lipophilic drugs by increasing the solubility (Chapter 13).

One model is discussed in this chapter, which describes the difference in the distribution and metabolism between genders. One simulated case study and two literature examples are presented in this chapter to illus-trate the utility of the model in the male and female studies. Additional literature examples of male and female studies can be found in the literature [1–19].

PHARMACOKINETIC MODEL

This section presents a model that is useful in describing the gender dif-ference in pharmacokinetics. The goal is to establish simple relationships between time constants and measurable parameters such as (1) mean resi-dence time, which is the sum of input and output times, and (2) area under the curves. The derivations of these relationships are straightforward and are discussed in Chapter 2.

Model 1: Difference in the Distribution and Metabolism between Genders

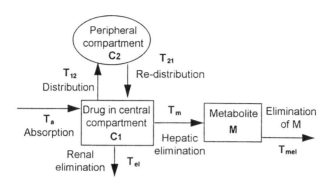

The key pharmacokinetic parameters that may be different between men and women include volume of distribution, absorption time constant, bioavailability, distribution time constants, hepatic elimination time constant, and renal elimination time constant. The same parameters may also be altered during pregnancy. Model 1 can be used to study the difference in these parameters between genders and the alteration of the parameters during pregnancy. The estimation of key time constants and pharmacokinetic parameters are described as follows.

The decay time constant T_z can be estimated by a partial area under the concentration curve and a curve-stripping technique (see Appendix 2):

$$\frac{1}{\text{Decay time } (T_z)} = \lambda_z = 2\frac{(t_{\text{ref}} - t_{\text{last}}) \ln (C_{t_{\text{ref}}}) - \text{AU} \ln C_{t_{\text{ref}}-t_{\text{last}}}}{(t_{\text{ref}} - t_{\text{last}})^2} \quad (16.1)$$

The mean residence time of the concentration curve is simply the sum of input and output times (see Chapter 2):

$$\text{Mean residence time of C following oral dose } (\bar{t}_{C,\text{po}}) = \frac{\text{AUMC}_{C1}}{\text{AUC}_{C1}}$$

$$= \text{Input time } (T_{c,\text{po,in}}) + \text{Output time } (T_{c,\text{po,out}}) = T_a + T_{\text{el},t} + T_{\text{el},t}\frac{T_{21}}{T_{12}}$$

$$(16.2)$$

$$\text{Mean residence time of M following oral dose } (\bar{t}_{M,po}) = \frac{AUMC_M}{AUC_M}$$

$$= \text{Input time } (T_{m,po,in}) + \text{Output time } (T_{m,po,out}) = T_a + T_{el,t} + T_{el,t}\frac{T_{21}}{T_{12}} + T_{mel}$$

$$(16.3)$$

where $T_{el,t} = 1/(1/T_{el} + 1/T_m + 1/T_{12})$. In a male versus female study and a pregnancy study, the mean residence time of a drug is most likely to be affected by the elimination time and the distribution time constants. The potential difference in metabolic rate between genders or between pregnant and nonpregnant women can be detected using the following ratio, assuming that there is no difference in the elimination time (T_{mel}) of the metabolite:

$$\frac{AUC_M}{AUC_C} = \frac{V_1 T_{mel}}{V_m T_m} = \frac{\text{Elimination clearance time of metabolite}}{\text{Formation clearance time toward metabolite}} \quad (16.4)$$

The renal clearance time may be different between genders or between pregnant and nonpregnant women as a result of different volume of distribution. The renal clearance time can be estimated from the cumulative urine recovery:

$$\text{Renal clearance time} \left(\frac{T_{el}}{V_1}\right) = \frac{AUC}{X_u} \quad (16.5)$$

The above equation applies to both the parent drug and the metabolite. The total clearance time may be affected by the heaptic elimination time or volume of distribution and can be estimated from the following equation:

$$\text{Apparent total clearance time} \left(\frac{T_{el,t}}{V_1}fF\right) = \frac{AUC_C}{X_0} \quad (16.6)$$

The apparent volume of distribution is frequently different between men and women and can be defined as follows:

$$\text{Apparent volume of distribution} \left(\frac{V_z}{fF}\right) = T_z\frac{X_0}{AUC_C} \quad (16.7)$$

The bioavailability of a drug may be different between pregnant and non-pregnant women due to altered gastrointestinal motility by the pregnancy and can be estimated from the total urine recovery of the drug, assuming the renal excretion is the predominant route of elimination.

$$\text{Fraction absorbed } (f) = \frac{X_{uc} + X_{um}}{X_0} \tag{16.8}$$

Following an intravenous administration, the mean residence time is equal to the output time.

$$\text{Mean residence time of C following iv dose } (\bar{t}_{iv}) = \frac{\text{AUMC}}{\text{AUC}}$$

$$= \text{Output time } (T_{iv,out}) = T_{el,t} + T_{el,t}\frac{T_{21}}{T_{12}} \tag{16.9}$$

The absorption time constant is then estimated from the difference in the mean residence time after oral and intravenous doses.

$$\text{Absorption time } (T_a) = \bar{t}_{po} - \bar{t}_{iv} \tag{16.10}$$

The relative bioavailability is estimated as follows:

$$\text{Bioavailability } (fF) = \frac{\text{AUC}_{po}}{\text{AUC}_{iv}} \tag{16.11}$$

CASE STUDY

Case 1: Difference in Volume of Distribution and Metabolism between Genders

Among the most common differences in the pharmacokinetics of drugs between men and women are differences in the volume of distribution and the rate of metabolism. The average body size of men is greater than that of women, which results in different volumes of distribution of both central and peripheral compartments between genders. The body mass composition (i.e., lean versus fat) is different between men and women [21], which affects the tissue binding of drugs and, consequently, the apparent volume of distribution. The metabolic rate may be different between men and women due to differences in hepatic enzyme activity [7,8], hormonal effects, or coadministration of oral contraceptives [1,10,13]. The pharmacokinetics of drugs in men and women can be described by Model 1.

Simulated plasma drug concentration profiles using the model are shown in Figure 16.1. In this example, the male subject has a larger volume of distribution in both central and peripheral compartments than the female subject, which results in a slightly lower maximum concentration in the male subject. However, the female subject has a faster metabolic rate, producing a much higher metabolite concentration than the male subject. The time to reach the maximum concentration is not much different between the subjects. This indicates that the hepatic metabolism does not dominate the drug elimination rate, since a change in the metabolic rate has a minor effect on the overall elimination.

The concentration profiles of the drug are similar between genders, while the metabolite concentration of the male subject is lower than that of the female. This indicates a difference in metabolism between genders, and therefore, the key time constant is the hepatic elimination time T_m. The estimated pharmacokinetic parameters of the above example using the time constant analysis are listed in Table 16.1, and the estimated time constants are presented in Figure 16.2. The areas under the concentration curve of the parent drug are not different between the male and the female subjects, while those of the metabolites are significantly different between the two subjects (70% higher in the female). The ratio of the area under the metabo-

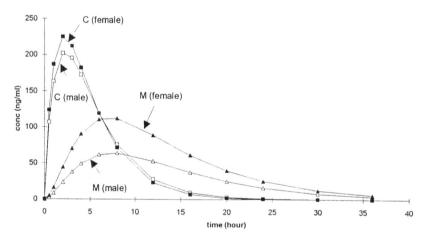

FIGURE 16.1. Simulated plasma drug concentration profiles for a man and woman using Model 1, illustrating gender difference in volume of distribution and metabolism. The time constant plot comparing the male and female is shown in Figure 16.2. The parameters used in this simulation are man: $X_0 = 10$ mg, $f^*F = 0.85$, $V_1 = 15$ L, $V_2 = 20$ L, $K_a = 0.5$ hr^{-1}, $K_{12} = 0.3$ hr^{-1}, $K_{21} = 1$ hr^{-1}, $K_{el} = 0.3$ hr^{-1}, $K_m = 0.09$ hr^{-1}, $K_{mel} = 0.12$ hr^{-1}; woman: $X_0 = 10$ mg, $f^*F = 0.8$, $V_1 = 12$ L, $V_2 = 18$ L, $K_a = 0.5$ hr^{-1}, $K_{12} = 0.3$ hr^{-1}, $K_{21} = 1$ hr^{-1}, $K_{el} = 0.3$ hr^{-1}, $K_m = 0.15$ hr^{-1}, $K_{mel} = 0.12$ hr^{-1}.

TABLE 16.1. The Estimated Time Constants of Model 1
for the Example in Figure 16.1.

Parameter	Male Time Constant Analysis	Male Model Value	Female Time Constant Analysis	Female Model Value	Equation
$\bar{t}_C$ (hr)	5.3	5.3	4.9	4.9	(16.2)
$\bar{t}_M$ (hr)	13.7	13.7	13.3	13.2	(16.3)
T_{zc} (hr)	3.70	3.57	3.23	3.23	(16.1)
T_{zm} (hr)	9.09	8.33	9.09	8.33	(16.1)
		(T_{mel})		(T_{mel})	
T_{el}/V_1 (hr/L)	0.22	0.22	0.27	0.27	(16.5)
T_{mel}/V_m (hr/L)	0.56	0.56	0.71	0.71	(16.5)
AUC_C (ng·hr/L)	1467	1452	1496	1481	
AUC_M (ng·hr/L)	1090	1089	1857	1851	
AUC_M/AUC_C	0.74	0.75	1.24	1.25	(16.4)
$X_{u,c}$ (μg)	6603	6538	5388	5333	
$X_{u,m}$ (μg)	1963	1961	2674	2666	
f	0.86	0.85	0.8	0.8	(16.8)
V_z (L)	22	21	18	17	(16.7)

lite concentration curve to that of the parent drug is much greater in the female than in the male, indicating a shorter hepatic elimination time in the female. However, the area under the parent drug concentration curve is barcly different between the two because the hepatic metabolism contributes only a small portion to the total elimination. The relatively large ratio (0.74 and 1.24 for the male and the female, respectively) of area under the metabolite concentration curve to that of parent drug is a result of a long T_{mel}, rather than a short T_m (shown in the time constant plot, Figure 16.2). The fact that the decay time (T_z) of the metabolite is much longer than that of the parent drug also indicates that the metabolite is eliminated more slowly than the parent drug. The mean residence time of both parent drug and metabolite is not much different between the two subjects, indicating again the small influence of the metabolism on the overall elimination rate. It is determined from the urinary excretion data that only 23% and 33% of the drug are converted to the metabolite in the male and the female subjects, respectively, which are relatively small values compared with the ratio of area under the curve AUC_M/AUC_C (74% and 124% for the male and the female, respectively). The renal clearance time of the metabolite is much longer than that of the parent drug, indicating that T_{mel} may be longer than T_{el} if the volume of distribution of the parent and the metabolite is similar.

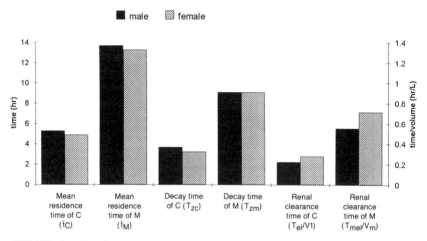

FIGURE 16.2. The time constant plot comparing pharmacokinetics of male and female in the example shown in Figure 16.1. The renal clearance time of the drug (T_{el}/V_1) and metabolite (T_{mel}/V_m) is longer in the female than in the male subject.

The apparent volume of distribution of the parent drug is greater in the male than the female due to the difference in the body size.

EXAMPLES

Example 1: Difference in Total Clearance Time between Genders

The pharmacokinetics of methylprednisolone were investigated in six men and six premenopausal women following the intravenous administration of 0.57 mg/kg methylprednisolone [11]. The plasma concentration of methylprednisolone for a selected male subject and a female subject is shown in Figure 16.3. The plasma concentration of methylprednisolone is higher in the male subject than in the female subject, due to a difference in either the dose or the elimination time.

The female subjects seem to have faster elimination of methylprednisolone than the male subjects, because the concentration of drug is lower and the decay time is shorter in the female subjects. However, metabolite and urine data are not available to identify the cause of the difference in elimination (hepatic or renal). Therefore, the key time constants in this example are the decay time and the total clearance time. The pharmacokinetic parameters of methylprednisolone are estimated using Model 1, and the two-

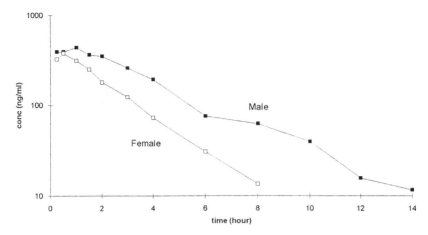

FIGURE 16.3. Plasma concentration profiles of methylprednisolone following an intravenous administration of 0.57 mg/kg methylprednisolone to a male subject and a female subject. (Reproduced from Reference [11] with permission.) The time constant plot comparing the two subjects is shown in Figure 16.4.

compartment model collapses to a one-compartment model. The estimated parameters are listed in Table 16.2, and the estimated time constants are presented in Figure 16.4. The average total body weight (TBW) of the male subjects is higher than that of the female subjects, resulting in a higher total dose per subject in males. The area under the concentration curve in the male subjects is 50% higher than that in the female subjects.

TABLE 16.2. The Estimated Pharmacokinetic Parameters of
Methylprednisolone in Six Male and Six Female Subjects Using Model 1.

Parameter*	Male	Female	Equation
T_z (hr)	3.72	2.48	(16.1)
$\bar{t}$ (hr)	3.8	2.4	(16.2)
$T_{el,t}/V_1$ (hr/L)	0.047	0.045	(16.6)
$T_{el,t}/V_1$*TBW (hr·kg/L)	3.70	2.50	
TBW (kg)	80.6	56.2	
X_0 (mg)	45.9	32.0	
AUC (ng·hr/ml)	2133	1443	
V_z (L)	80.0	54.9	(16.7)
V_z/TBW (L/kg)	0.99	0.98	
f_u (%)	23.1	24.7	

*Parameters estimated from the concentration profiles or the mean reported values.
TBW: Total body weight.

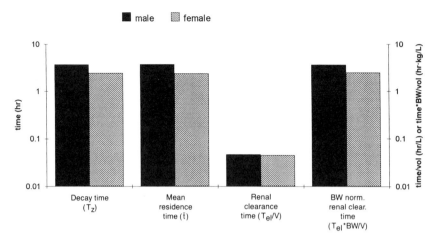

FIGURE 16.4. The time constant plot (logarithm) of methylprednisolone comparing a male and a female subject using Model 1. The decay time (T_z) of the concentration curve is longer in the male subjects than in the female subjects, indicating a slower rate of elimination in the former.

Now let us examine the time constant plot (Figure 16.4). The decay time of the concentration curve is longer in the male subjects than in the female subjects, indicating a slower rate of elimination in the former. In addition, the mean residence time is close to the value of the decay time, indicating that the decay time constant represents the elimination time (i.e., very little distribution is involved). The total clearance time is not different between the male and female subjects, while the body weight normalized clearance time $(T_{el,r}/V_1*BW)$ is longer in the male subjects than the female subjects. The volume of distribution seems to be proportional to the total body weight. The fraction of unbound drug (f_u) in the plasma is similar between the male and female subjects, indicating that the protein binding is not responsible for the difference in the volume of distribution. To summarize, the concentration of methylprednisolone is lower in the female when the dosage is based on the total body weight, due to a faster elimination in the female. However, women are more sensitive to the drug in terms of cortisol suppression [11], which may compensate for the low concentration, and the body weight normalized dose produces similar responses in both genders.

Example 2: Change in Elimination during Pregnancy

The pharmacokinetics of cephradine were studied in twelve women after oral and intravenous administration of 0.5 g cephradine during and after pregnancy [16]. The mean concentration profiles of cephradine after the four treatments are shown in Figure 16.5. Following the intravenous dose, the plasma concentration of cephradine after the pregnancy is higher than that during the pregnancy.

Cephradine is only 14% bound to the protein and is eliminated predominantly through the renal route [16]. Therefore, a change in protein binding during pregnancy may not affect the drug plasma concentration, while a change in renal excretion may affect the elimination. The decay time can be used as the key time constant for the assessment of renal excretion, since there is no other competitive elimination route. The pharmacokinetic parameters of cephradine are estimated using Model 1, and the two-compartment model collapses to a one-compartment model, since the terminal phase is monoexponential. The estimated pharmacokinetic parameters are listed in Table 16.3, and the estimated time constants are presented in Figure 16.6. The areas under the curve are smaller during the pregnancy than after the pregnancy for both oral and intravenous doses, which can be due to altered elimination time, volume of distribution, or extent of absorption (for the oral dose).

Now let us examine the time constant plot (Figure 16.6). The decay time of the concentration profiles following the oral and intravenous doses is shorter during the pregnancy than those after the pregnancy, indicating an increased elimination rate during the pregnancy. The mean residence time

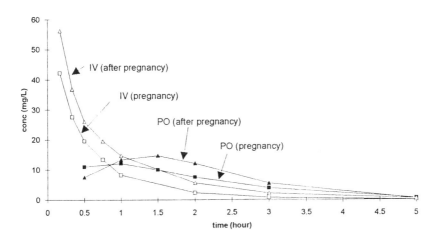

FIGURE 16.5. Mean plasma concentration profiles of cephradine after oral and intravenous administration of 0.5 g cephradine to twelve women during and after pregnancy. (Reproduced from Reference [16] with permission.) The time constant plot comparing the two treatments in the two populations is shown in Figure 16.6.

TABLE 16.3. Estimated Pharmacokinetic Parameters of Cephradine of the Example in Figure 16.3 Using Model 1.

Parameter*	Intravenous—Pregnancy	Intravenous—after Pregnancy	Oral—Pregnancy	Oral—after Pregnancy	Equation
T_z (hr)	0.72	0.97	0.85	0.97	(16.1)
$\bar{t}$ (hr)	0.84	1.06	1.69	1.82	(16.2)
$T_{el,t}/V_1$ (hr/L)	0.045	0.071			(16.6)
$T_{el,t}/V_1*BW$ (hr·kg/L)	2.79	4.29			
T_a (hr)			0.85	0.76	(16.10)
BW (kg)	62.9	61.0			
AUC (mg·hr/L)	24.3	38.9	25.3	31.9	
V_z (L)	15.6	13.2			(16.7)
V_z/BW (L/kg)	0.251	0.221			
$f*F$			1.049	0.846	(16.11)

*Parameters estimated from the mean concentration profiles or the reported mean values.
BW: Body weight.

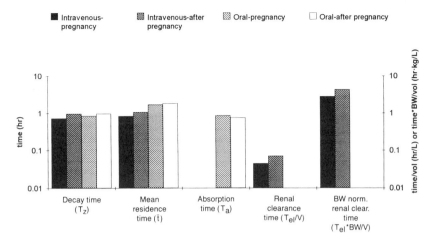

FIGURE 16.6. The time constant plot of cephradine comparing oral and intravenous administration of cephradine to twelve women during and after pregnancy using Model 1. Both total clearance time ($T_{el,t}/V$) and the body weight normalized clearance time ($T_{el,t}/V^*$BW) decrease during the pregnancy.

decreases during the pregnancy, consistent with the decrease in the elimination time. Both total clearance time and the body weight normalized clearance time decrease during the pregnancy, which is likely caused by a decrease in the elimination time since the volume of distribution (V_z) does not change much during the pregnancy. The extent of absorption increases while the absorption time is prolonged during pregnancy, probably due to a decrease in the gastrointestinal motility. Notice that the absorption time constant after the oral dose during pregnancy ($T_a = 0.85$) is very close to the decay time ($T_z = 0.85$), suggesting a possible flip-flop, where the absorption time is longer than the elimination time. To summarize, the concentration of cephradine decreases during pregnancy, probably due to an increase in renal clearance, and the dosage of the drug may need to be increased when treating pregnant women, as suggested in Reference [16].

REFERENCES

1. Back D. J., "Pharmacokinetic drug interactions with oral contraceptives," *Clin. Pharmacokinet.*, 1990; 18:472–484.
2. Barbhaiya R. H., Knupp C. A., and Pittman K. A., "Effects of age and gender on pharmacokinetics of cefepime," *Antimicrobial Agents and Chemotherapy*, 1992; 36(6):1181–1185.
3. Blychert E., Edgar B., Elmfeldt D., and Hedner T., "A population study of the pharmacokinetics of felodipine," *Br. J. Clin. Pharmac.*, 1991; 31:15–24.

4. Bonate P., "Gender-related differences in xenobiotic metabolism," *J. Clin. Pharmacol.*, 1991; 31:684–690.

5. Divoll M., Greenblatt D. J., Harmatz J. S., and Shader R. I., "Effects of age and gender on disposition of temazepam," *Journal of Pharmaceutical Sciences*, 1981; 70(10):1104–1107.

6. Gaudry S. E., Sitar D. S., Smyth D. D., McKenzie J. K., and Aoki F. Y., "Gender and age as factors in the inhibition of renal clearance of amantadine by quinine and quinidine," *Clinical Pharmacology & Therapeutics*, 1993; 54(1):23–27.

7. Greenblatt D. J., Divoll M., Harmatz J. S., and Shader R. I., "Oxazepam kinetics: Effects of age and sex," *Journal of Pharmacology and Experimental Therapeutics*, 1980; 215(1):86–91.

8. Hogstedt S., Lindberg B., Peng D. R., Regardh C., and Rane A., "Pregnancy-induced increases in metoprolol metabolism," *Clin. Pharmacol. Ther.*, 1985; 37(6):688–692.

9. Hogstedt S., Lindberg B., and Rane A., "Increased oral clearance of metoprolol in pregnancy," *Eur. J. Clin. Pharmacol.*, 1983; 24:217–220.

10. Jochemsen R., "Influence of sex, menstrual cycle and oral contraception on the disposition of nitrazepam," *Br. J. Clin. Pharmacol.*, 1982; 13:319–24.

11. Lew K. H., Ludwig E. A., Milad M. A., Donovan K., Middleton, E. Jr., Ferry J. J., and Jusko W. J., "Gender-based effects on methylprednisolone pharmacokinetics and pharmacodynamics," *Clinical Pharmacology & Therapeutics*, 1993; 54(4):402–414.

12. Luxford A. M. E. and Kellaway G. S. M., "Pharmacokinetics of digoxin in pregnancy," *Eur. J. Clin. Pharmacol.*, 1983; 25:117.

13. MacDonald J. I., "Sex difference and the effect of smoking and oral contraceptive steroids on the kinetics of diflunisal," *Eur. J. Clin. Pharmacol.*, 1990; 38:175–179.

14. Minerd J. O., Attwood J., and Birkett D. J., "Influence of sex and oral contraceptive steroids on paracetamol metabolism," *Br. J. Clin. Pharmacol.*, 1983; 16:503–509.

15. Nakatsu K., Brien J. F., Savard G., Toffelmire E. B., Abdollah H., Bennett B. H., and Marks G. S., "Plasma disposition and dynamic effects of a single oral dose of isosorbide dinitrate in human males and females," *Biopharmaceutics & Drug Disposition*, 1992; 13:357–367.

16. Philipson A., Stiernstedt G., and Ehrnebo M., "Comparison of the pharmacokinetics of cephradine and cefazolin in pregnant and non-pregnant women," *Clinical Pharmacokinetics*, 1987; 12:136–144.

17. Philipson A., "Pharmacokinetics of ampicillin during pregnancy," *Journal of Infectious Diseases*, 1977; 136(3):370–376.

18. Sasaki M., Tateishi T., and Ebihara A., "The effect of age and gender on the stereoselective pharmacokinetics of verapamil," *Clinical Pharmacology & Therapeutics*, 1993; 54(3):278–285.

19. von Bahr C., Wiesel F. A., Movin G., Eneroth P., Jansson P., Nilsson L., and Ogenstad S., "Neuroendocrine response to single oral doses of remoxipride and sulpiride in healthy female and male volunteers," *Psychopharmacology*, 1991: 103:443–448.

20. Nimmo, W. S., "Drugs, diseases and altered gastric emptying," *Clin. Pharmacokinet.*, 1976; 27:73–79.

21. Crook J., O'Malley K., and Stevenson I. H., "Pharmacokinetics in the elderly," *Clin. Pharmacokinet.*, 1976; 1:280–296.

CHAPTER 17

Special Pharmacokinetic Considerations in Renal Impairment

INTRODUCTION

The effects of deteriorating renal function on the drug pharmacokinetics can be determined by the renal impairment study. In renal-impaired patients, the creatinine clearance declines, which reflects decreased renal elimination rates. Due to the reduced elimination rate, drugs and their metabolites may accumulate in the body. Plasma protein binding may also decrease in patients with renal impairment [2,6], due to either a decrease in plasma protein concentration or an accumulation of inhibitors of the binding. Change in protein binding can affect the volume of distribution, the distribution time, or the hepatic and the renal elimination times. Metabolism in renal-impaired patients may also be inhibited because of an accumulation of metabolic inhibitors [11,15]. However, the inhibitors of protein binding and metabolism may be removed by dialysis. Thus, renal-impaired patients with dialysis may have different pharmacokinetics than patients without dialysis. To summarize, the key time constants and parameters in a renal impairment study are the renal elimination time, the hepatic elimination time, the distribution time, and the volume of distribution.

Some common themes in the time constant view can be observed in the renal impairment study as well as other studies. The first common factor is the predominant elimination route. If the predominant route of elimination is renal elimination, then plasma drug concentrations will be significantly affected by renal impairment and other clinical conditions involving a change in renal function, such as age (Chapter 15) and drug interaction (Chapter 14). If the renal excretion of a drug is insignificant compared with other elimination routes, the plasma concentration will only be slightly

407

affected by a change in the renal elimination time. A second common factor often observed in the renal impairment study is protein binding. The time constants that may be affected by a change in protein binding include the distribution time, the redistribution time, and the decay time. The distribution time may decrease, and the redistribution time may increase with a reduced protein binding in renal impaired patients. A change in these time constants may also be observed in other studies involving reduced or increased protein binding, such as the age study (Chapter 15), gender study (Chapter 16), drug interaction study (Chapter 14), and inflammatory diseases studies (Chapter 19). One of the typical changes in descriptive pharmacokinetic parameters as a result of increased protein binding, which may be commonly observed in the above-mentioned studies, involves a decrease in the maximum concentration and an increase in the decay time. Another common factor relevant to the renal impairment study is the pK_a value of the drug. The pK_a value determines to which plasma protein the drug may bind: acidic drugs tend to bind with albumin and basic drugs with α_1-acid glycoprotein. The effect of urine pH on renal elimination time also depends on the pK_a of the drug: high pH of urine may facilitate the excretion of acidic drugs, while low pH may improve the excretion of basic drugs.

Two pharmacokinetic models are described in this chapter for the estimation of time constants in renal impairment studies: (1) the first model describes the drugs with a monoexponential terminal phase, and (2) the second model describes the drugs with a biexponential terminal phase. Three stimulated case studies are considered in this chapter: (1) decreased renal elimination of parent drugs and metabolites, (2) decreased renal excretion and inhibited metabolism, and (3) decreased renal excretion and reduced protein binding. In addition, three literature examples are presented to illustrate the utility of the models in renal impairment studies. Additional examples of renal impairment studies can be found in the literature [1–17].

PHARMACOKINETIC MODELS

This section presents two models that are useful in determining effects of renal impairment on pharmacokinetics. The goal is to establish simple relationships between time constants and measurable parameters such as (1) mean residence time, which is the sum of input and output times, and (2) area under the curves. The derivations of these relationships are straightforward and are discussed in Chapter 2.

Model 1: Monoexponential Terminal Phase with Metabolism

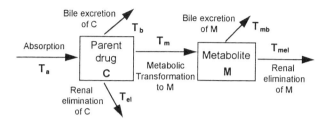

The elimination of drugs in patients with renal impairment may rely significantly on the nonrenal routes, such as metabolism or bile excretion. Therefore, the nonrenal elimination must be emphasized in the pharmacokinetics of drugs in the renal impaired patients as described in Model 1. In addition, the metabolic rate may also be affected in patients with renal disease due to an accumulation of metabolic inhibitors.

The mean residence time of the concentration curve in this model is simply the sum of input and output times:

$$\text{Mean residence time of C } (\bar{t}_{\text{C}}) = \frac{\text{AUMC}_{\text{C}}}{\text{AUC}_{\text{C}}}$$

$$= \text{Input time } (T_{\text{c,in}}) + \text{Output time } (T_{\text{c,out}}) = T_{\text{a}} + T_{\text{el},t} \quad (17.1)$$

$$\text{Mean residence time of M } (\bar{t}_{\text{M}}) = \frac{\text{AUMC}_{\text{M}}}{\text{AUC}_{\text{M}}}$$

$$= \text{Input time } (T_{\text{m,in}}) + \text{Output time } (T_{\text{m,out}}) = T_{\text{a}} + T_{\text{el},t} + T_{\text{mel},t}$$

$$(17.2)$$

where $T_{\text{el},t} = 1/(1/T_{\text{el}} + 1/T_{\text{m}} + 1/T_{\text{b}})$ and $t_{\text{mel},t} = 1/(1/T_{\text{mel}} + 1/T_{\text{mb}})$. The mean residence time of a drug in patients with renal diseases may increase due to an increase in the renal and hepatic elimination time constants. The total elimination time constant of the metabolite can be calculated from the difference in the mean residence times of the metabolite and the drug:

$$\text{Total elimination time of metabolite } (T_{\text{mel},t}) = \bar{t}_{\text{M}} - \bar{t}_{\text{C}} \quad (17.3)$$

The ratio of the area under the metabolite concentration curve to the area under the drug concentration curve gives the ratio of the total clearance time of the metabolite to the hepatic clearance time of the drug:

$$\frac{AUC_M}{AUC_C} = \frac{T_{mel,t}V_c}{T_m V_m} = \frac{\text{Total clearance time of metabolite}}{\text{Hepatic clearance time toward metabolite}} \quad (17.4)$$

The hepatic clearance time of the drug may be affected by the renal diseases due to an accumulation of metabolic inhibitors. The hepatic elimination time can be estimated by combining Equations (17.3) and (17.4):

$$\text{Normalized hepatic elimination time} \left(T_m \frac{V_m}{V_c} \right)$$

$$= T_{mel,t} \frac{AUC_C}{AUC_M} = (\bar{t}_M - \bar{t}_C) \frac{AUC_C}{AUC_M} \quad (17.5)$$

The renal clearance time of the drug and its metabolite can be estimated by the following two equations:

$$\text{Renal clearance time of C} \left(\frac{T_{el}}{V_c} \right) = \frac{AUC_C}{X_{uc}} \quad (17.6)$$

$$\text{Renal clearance time of M} \left(\frac{T_{mel}}{V_m} \right) = \frac{AUC_M}{X_{um}} \quad (17.7)$$

The total apparent clearance time of a drug may also increase in renal-impaired patients, and it is defined as the area under the concentration curve divided by the dose.

$$\text{Apparent total clearance time} \left(\frac{T_{el,t}}{V_c} fF \right) = \frac{AUC_C}{X_0} \quad (17.8)$$

The volume of distribution may also be affected by renal diseases due to a decrease in the plasma protein binding. The steady-state volume of distribution is defined as follows:

$$\text{Steady-state volume of distribution } (V_{ss}) = \frac{\bar{t}_C}{T_{el,t}} \frac{V_c}{fF} = \bar{t}_C \frac{X_0}{AUC_C} \quad (17.9)$$

Model 2: Biexponential Terminal Phase with Metabolism

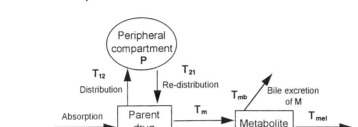

Frequently, protein binding of drugs decreases in patients with renal diseases [2,6]. As a result of the decreased protein binding, the free fraction of the drug in the plasma increases, and more free drug is available for tissue distribution and for metabolism. Therefore, the volume of distribution may increase and the distribution and metabolite time constants may decrease in the patients. A two-compartment model, Model 2, can be used to describe the effects of a decreased protein binding. In this model, compartment P represents the peripheral compartment to account for the change in distribution in renal-impaired patients.

The mean residence time of the concentration curves in this model is the sum of input and output times (see Chapter 2):

$$\text{Mean residence time of C } (\bar{t}_{\text{C}}) = \frac{\text{AUMC}_{\text{C}}}{\text{AUC}_{\text{C}}}$$

$$= \text{Input time } (T_{\text{c,in}}) + \text{Output time } (T_{\text{c,out}}) = T_{\text{a}} + T_{\text{el},t} + T_{\text{el},t}\frac{T_{21}}{T_{12}}$$

$$(17.10)$$

$$\text{Mean residence time of M } (\bar{t}_{\text{M}})$$

$$= \text{Input time } (T_{\text{m,in}}) + \text{Output time } (T_{\text{m,out}}) = \bar{t}_{\text{C}} + T_{\text{mel},t}$$

$$(17.11)$$

where $T_{\text{el},t} = 1/(1/T_{\text{el}} + 1/T_{\text{m}} + 1/T_{\text{b}})$ and $T_{\text{mel},t} = 1/(1/T_{\text{mel}} + 1/T_{\text{mb}})$. The ratio of the area under the metabolite concentration curve to the area under the drug concentration curve may be affected in the renal diseases due to altered hepatic clearance time or altered total clearance time of the metabolite.

$$\frac{AUC_M}{AUC_C} = \frac{T_{mel,t}V_c}{T_mV_m} = \frac{\text{Total clearance time of metabolite}}{\text{Hepatic clearance time toward metabolite}} \quad (17.12)$$

By combining Equations (17.11) and (17.12), the hepatic clearance time can be estimated according to the following equation:

$$\text{Normalized hepatic elimination time} \left(T_m \frac{V_m}{V_c} \right)$$

$$= T_{mel,t} \frac{AUC_C}{AUC_M} = (\bar{t}_M - \bar{t}_C) \frac{AUC_C}{AUC_M} \quad (17.13)$$

The renal clearance time is estimated from the cumulative urine recovery:

$$\text{Renal clearance time of C} \left(\frac{T_{el}}{V_c} \right) = \frac{AUC_C}{X_{uc}} \quad (17.14)$$

$$\text{Renal clearance time of M} \left(\frac{T_{mel}}{V_m} \right) = \frac{AUC_M}{X_{um}} \quad (17.15)$$

The apparent clearance time of the drug is defined as the ratio of the area under the curve to the dose:

$$\text{Apparent total clearance time} \left(\frac{T_{el,t}}{V_c} fF \right) = \frac{AUC_C}{X_0} \quad (17.16)$$

The steady-state volume of distribution is defined as follows

$$\text{Steady-state volume of distribution} (V_{ss}) = \frac{\bar{t}_C}{T_{el,t}} \frac{V_C}{fF} = \bar{t}_C \frac{X_0}{AUC_C}$$

$$(17.17)$$

CASE STUDIES

Case 1: Renal Excretion Is Not the Predominant Route of Elimination

The influence of renal impairment on the half-life of a drug in the blood depends on the relative importance of the renal and nonrenal elimination rates of the drug. If the drug is predominantly eliminated by the kidney, renal impairment will result in an accumulation of the drug in the body . On the other hand, if a drug can be eliminated through hepatic metabolism or bile excretion, as well as by renal elimination, the half-life of the drug may be affected by renal impairment to a small degree. The determination of metabolite concentrations in the plasma and urine is important in a renal impairment study in order to identify alternative routes of elimination in addition to the kidney. An example of plasma concentration profiles simulated by Model 1 is shown in Figures 17.1 and 17.2. In this example, the

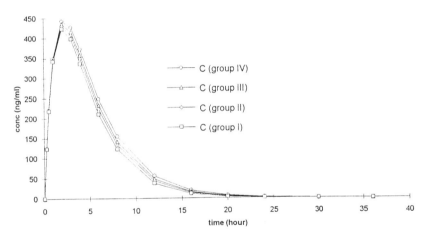

FIGURE 17.1. Simulated plasma drug concentration profiles using Model 1 for different degrees of renal-impaired patients. The renal excretion is not the predominant route of elimination. The time constant plot comparing the different patient groups is shown in Figure 17.3. The parameters used in this simulation are as follows: group 1: Cl_{cr} = 80 ml/min, X_0 = 10 mg, $f^{*}F$ = 0.8, V_c = 10 L, K_a = 0.7 hr^{-1}, K_{el} = 0.05 hr^{-1}, K_b = 0.05 hr^{-1}, V_m = 10 L, K_m = 0.2 hr^{-1}, K_{mel} = 0.3 hr^{-1}, K_{mb} = 0.05 hr^{-1}; group II: Cl_{cr} = 60 ml/min, X_0 = 10 mg, $f^{*}F$ = 0.8, V_c = 10 L, K_a = 0.7 hr^{-1}, K_{el} = 0.035 hr^{-1}, K_b = 0.05 hr^{-1}, V_m = 10 L, K_m = 0.2 hr^{-1}, K_{mel} = 0.24 hr^{-1}, K_{mb} = 0.05 hr^{-1}; group III: Cl_{cr} = 40 ml/min, X_0 = 10 mg, $f^{*}F$ = 0.8, V_c = 10 L, K_a = 0.7 hr^{-1}, K_{el} = 0.025 hr^{-1}, K_b = 0.05 hr^{-1}, V_m = 10 L, K_m = 0.2 hr^{-1}, K_{mel} = 0.15 hr^{-1}, K_{mb} = 0.05 hr^{-1}; group IV: Cl_{cr} = 20 ml/min, X_0 = 10 mg, $f^{*}F$ = 0.8, V_c = 10 L, K_a = 0.7 hr^{-1}, K_{el} = 0.01 hr^{-1}, K_b = 0.05 hr^{-1}, V_m = 10 L, K_m = 0.2 hr^{-1}, K_{mel} = 0.06 hr^{-1}, K_{mb} = 0.05 hr^{-1}.

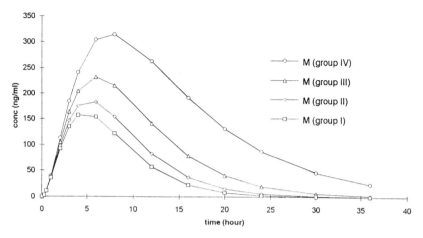

FIGURE 17.2. Simulated plasma metabolite concentration profiles of the example in Figure 17.1 for different degrees of renal-impaired patients.

subjects are divided into four groups based on their creatinine clearance. The renal elimination rate constants of the parent drug and the metabolite decrease proportionally with the creatinine clearance. The parent drug concentration profiles do not differ much between patients with various degrees of renal impairment, indicating that the renal excretion is not the dominant route of the elimination of the drug. On the other hand, the plasma metabolite concentration increases with the severity of renal impairment, indicating that the metabolite is eliminated through the kidney to a significant degree. The time to reach the maximum concentration of the metabolite is delayed in the renal-impaired patients, reflecting a decrease in the total elimination rate of the metabolite in these subjects.

The key time constant that may be affected by impaired renal function is the renal elimination time of the drug and the metabolite. However, a change in the renal elimination time of the drug may not affect the drug concentration if hepatic metabolism is the predominant elimination route. In addition, the hepatic elimination time may also be affected by the renal impairment. The estimated pharmacokinetic parameters of the above example using the time constant analysis are listed in Table 17.1, and the estimated time constants are presented in Figure 17.3. The area under the concentration curve of the parent drug does not differ much between the four groups, indicating the renal excretion does not dominate the elimination of the drug. On the other hand, the area under the metabolite concentration curve increases with the severity of the renal impairment, and the difference between groups III and IV is more significant than the difference between groups I and II.

TABLE 17.1. The Estimated Pharmacokinetic Parameters Using the Time Constant Analysis for the Example Shown in Figure 17.1.

Parameter	Group I TCA	Group I Model Value	Group II TCA	Group II Model Value	Group III TCA	Group III Model Value	Group IV TCA	Group IV Model Value	Equation
T_{zc} (hr)	3.33	3.33 ($T_{el,r}$)	3.52	3.51 ($T_{el,r}$)	3.64	3.64 ($T_{el,r}$)	3.85	3.85 ($T_{el,r}$)	
T_{zm} (hr)	3.57	3.33 ($T_{el,r}$)	4.17	3.51 ($T_{el,r}$)	5.56	5.0 ($T_{mel,r}$)	10.0	9.1 ($T_{mel,r}$)	
$\bar{t}_C$ (hr)	4.7	4.8	4.9	4.9	5	5.1	5.2	5.3	(17.1)
$\bar{t}_M$ (hr)	7.6	7.6	8.3	8.4	10	10.1	14.4	14.4	(17.2)
T_{el}/V_c (hr/L)	2.0	2.0	2.86	2.86	4.0	4.0	10.0	10.0	(17.6)
T_{mel}/V_m (hr/L)	0.33	0.33	0.42	0.42	0.67	0.67	1.67	1.67	(17.7)
$T_{mel,r}$ (hr)	2.78	2.86	3.45	3.45	5.0	5.0	9.09	9.09	(17.3)
T_m*V_m/V_c (hr)	5.0	5.0	5.0	5.0	5.0	5.0	5.0	5.0	(17.5)
AUC_C (ng·hr/L)	2699	2666	2840	2807	2943	2909	3111	3078	
AUC_M (ng·hr/L)	1536	1523	1947	1935	2918	2919	5607	5594	
X_{uc} (µg)	1349	1333	994	982	735	727	311	307	
X_{um} (µg)	4609	4571	4674	4646	4377	4363	3364	3356	
X_{uc}/X_0	0.13	0.13	0.1	0.1	0.07	0.07	0.03	0.03	
X_{um}/X_0	0.46	0.46	0.47	0.46	0.44	0.44	0.33	0.34	
AUC_M/AUC_C	0.57	0.57	0.69	0.69	0.99	1	1.8	1.8	(17.4)

TCA: Time constant analysis.

415

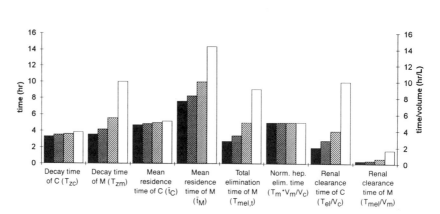

FIGURE 17.3. The time constant plot comparing different degrees of renal impairment in the example shown in Figure 17.1. The mean residence time of the parent drug ($\bar{t}_C$) does not change much with renal impairment, reflecting insignificant influence of the disease on the elimination of the drug. On the other hand, the mean residence time of the metabolite ($\bar{t}_M$) increases with the severity of the disease, reflecting the predominant role of the renal excretion in the elimination of the metabolite.

Now let us examine the time constant plot (Figure 17.3). The decay time of the metabolite is the same as that of the parent drug in groups I and II, indicating the elimination of the metabolite is faster than that of the parent drug in these groups. However, in more severe patients (groups III and IV), the decay time of the metabolite becomes longer than that of the parent drug, indicating that the metabolite elimination is affected by the renal impairment and becomes slower than the elimination of the parent drug. The mean residence time of the parent drug does not change much with renal impairment, reflecting insignificant influence of the disease on the elimination of the drug. On the other hand, the mean residence time of the metabolite increases with the severity of the disease, reflecting the predominant role of the renal excretion in the elimination of the metabolite. The urine recovery of the parent drug is much smaller than that of the metabolite, indicating again the insignificance of the renal elimination of the parent drug. The total urine recovery (parent + metabolite) decreases with the severity of the disease between groups I and II; however, the urine recovery of the metabolite is similar between the two groups because more of the drug is converted into the metabolite in group II than in group I. The total urine recovery decreases in the more severe patients, indicating more drug is eliminated through the nonrenal route (bile excretion) in these patients.

Renal clearance times of both parent drug and metabolite are proportional to the creatinine clearance time in the patients (Figure 17.4). The ratio of the area under the curve of the metabolite to that of the parent drug increases with the severity of the disease, not because the hepatic clearance time decreases, but because the total clearance time of the metabolite increases. The steady-state volume of distribution of the parent drug remains constant between the groups.

Case 2: Renal Impairment Affects Hepatic and Renal Eliminations

The rate of metabolism may be affected by the renal impairment due to an accumulation of metabolism inhibitors. In this case, the causes for prolonged half-life and increased accumulation may be due to the impaired renal function or the inhibited metabolism. A simulated example using Model 1 is illustrated in Figures 17.5 and 17.6. In this example, the renal elimination rates of the parent and metabolite and the metabolic rate decrease with the severity of the renal impairment. The plasma concentrations of both parent drug and metabolite increase with the decreasing creatinine clearance. The absorption phase of the parent drug in all four groups overlaps, indicating that the absorption is not affected by the disease. The time to reach the maximum concentration of the parent drug does not differ much between the groups, suggesting the renal excretion may not be the predominant route of elimination. However, the time to reach the

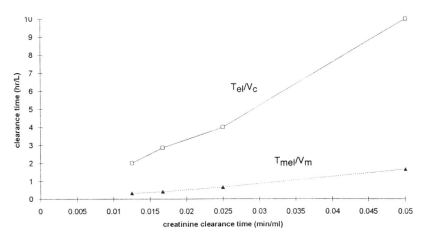

FIGURE 17.4. Renal clearance times of the drug and its metabolite in the example in Figure 17.1 as functions of creatinine clearance time.

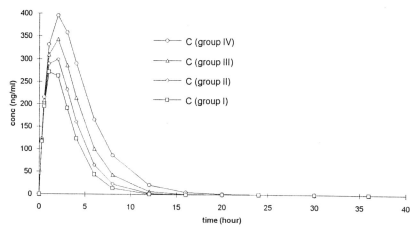

FIGURE 17.5. Simulated plasma drug concentration profiles using Model 1 for different degrees of renal-impaired patients, with the renal impairment affecting hepatic and renal eliminations. The time constant plot comparing the different degrees of patient groups is shown in Figure 17.7. The parameters used in this simulation are as follows: group 1: Cl_{cr} = 80 ml/min, X_0 = 10 mg, f^*F = 0.8, V_c = 10 L, K_a = 0.7 hr^{-1}, K_{el} = 0.4 hr^{-1}, K_b = 0.05 hr^{-1}, V_m = 10 L, K_m = 0.3 hr^{-1}, K_{mel} = 0.3 hr^{-1}, K_{mb} = 0.05 hr^{-1}; group II: Cl_{cr} = 60 ml/min, X_0 = 10 mg, f^*F = 0.8, V_c = 10 L, K_a = 0.7 hr^{-1}, K_{el} = 0.032 hr^{-1}, K_b = 0.05 hr^{-1}, V_m = 10 L, K_m = 0.25 hr^{-1}, K_{mel} = 0.24 hr^{-1}, K_{mb} = 0.05 hr^{-1}; group III: Cl_{cr} = 40 ml/min, X_0 = 10 mg, f^*F = 0.8, V_c = 10 L, K_a = 0.7 hr^{-1}, K_{el} = 0.024 hr^{-1}, K_b = 0.05 hr^{-1}, V_m = 10 L, K_m = 0.2 hr^{-1}, K_{mel} = 0.15 hr^{-1}, K_{mb} = 0.05 hr^{-1}; group IV: Cl_{cr} = 20 ml/min, X_0 = 10 mg, f^*F = 0.8, V_c = 10 L, K_a = 0.7 hr^{-1}, K_{el} = 0.16 hr^{-1}, K_b = 0.05 hr^{-1}, V_m = 10 L, K_m = 0.15 hr^{-1}, K_{mel} = 0.06 hr^{-1}, K_{mb} = 0.05 hr^{-1}.

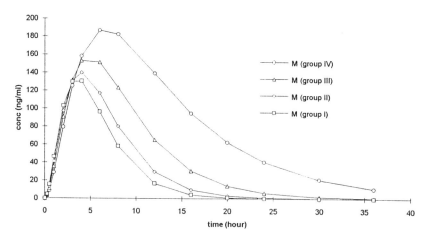

FIGURE 17.6. Simulated plasma metabolite concentration profiles of the example in Figure 17.5 for different degrees of renal-impaired patients.

418

TABLE 17.2. The Estimated Pharmacokinetic Parameters Using the Time Constant Analysis for the Example Shown in Figure 17.5.

Parameter	Group I		Group II		Group III		Group IV		Equation
	TCA	Model Value	TCA	Model Value	TCA	Model Value	TCA	Model Value	
T_{zc} (hr)	1.49	1.43 (T_a)	1.67	1.61 $(T_{el,r})$	2.04	2.04 $(T_{el,r})$	2.78	2.78 $(T_{el,r})$	(17.1)
T_{zm} (hr)	2.86	2.86 $(T_{mel,r})$	3.45	3.45 $(T_{mel,r})$	5.0	5.0 $(T_{mel,r})$	9.09	9.09 $(T_{mel,r})$	(17.2)
$\bar{t}_c$ (hr)	2.8	2.8	3.1	3.0	3.5	3.5	4.2	4.2	(17.6)
$\bar{t}_M$ (hr)	5.6	5.6	6.4	6.5	8.4	8.5	13.3	13.3	(17.7)
T_{el}/V_c (hr/L)	0.25	0.25	0.31	0.31	0.42	0.42	0.63	0.63	(17.6)
T_{mel}/V_m (hr/L)	0.33	0.33	0.42	0.42	0.67	0.67	1.67	1.67	(17.7)
$T_{mel,r}$ (hr)	2.78	2.86	3.33	3.45	5.0	5.0	9.09	9.09	(17.3)
$T_m * V_m / V_c$ (hr)	3.23	3.33	3.85	4.0	5.0	5.0	6.67	6.67	(17.5)
AUC_C (ng·hr/L)	1077	1066	1305	1290	1653	1632	2251	2222	
AUC_M (ng·hr/L)	928	914	1126	1112	1643	1632	3034	3030	
X_{uc} (μg)	4310	4266	4177	4129	3968	3918	3601	3555	
X_{um} (μg)	2784	2742	2702	2669	2465	2448	1820	1818	
X_{uc}/X_0	0.43	0.43	0.42	0.41	0.40	0.39	0.36	0.36	
X_{um}/X_0	0.28	0.27	0.27	0.27	0.25	0.24	0.18	0.18	
AUC_M/AUC_C	0.86	0.86	0.86	0.86	0.99	1	1.3	1.4	(17.4)

TCA: Time constant analysis.

maximum concentration of the metabolite increases significantly with the severity of the disease, indicating the importance of the renal excretion to the elimination of the metabolite.

The estimated pharmacokinetic parameters of the above example using the time constant analysis are listed in Table 17.2, and the estimated time constants are presented in Figure 17.7. The area under the curve of both parent drug and metabolite increases with the severity of renal impairment.

Now let us examine the time constant plot (Figure 17.7). The decay time of the metabolite is longer than that of the parent drug, indicating that the elimination time of the metabolite is longer than that of the parent drug. The mean residence times of the parent drug and metabolite increase with the disease, and the increase is especially pronounced for the metabolite. This indicates that the renal excretion is the predominant route of elimination for the metabolite. The urine recovery of both parent drug and metabolite decreases with the severity of the disease, and the renal clearance time of the drug is linearly related to the creatinine clearance time (Figure 17.8). The hepatic clearance time also increases with the disease, which shares a part of the reason for the accumulation of the drug and the prolongation of the half-life.

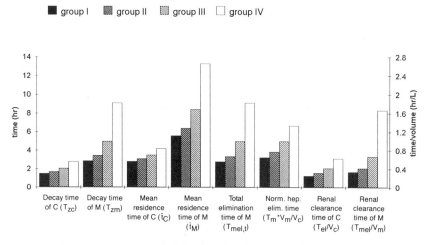

FIGURE 17.7. The time constant plot comparing the different degrees of renal-impaired patient groups in the example shown in Figure 17.5. The renal clearance time (T_{el}/V_c) of the drug is linearly related to the creatinine clearance time. The hepatic clearance time (T_m*V_m/V_c) also increases with the disease, which shares a part of the reason for the accumulation of the drug and the prolongation of the half-life.

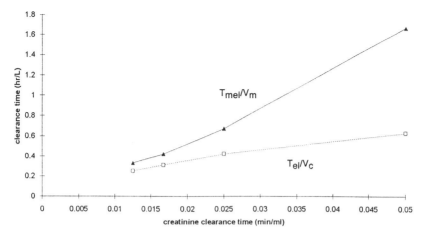

FIGURE 17.8. Renal clearance times of the drug and its metabolite in the example in Figure 17.5 as functions of creatinine clearance time.

Case 3: Renal Impairment Affects Protein Binding

Protein binding of a drug may decrease in renal impairment due to an accumulation of protein binding inhibitors. A decrease in protein binding may affect the distribution of the drug in the body. The degree of influence of protein binding on the volume of distributions of a drug may depend on whether the drug readily penetrates into the tissue compartment. If a drug is lipophilic and/or readily penetrates into the tissue compartment, the volume of distribution may increase significantly as its protein binding decreases (which increases the free fraction of the drug in plasma). In addition, the effects of a change in protein binding on the volume of distribution also depend on the percentage amount of the drug bound to the plasma proteins. If a drug is highly bound to the plasma proteins, a slight change in the protein binding may result in a significant change in the free drug concentration and thus in the volume of distribution. An example is simulated by Model 2 and shown in Figures 17.9 and 17.10. In the example, the renal elimination rates of both parent drug and metabolite decrease with the severity of the disease, and the distribution rate constant (K_{12}) and the volume of the central compartment increase in the patients. The plasma concentration of the parent drug decreases with the severity of renal impairment due to the reduced protein binding in the patients. In addition, the drug is predominantly eliminated by the hepatic metabolism, and thus the renal impairment does not cause an accumulation of the drug. On the other hand, the metabo-

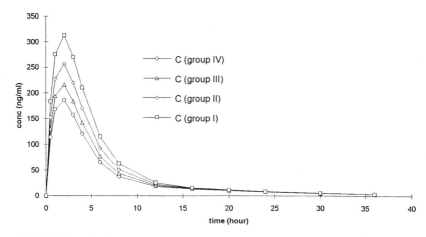

FIGURE 17.9. Simulated plasma drug concentration profiles using Model 2 for different degrees of renal-impaired patients, with the renal impairment affecting protein binding. The time constant plot comparing the different degrees of renal impairment is shown in Figure 17.11. The parameters used in this simulation are as follows: group I: Cl_{cr} = 80 ml/min, X_0 = 10 mg, f^*F = 0.7, V_c = 10 L, V_p = 20 L, K_a = 0.7 hr^{-1}, K_{el} = 0.01 hr^{-1}, K_b = 0.05 hr^{-1}, K_{12} = 0.1 hr^{-1}, K_{21} = 0.1 hr^{-1}, V_m = 10 L, K_m = 0.3 hr^{-1}, K_{mel} = 0.08 hr^{-1}, K_{mb} = 0.05 hr^{-1}; group II: Cl_{cr} = 60 ml/min, X_0 = 10 mg, f^*F = 0.7, V_c = 12 L, V_p = 20 L, K_a = 0.7 hr^{-1}, K_{el} = 0.007 hr^{-1}, K_b = 0.05 hr^{-1}, K_{12} = 0.12 hr^{-1}, K_{21} = 0.1 hr^{-1}, V_m = 10 L, K_m = 0.3 hr^{-1}, K_{mel} = 0.06 hr^{-1}, K_{mb} = 0.05 hr^{-1}; group III: Cl_{cr} = 40 ml/min, X_0 = 10 mg, f^*F = 0.7, V_c = 14 L, V_p = 20 L, K_a = 0.7 hr^{-1}, K_{el} = 0.004 hr^{-1}, K_b = 0.05 hr^{-1}, K_{12} = 0.14 hr^{-1}, K_{21} = 0.1 hr^{-1}, V_m = 10 L, K_m = 0.3 hr^{-1}, K_{mel} = 0.04 hr^{-1}, K_{mb} = 0.05 hr^{-1}; group IV Cl_{cr} = 20 ml/min, X_0 = 10 mg, f^*F = 0.7, V_c = 16 L, V_p = 20 L, K_a = 0.7 hr^{-1}, K_{el} = 0.001 hr^{-1}, K_b = 0.05 hr^{-1}, K_{12} = 0.16 hr^{-1}, K_{21} = 0.1 hr^{-1}, V_m = 10 L, K_m = 0.3 hr^{-1}, K_{mel} = 0.02 hr^{-1}, K_{mb} = 0.05 hr^{-1}.

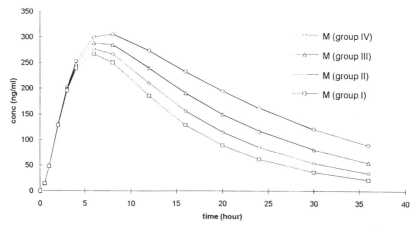

FIGURE 17.10. Simulated plasma metabolite concentration profiles of the example in Figure 17.9 for different degrees of renal-impaired patients.

422

TABLE 17.3. The Estimated Pharmacokinetic Parameters Using the Time Constant Analysis for the Example Shown in Figure 17.9.

Parameter	Group I		Group II		Group III		Group IV		Equation
	TCA	Model Value	TCA	Model Value	TCA	Model Value	TCA	Model Value	
T_{z1c} (hr)	13.2	13.5	14.1	14.3	14.7	14.9	15.4	15.6	
T_{z1m} (hr)	11.4	na	13.3	14.3	16.4	14.9	20.8	na	
$\bar{T}_{z2c}$ (hr)	2.08	2.04	2.0	1.96	1.96	1.92	1.92	1.82	
$\bar{t}_C$ (hr)	6.7	6.9	7.3	7.6	7.9	8.2	8.5	8.8	(17.10)
$\bar{t}_M$ (hr)	14.3	14.7	16.5	16.7	19.5	19.3	24.5	23.1	(17.11)
T_{el}/V_c (hr/L)	10.0	10.0	11.9	11.9	17.9	17.9	62.5	62.5	(17.14)
T_{mel}/V_m (hr/L)	1.25	1.25	1.67	1.67	2.5	2.5	5.0	5.0	(17.15)
$T_{mel,r}$ (hr)	7.69	7.69	9.09	9.09	11.63	11.11	16.13	14.3	(17.11)
T_m*V_m/V_c (hr)	3.33	3.33	2.86	2.78	2.5	2.38	2.27	2.08	(17.13)
AUC_C (ng·hr/L)	1950	1944	1637	1633	1413	1412	1246	1246	
AUC_M (ng·hr/L)	13,083	13,580	11,929	12,403	11,141	11,593	10,583	11,013	
X_{uc} (µg)	195	194	137	137	79	79	19	19	
X_{um} (µg)	3571	3589	3199	3208	2648	2636	1750	1709	
AUC_M/AUC_C	2.3	2.3	3.3	3.3	4.7	4.7	7.0	6.9	(17.12)
V_{ss} (L)	34	35	44	46	55	58	68	70	(17.17)

na: Not available.

423

lite is eliminated predominantly by the kidney, and its plasma concentration increases with the severity of the disease.

The drug concentration decreases in the renal-impaired patients, implying the possibility of decreased protein binding. Therefore, the key parameter in this example is the volume of distribution. The estimated pharmacokinetic parameters of the above example using the time constant analysis are listed in Table 17.3, and the estimated time constants are presented in Figure 17.11. The area under the curve of the parent drug and the metabolite is reduced with the severity of the disease. The difference in the area under the curve of the metabolite between groups III and IV is not significant, indicating that the elimination is dominated by the nonrenal route in these two groups.

Now let us examine the time constant plot (Figure 17.11). The first and second decay time of the parent drug concentration curves do not differ much between the groups; therefore, the decay times are not good indicators for the systemic clearance in this example. On the other hand, the mean residence time shows a stronger trend in relation to the creatinine clearance time. The urine recovery data indicate that the drug is predominantly eliminated by the hepatic metabolism. The clearance time of the drug is linearly related to the creatinine clearance time (Figure 17.12). There is an increase in the total elimination time of the metabolite with the severity of

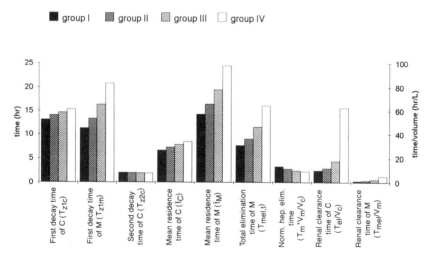

FIGURE 17.11. The time constant plot comparing different degrees of renal impairment in the example shown in Figure 17.9. There is an increase in the total elimination time $(T_{mel,t})$ of the metabolite with the severity of the disease. The hepatic elimination time (T_m) increases with the increased creatinine clearance time.

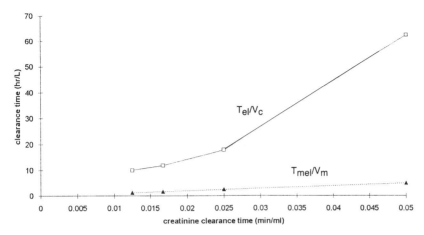

FIGURE 17.12. Renal clearance times of the drug and its metabolite in the example in Figure 17.9 as functions of creatinine clearance time.

the disease. The hepatic elimination time T_m*V_m/V_c decreases with the increased creatinine clearance time, probably due to an increase in the volume of distribution. This is consistent with the increase in the steady-state volume of distribution in the more severe patients.

EXAMPLES

Example 1: Renal Impairment Affects Renal and Hepatic Eliminations

The pharmacokinetics of meropenem and its metabolite were studied in five healthy subjects and eighteen patients with various degrees of renal impairment after the administration of 500 mg of meropenem intravenously as a 30-minute infusion [5]. The subjects were divided into four groups with glomerular filtration rates (GFR) of > 80, 30 to 80, 5 to 29, or < 5 ml/min. The mean plasma concentration profiles of meropenem and its metabolite are shown in Figures 17.13 and 17.14. The plasma concentrations of meropenem and the metabolite increases in the patients with the severity of renal impairment. In the most severe patients (GFR < 5 ml/min), the elimination of the metabolite is extremely slow, resulting in a very long decay time of the concentration curve.

In healthy subjects, approximately 70% of meropenem is excreted unchanged in urine, and 20% is eliminated by the liver. Therefore, both

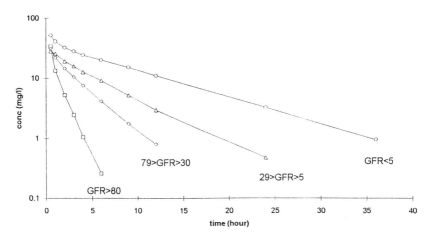

FIGURE 17.13. Mean plasma concentration of meropenem in five healthy subjects and eighteen patients with various degrees of renal impairment after the administration of 500 mg of meropenem intravenously as a 30-minute infusion. (Reproduced from Reference [5] with permission.) The time constant plot comparing the various degrees of renal impairment is shown in Figure 17.15.

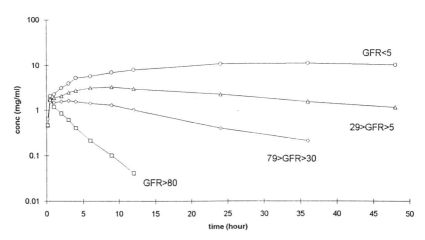

FIGURE 17.14. Mean plasma concentration of the metabolite of meropenem in five healthy subjects and eighteen patients with various degrees of renal impairment after the administration of 500 mg of meropenem intravenously as a 30-minute infusion. (Reproduced from Reference [5] with permission.)

426

TABLE 17.4. *The Estimated Pharmacokinetic Parameters of Meropenem and Its Metabolite Using Model 1.*

Parameter*	GFR > 80	80 > GFR > 30	29 > GFR > 5	GFR > 5	Equation
T_{zc} (hr)	1.30	3.29	5.03	9.80	
T_{zm} (hr)	3.33	12.82	34.48		
$\bar{t}_C$ (hr)	1.24	3.27	5.37	9.36	
$\bar{t}_M$ (hr)	3.32	14.80	37.72		
T_{el}/V_c (min/ml)	0.0070	0.0244	0.0435		(17.1)
T_{mel}/V_m (min/ml)	0.0023	0.0287	0.0344		(17.2)
$T_{el,t}/V_c$ (min/ml)	0.0054	0.0135	0.0187	0.0526	(17.6)
					(17.7)
					(17.8)
T_{nr}/V_c (min/ml)	0.0227	0.0286	0.0345		$\dfrac{1}{V_c/T_{el,t} - C_c/T_{el}}$
$T_{mel,t}$ (hr)	2.08	11.49	32.26		(17.3)
T_m*V_m/V_c (hr)	16.13	33.33	34.48		(17.5)
V_{ss} (L/kg)	0.21	0.20	0.23	0.17	(17.9)
AUC_c (mg·hr/L)	36	89.8	156	393	
AUC_M (mg·hr/L)	4.63	31	144		
X_{uc} (% dose)	77	53	38		
X_{um} (% dose)	22	13	6		
AUC_M/AUC_c	0.129	0.345	0.923		(17.4)

*Parameters estimated from the mean concentration profiles or the mean reported values.

hepatic elimination time and renal elimination time may potentially be affected by renal impairment and may result in significant change in plasma drug concentration. The pharmacokinetic parameters of meropenem are estimated using Model 1 since the terminal phase exhibits a monoexponential decay. The estimated parameters are listed in Table 17.4, and the estimated time constants are presented in Figure 17.15. The area under the meropenem concentration curve increases with the severity of the disease, indicating the renal excretion accounts for a substantial part of its elimination. The area under the metabolite concentration curve also increases in the patients significantly.

Now let us examine the time constant plot (Figure 17.15). The decay times of meropenem and the metabolite increase with the severity of renal impairment, indicating an increase in total elimination time in the patients. The increase in the elimination time is also evidenced from the increase in the mean residence time in the patients. The renal clearance time of meropenem increases 2.5-fold from group I (GFR > 80) to II (80 > GFR > 30) and increases by another 38% in group III (29 > GFR > 5). The increase in the renal clearance time of the metabolite is even more significant than that of meropenem, prolonged thirteenfold from group I to II and

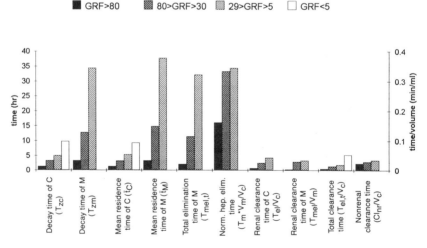

FIGURE 17.15. The time constant plot of meropenem comparing the various degrees of renal impairment using Model 1. The renal clearance time of meropenem (T_{el}/V_c) increases 2.5-fold from group I (GFR > 80) to II (80 > GFR > 30) and increases by another 38% in group III (29 > GFR > 5). The increase in the renal clearance time of the metabolite (T_{mel}/V_m) is even more significant than that of meropenem, prolonged thirteenfold from group I to II and another tenfold from group II to III. The increase in the hepatic elimination time ($T_m * V_m/V_c$) is only twofold from group I to group III.

another tenfold from group II to III. The total clearance time and the nonrenal clearance time also increase in the patients. The total elimination time of the metabolite $(T_{mel,t})$ increases fifteenfold from group I to III. Although the AUC_M/AUC_C ratio increases sevenfold, the increase in the hepatic elimination time is only twofold from group I to group III. The increase in the hepatic elimination time is probably due to an accumulation of metabolic inhibitors. However, there is no change in the hepatic elimination time between groups II and III. The apparent volume of distribution remains about the same in the patients. To summarize, the plasma concentration of meropenem increases with the severity of renal impairment, due to increases in both renal and hepatic elimination time. Therefore, dosage of the drug should be based on the severity of renal disease, as indicated in Reference [5].

Example 2: Different Metabolic Pathways Are Affected by Renal Impairment to Different Degrees

The pharmacokinetics of perindopril and its metabolites perindoprilat and perindoprilat glucuronide were studied in twenty-six hypertensive patients with various degrees of renal insufficiency following an oral dose of 4 mg perindopril [15]. The patients were divided into five groups with creatinine clearance (normalized by body surface area) > 100, 31 to 80, 15 to 30, < 15 ml/min^{-1} 1.73 m^{-2}, and end-stage renal impairment. The mean plasma concentrations of perindopril and its metabolites are shown in Figures 17.16–17.18. Perindopril is quickly absorbed and eliminated in the blood. Both metabolites, perindoprilat and perindoprilat glucuronide, appear rapidly in the blood, indicating a fast metabolic rate. The metabolites remain much longer in the blood than perindopril, indicating that the elimination of the metabolites is slower than that of perindopril.

The renal clearance of perindopril is only 10% of the total clearance; as a result, change in the hepatic elimination time be renal impairment may affect the drug concentration more significantly than the change in renal elimination time. Therefore, the key time constants in this example are the hepatic and renal elimination times. The concentration profile of perindopril exhibits a biexponential terminal phase; therefore, the pharmacokinetic parameters are estimated using Model 2 with the addition of a second metabolite parallel to the first one. The estimated pharmacokinetic parameters are listed in Table 17.5, and the estimated time constants are presented in Figure 17.19. The area under the concentration curves of perindopril and its metabolites increases with the severity of the disease: periodopril by 2.5 times, perindoprilat by 11.9 times, and perindoprilat glucuronide by 6.6 times from group I ($Cl_{cr} > 100$) to group IV ($Cl_{cr} < 15$). The increase in the

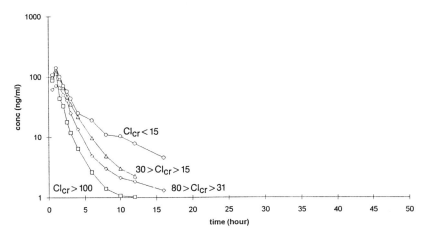

FIGURE 17.16. Mean plasma concentration of perindopril in twenty-six hypertensive patients with various degrees of renal insufficiency following an oral dose of 4 mg perindopril. (Reproduced from Reference [15] with permission from Blackwell Science Ltd.) The time constant plot comparing the different degrees of renal impairment is shown in Figure 17.19.

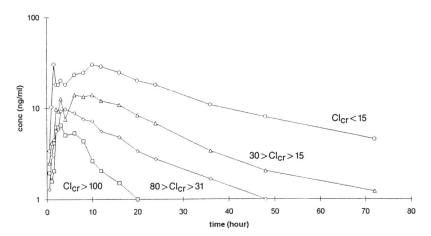

FIGURE 17.17. Mean plasma concentration of perindoprilat in twenty-six hypertensive patients with various degrees of renal insufficiency following an oral dose of 4 mg perindopril. (Reproduced from Reference [15] with permission from Blackwell Science Ltd.)

430

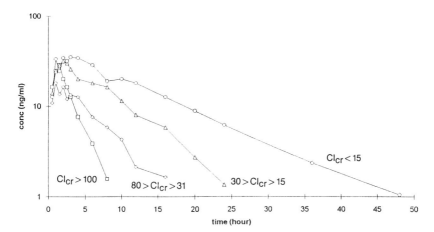

FIGURE 17.18. Mean plasma concentration of perindoprilat glucuronide in twenty-six hypertensive patients with various degrees of renal insufficiency following an oral dose of 4 mg perindopril. (Reproduced from Reference [15] with permission from Blackwell Science Ltd.)

area under the curve of perindopril is not as significant as those of its metabolites in the patients, indicating that the renal excretion is not the predominant route of the elimination of perindopril.

Now let us examine the time constant plot (Figure 17.19). The decay time of perindopril changes only slightly in the patients, another indication that the renal excretion is not the predominant route of elimination. On the other hand, the decay times of perindoprilat and perindoprilat glucuronide increase significantly in the patients. Based on the mean residence time, perindopril appears earliest in the blood, followed by perindoprilat glucuronide and perindoprilat. The total clearance time of perindopril increases 2.5-fold from group I to group IV. The increase in the total elimination times of the metabolites is more substantial than that of the parent drug: 4.4-fold in perindoprilat and 8.6-fold in perindoprilat glucuronide from group I to IV. The hepatic elimination time $(T_m * V_m / V_c)$ toward perindoprilat does not change much in the patients, while that toward perindoprilat glucuronide increases substantially. The apparent volume of distribution is not affected by the renal impairment. To summarize, the elimination of perindopril is only slightly affected by renal failure, while the eliminations of perindoprilat and perindoprilat glucuronide are significantly affected by renal impairment. The formation of perindoprilat glucuronide is reduced by renal impairment, while that of perindoprilat is not. Since the total elimination time of the active metabolite perinoprilat is prolonged in renal-

TABLE 17.5. *The Estimated Pharmacokinetic Parameters of Perindopril and Its Metabolites Using Model 2.*

Parameter*	$Cl_{cr} > 100$	$80 > Cl_{cr} > 31$	$30 > Cl_{cr} > 15$	$Cl_{cr} < 15$	Equation
T_{zc} (hr)	1.30	2.0	2.33	1.01	
T_{zm1} (hr)	7.14	9.09	19.23	40.0	
T_{zm2} (hr)	2.56	4.0	6.67	11.11	
$\bar{t}_C$ (hr)	1.9	3.0	2.7	3.9	(17.10)
$\bar{t}_{M1}$ (hr)	9.7	15.9	22.6	38.5	(17.11)
$\bar{t}_{M2}$ (hr)	2.9	6.0	8.1	13.2	(17.11)
$T_{el,r}*f*F/V_c$ (hr/L)	0.045	0.053	0.076	0.112	(17.16)
$T_{mel1,r}$ (hr)	7.81	12.99	20.0	34.48	(17.11)
$T_{mel2,r}$ (hr)	1.05	2.94	5.26	9.09	(17.11)
$T_{m1}*V_{m1}/V_c$ (hr)	15.38	12.5	15.15	13.89	(15.13)
$T_{m2}*V_{m2}/V_c$ (hr)	2.46	5.26	6.10	8.13	(17.13)
AUC_C (ng·hr/L)	182	210	302	448	
AUC_{M1} (ng·hr/L)	93	217	398	1106	
AUC_{M2} (ng·hr/L)	78	119	266	513	
AUC_{M1}/AUC_C	0.51	1.03	1.32	2.47	(17.12)
AUC_{M2}/AUC_C	0.43	0.57	0.88	1.15	(17.12)
$V_{ss}/f/F$ (L)	41.2	57.1	35.8	35.2	(17.17)

*Parameters estimated from the mean concentration profiles or the mean reported values.
c: perindopril, m1: perindoprilat, m2: perindoprilat glucuronide.

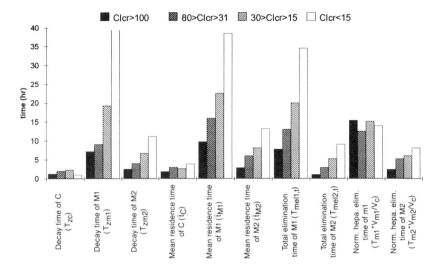

FIGURE 17.19. The time constant plot of perindopril comparing various degrees of renal insufficiency using Model 2. The hepatic elimination time toward perindoprilat ($T_{m1}*V_{m1}/V_c$) does not change much in the patients, while that toward perindoprilat glucuronide ($T_{m2}*V_{m2}/V_c$) increases substantially.

impaired patients, a dose reduction in these patients may be necessary, as suggested in Reference [15].

Example 3: Renal Impairment Affects Volume of Distribution

The pharmacokinetics of flurbiprofen and its metabolite were studied in eight end-stage renal disease subjects and nine subjects with normal renal function following a 100-mg oral dose of racemic flurbiprofen [3]. The plasma concentration profiles of the R-isomer of flurbiprofen and its metabolite are shown in Figures 17.20 and 17.21. The most interesting observation from the concentration profiles is that the concentration of flurbiprofen is lower in the end-stage renal disease patients than in the normal subjects. This may be the result of a decreased absorption or an increased volume of distribution. On the other hand, the concentration of the metabolite increases in the patients, indicating an accumulation due to poor renal elimination.

The plasma concentration of flurbiprofen decreases in the renal-impaired patients, implying the possibility of decreased protein binding in the patients. This hypothesis is supported by the fact that flurbiprofen is extensively bound ($>90\%$) to the plasma proteins [3]. Therefore, the key param-

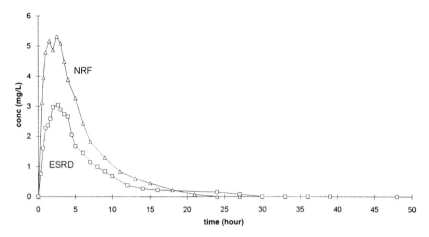

FIGURE 17.20. Mean plasma concentration profiles of flurbiprofen (R-isomer) in eight end-stage renal disease (ESRD) subjects and nine subjects with normal renal function (NRF) following 100 mg oral dose of racemic flurbiprofen. (Reproduced from Reference [3] with permission.) The time constant plot comparing the various degrees of renal impairment is shown in Figure 17.22.

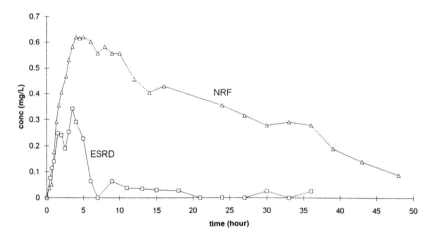

FIGURE 17.21. Mean plasma concentration profiles of the metabolite of flurbiprofen (R-isomer) in eight end-stage renal disease (ESRD) subjects of nine subjects with normal renal function (NRF) following a 100-mg oral dose of racemic flurbiprofen. (Reproduced from Reference [3] with permission.)

434

eters in this example include volume of distribution, as well as hepatic and renal elimination times. The pharmacokinetic parameters of flurbiprofen and its metabolite are estimated using Model 2 and listed in Table 17.6, and the estimated time constants are presented in Figure 17.22. The area under the flurbiprofen concentration curve decreases in the patients while the area under the metabolite concentration curve increases in the patients.

Now let us examine the time constant plot (Figure 17.22). The decay time and the mean residence time of flurbiprofen change only slightly in the patients, indicating that the total elimination of flurbiprofen is only slightly affected by renal impairment. The urine recovery of flurbiprofen accounts for 20% of the dose, indicating that renal excretion of flurbiprofen cannot be ignored. The hepatic elimination time (T_m*V_m/V_c) decreases by 39%, indicating that an increase in the hepatic elimination may have compensated for the decrease in the renal elimination of flurbiprofen in the patients. In addition, the apparent volume of distribution (V_{ss}/fF) increases twofold, which may result in an increase in the distribution rate and may compensate for the decrease in the renal elimination rate. Therefore, the combined effects of an increase in the metabolic rate and a possible increase in the distribution rate may have compensated for the decrease in the renal elimination rate in the patients and result in only a small change in the decay time and the mean residence time of flurbiprofen. The increase in the apparent

TABLE 17.6. The Estimated Pharmacokinetic
Parameters of Flurbiprofen and
Its Metabolite Using Model 2.

Parameter*	NRF	ESRD	Equation
T_{zc} (hr)	5.56	4.35	
$\bar{t}_C$ (hr)	5.3	6.5	(17.10)
$\bar{t}_M$ (hr)	7.4	19.0	(17.11)
T_{el}/V_c (hr/L)	1.82	22.22	(17.14)
T_{mel}/V_m (hr/L)	0.086	6.25	(17.15)
$T_{el,t}*f*F/V_c$ (hr/L)	0.36	0.22	(17.16)
$T_{mel,t}$ (hr)	2.07	12.5	(17.11)
T_m*V_m/V_c (hr)	24.4	14.9	(17.13)
AUC_C (mg·hr/L)	36.4	22.1	
AUC_M (mg·hr/L)	3.1	18.6	
X_{uc} (% dose)	20	1	
X_{um} (% dose)	36	3	
AUC_M/AUC_C	0.085	0.84	(17.12)
$V_{ss}/f/F$ (L/kg)	14.6	29.5	(17.17)

*Parameters estimated from the mean concentration profiles or the mean reported values.

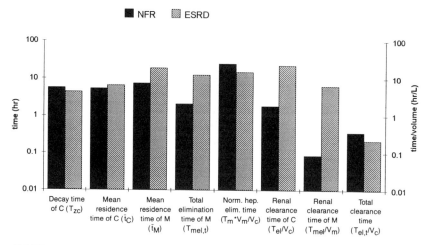

FIGURE 17.22. The time constant plot of flurbiprofen comparing the various degrees of renal impairment using Model 2. The hepatic elimination time (T_m*V_m/V_c) decreases by 39%, indicating that an increase in the hepatic elimination may have compensated for the decrease in the renal elimination of flurbiprofen in the patients.

volume of distribution may also explain the decrease in the area under the flurbiprofen concentration curve in the patients; however, a decrease in the extent of absorption is also possible.

REFERENCES

1. Bevan E. G., McInnes G. T., Aldigier J. C., Conte J. J., Grunfeld J. P., Harper S. J., Meyer B. H., Pauly N., and Wilkinson R., "Effect of renal function on the pharmacokinetics and pharmacodynamics of trandolapril," *Br. J. Clin. Pharmac.*, 1993; 35:128–135.

2. Boobis S. W., "Alteration of plasma albumin in relation to decreased drug binding in uremia," *Clin. Pharmacol. Ther.*, 1977; 22:147–153.

3. Cefali E. A., Poynor W. J., Sica D., and Cox S., "Pharmacokinetic comparison of flurbiprofen in end-stage renal disease subjects and subjects with normal renal function," *J. Clin. Pharmacol.*, 1991; 31:808–814.

4. Chimata M., Nagase M., Suzuki Y., Shimomura M., and Kakuta S., "Pharmacokinetics of meropenem in patients with various degrees of renal function, including patients with end-stage renal disease," *Antimicrobial Agents and Chemotherapy*, 1993; 37(2):229–233.

5. Christensson B. A., Nilsson-Ehle I., Hutchison M., Haworth S. J., Oqvist B., and Norrby S. R., "Pharmacokinetics of meropenem in subjects with various degrees of renal impairment," *Antimicrobial Agents and Chemotherapy*, 1992; 36(7):1532–1537.

6. Craig W. A., Evenson M. A., and Ramgopal V., "The effect of uremia, cardiopul-

monary bypass and bacterial infection on serum protein binding," in *The Effect of Disease States on Drug Pharmacokinetics,* L. Z. Benet, American Pharmaceutical Association, Washington, D.C., 1976; pp. 125–136.

7. Granneman G . R., Braeckman R., Kraut J., Shupien S., and Craft J. C., "Temafloxacin pharmacokinetics in subjects with normal and impaired renal function," *Antimicrobial Agents and Chemotherapy,* 1991; 35(11):2345–2351.

8. Halstenson C. E., Opshal J. A., Rachael K., Olson S. C., Horvath A. M., Abraham P. A., and Posvar E. L., "The pharmacokinetics of quinapril and its active metabolite, quinaprilat, in patients with various degrees of renal function," *J. Clin. Pharmacol.,* 1992; 32:344–350.

9. Hui K. K., Duchin K. L., Kripalani K. L., Chan D., Kramer P. K., Yanagawa N., "Pharmacokinetics of fosinopril in patients with various degrees of renal function," *Clin. Pharmacol. Ther.,* 1991; 49(4):457–467.

10. Oguchi H., Miyasaka M., Koiwai T., Tokunaga S., Hora K., Sato K., Yoshie T., Shioya H., and Furuta S., "Pharmacokinetics of temocapril and enalapril in patients with various degrees of renal insufficiency," *Clin. Pharmacokinet.,* 1993; 24(5):421–427.

11. Osborne R. J., Joel S. P., and Slevin M. L., "Morphine intoxication in renal failure: The role of morphine-6-glucuronide," *Br. Med. J.,* 1986; 292:1548.

12. Prescott L. F., Freestone S., and McAuslane J. A. N., "The concentration-dependent disposition of intravenous *p*-aminohippurate in subjects with normal and impaired renal function," *Br. J. Clin. Pharmac.,* 1993; 35:20–29.

13. Shyu W. C., Pittman K. A., Wilber R. B., Matzke G. R., and Barhaiya R. H., "Pharmacokinetics of cefprozil in healthy subjects and patients with renal impairment," *J. Clin. Pharmacol.,* 1991; 31:362–371.

14. St. Peter J. V., Borin M. T., Hughes G. S., Keloway J. S., Shapiro B. E., and Halstenson C. E., "Disposition of cefpodoxime proxetil in healthy volunteers and patients with impaired renal function," *Antimicrobial Agents and Chemotherapy,* 1992; 36(1):126–131.

15. Verpooten G. A., Genissel P. M., Thomas J. R., and De Broe M. E., "Single dose pharmacokinetics of perindopril and its metabolites in hypertensive patients with various degrees of renal insufficiency," *Br. J. Clin. Pharmac.,* 1991; 32:187–192.

16. Verbeeck R. K., Branch R. A., and Wilkinson G. R., "Drug metabolism in renal failure: Pharmacokinetic and clinical implication," *Clin. Pharmacokinet.,* 1981; 6:329.

17. Zazgornik J., Huang M. L., Van Peer A., Woestenboughs R., Heykants J., and Stephen A., "Pharmacokinetics of orally administered levocabastine in patients with renal insufficiency," *J. Clin. Pharmacol.,* 1993; 33:1214–1218.

Special Pharmacokinetic Considerations in Hepatic Impairment

INTRODUCTION

The effects of liver diseases on pharmacokinetics of the drugs can be assessed in the hepatic impairment study. The major influence of liver diseases on drug pharmacokinetics is a decrease in liver enzyme activities [3], which affects the first pass metabolism, as well as the hepatic elimination time. Protein binding may sometimes be reduced in alcoholic cirrhosis and other liver dysfunction [4] and results in an increased free fraction of the drug in plasma and an increased apparent volume of distribution. The decrease in protein binding may result in an increased unbound fraction and improve the hepatic elimination. Overall, the hepatic clearance should be more sensitive to the changes in hepatic enzyme activities than the change in protein binding in patients with liver diseases. Cirrhosis and other liver dysfunctions also affect liver blood flow, which in turn influences hepatic clearance of drugs with high hepatic extraction ratios [11]. On the other hand, hepatic impairment exerts influence on the drugs with intermediate extraction ratio by decreasing the intrinsic clearance [11]. If ascites or fluid retention occur in the hepatic-impaired patient, the volume of distribution of drugs may increase [9]. When bilirubinemia develops [4], the accumulated bilirubin in the blood may displace the drugs from plasma protein binding sites or compete with the drug for glucuronidation metabolism. Consequently, the key pharmacokinetic parameters in a hepatic impairment study are the hepatic elimination time constant, first pass bioavailability, and volume of distribution. If the elimination of a drug is dominated by hepatic metabolism, then hepatic impairment will likely prolong the total clearance time.

Some common themes in the time constant view can be observed in the renal impairment study as well as other studies. One common factor is the predominant route of elimination. If renal excretion dominates the total clearance of a drug, then the decrease in the metabolic elimination due to hepatic impairment may be compensated for by an increase in the renal clearance secondary to an increase in the unbound fraction in the plasma. At the same time, if renal excretion dominates the elimination, change in renal elimination time due to age difference (Chapter 15) or renal impairment (Chapter 17) will have significant effects on the plasma concentration. Another common factor is volume of distribution. A change in apparent volume of distribution can be attributed to some fundamental changes in physiology: (1) altered protein binding, such as in hepatic impairment, renal impairment (Chapter 17), different age groups (Chapter 15), different genders (Chapter 16), and inflammatory diseases (Chapter 19); (2) altered lean to fat ratio, such as in different age groups (Chapter 15) and different genders (Chapter 16); and (3) altered peripheral to central compartment ratio, such as in pregnancy (Chapter 16) and obesity. The effects of a decrease in protein binding on the apparent volume of distribution of a drug may depend on the ability of the drug to penetrate into the tissue compartment. If a drug readily penetrates into the tissue compartment (usually indicated by a biexponential elimination phase, long half-life, or $V_z > 0.65$ L/kg), an increase in the unbound fraction in the plasma may result in a greater apparent volume of distribution. The effects of lean to fat ratio and peripheral to central compartment ratio on the apparent volume of distribution also depend, more or less, on the ability of the drug to penetrate into the tissue.

Two models are discussed in this chapter to describe the pharmacokinetics in hepatic-impaired patients for (1) drugs with low first pass elimination and (2) drugs with high first pass elimination. Three simulated case studies and three literature examples are presented in this chapter to illustrate the utility of these models in hepatic impairment studies. Additional examples of hepatic impairment studies can be found in the literature [1–10].

PHARMACOKINETIC MODELS

This section presents two models that are useful in describing the pharmacokinetics in hepatic-impaired patients. The goal is to establish simple relationships between time constants and measurable parameters such as (1) mean residence time, which is the sum of input and output times, and (2) area under the curves. The derivations of these relationships are straightforward and are discussed in Chapter 2.

Model 1: Drugs with Low First Pass Elimination

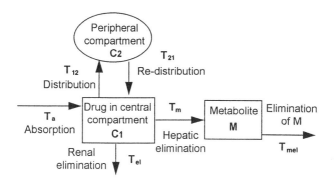

The most likely effect of hepatic diseases on pharmacokinetics of a drug is a decrease in the metabolic rate due to the impaired hepatic functions. In addition, protein binding of drugs in patients with liver disease may also decrease [4] and may result in an increase in the volume of distribution. The combined effects of decreased metabolism and protein binding can be described by Model 1. In this model, an impaired hepatic function in patients with liver disease is reflected by an increased T_m, and a decreased protein binding increases V_1 and decreases T_{12} and T_{el}.

The mean residence time of the concentration profile can be estimated from the ratio of area under the first moment curve to the area under the concentration curve. Following an oral administration, the mean residence time of the drug and its metabolite is simply the sum of input and output times (see Chapter 2):

$$\text{Mean residence time of C following oral dose } (\bar{t}_{C,po}) = \frac{\text{AUMC}_C}{\text{AUC}_C}$$

$$= \text{Input time } (T_{c,po,in}) + \text{Output time } (T_{c,po,out}) = T_a + T_{el,t} + T_{el,t}\frac{T_{21}}{T_{12}}$$

$$(18.1)$$

$$\text{Mean residence time of M following oral dose } (\bar{t}_{M,po})$$

$$= \text{Input time } (T_{m,po,in}) + \text{Output time } (T_{m,po,out}) = T_a + T_{el,t} + T_{el,t}\frac{T_{21}}{T_{12}} + T_{mel}$$

$$(18.2)$$

where $T_{el,t} = 1/(1/T_m + 1/T_{el})$. Liver diseases may affect the mean residence time by altering hepatic elimination time T_m, renal elimination time T_{el}, and distribution time T_{12}. The decay time constant can be estimated from a partial area under the curve (see Appendix 2).

$$\frac{1}{\text{Decay time } (T_z)} = \lambda_z = 2\frac{(t - t_{last}) \ln (C_t) - AU \ln C_{t-t_{last}}}{(t - t_{last})^2} \qquad (18.3)$$

A clearance time is defined as the amount of time required to clear up the drug in one unit volume of blood (Chapter 2). The ratio of the area under the metabolite concentration to the area under the drug concentration results in the ratio of renal clearance time of the metabolite to the hepatic clearance time of the drug.

$$\frac{AUC_M}{AUC_C} = \frac{T_{mel}V_1}{T_m V_m} = \frac{\text{Renal clearance time of metabolite}}{\text{Hepatic clearance time of the drug}} \qquad (18.4)$$

The above ratio can be used to detect a change in hepatic clearance time T_m/V_1 in patients with liver disease. However, this equation is useful for comparing the hepatic clearance time in healthy subjects and patients only when the renal clearance time of the metabolite is not affected by the disease. The renal clearance time of the metabolite can be estimated from the following equation:

$$\text{Renal clearance time}\left(\frac{T_{mel}}{V_m}\right) = \frac{AUC_M}{X_{um}} \qquad (18.5)$$

Then the hepatic clearance time can be obtained from Equations (18.4) and (18.5) as follows:

$$\text{Hepatic clearance time}\left(\frac{T_m}{V_1}\right) = \frac{AUC_C}{X_{um}} \qquad (18.6)$$

The important assumption of this equation is that the renal clearance is the predominant route for the elimination of the metabolite. If this assumption does not hold, the hepatic clearance time of the drug will be overestimated. The total clearance time of the drug can be determined as the ratio of the area under the curve to dose

$$\text{Apparent total clearance time}\left(\frac{T_{el,t}}{V_1}fF\right) = \frac{AUC_C}{X_0} \qquad (18.7)$$

The fraction absorbed can be determined from the urine recovery

$$\text{Fraction absorbed } (f) = \frac{X_{uc} + X_{um}}{X_0} \tag{18.8}$$

If the renal clearance time and the hepatic clearance time are known, the first pass effect can be determined by substituting $1/T_{el,t} = 1/T_m + 1/T_{el}$ into Equation (18.7):

$$\text{Bioavailability } (f*F) = \frac{\text{AUC}_C}{V_1/T_m + V_1/T_{el}} \tag{18.9}$$

The apparent volume of distribution can be estimated in the following two ways:

$$\text{Apparent volume of distribution } (V_z) = T_z \frac{V_1}{T_{el,t}} \tag{18.10}$$

$$\text{Steady-state volume of distribution } (V_{ss}) = \bar{t} \frac{V_1}{T_{el,t}} \tag{18.11}$$

Following an intravenous dose, the mean residence time of the concentration profile is the sum of input and output times:

$$\text{Mean residence time of C following iv dose } (\bar{t}_{C,iv}) = \frac{\text{AUMC}}{\text{AUC}}$$

$$= \text{Input time } (T_{c,iv,in}) + \text{Output time } (T_{c,iv,out}) = T_{el,t} + T_{el,t} \frac{T_{21}}{T_{12}} \tag{18.12}$$

$$\text{Mean residence time of M following iv dose } (\bar{t}_{M,iv})$$

$$= \text{Input time } (T_{m,iv,in}) + \text{Output time } (T_{m,iv,out}) = T_{el,t} + T_{el,t} \frac{T_{21}}{T_{12}} + T_{mel} \tag{18.13}$$

The absorption time constant can be estimated from the difference in the mean residence times between the oral and the intravenous administrations:

$$\text{Absorption time } (T_a) = \bar{t}_{po} - \bar{t}_{iv} \tag{18.14}$$

The bioavailability can be determined from the ratio of the area under the concentration curve after the oral dose to that after the intravenous dose:

$$\text{Bioavailability } (fF) = \frac{\text{AUC}_{po}}{\text{AUC}_{iv}} \qquad (18.15)$$

The volume of the central compartment can be estimated from the extrapolated initial concentration:

$$\text{Volume of central compartment } (V_c) = \frac{X_0}{C_0} \qquad (18.16)$$

Model 2: Drugs with High First Pass Elimination

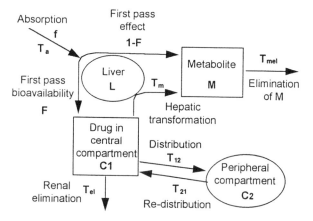

Liver diseases may reduce the first pass effect as well as the metabolic rate of a drug by altering the heaptic extraction ratio. The combined effects of altered first pass effect, metabolic rate, and protein binding can be described by Model 2.

Following an oral dose, the mean residence time of the drug concentration curve in the central compartment C_1 is the sum of input and output times (see Chapter 2):

$$\text{Mean residence time of C following oral dose } (\bar{t}_{C,po}) = \frac{\text{AUMC}_C}{\text{AUC}_C}$$

$$= \text{Input time } (T_{c,po,in}) + \text{Output time } (T_{c,po,out}) = T_a + T_{el,t} + T_{el,t}\frac{T_{21}}{T_{12}}$$

$$(18.17)$$

where $T_{el,t} = 1/(1/T_m + 1/T_{el})$. The ratio of the area under the metabolite concentration curve to the area under the parent drug concentration decreases with a decrease in the first pass effect as shown in the following equation:

$$\frac{AUC_M}{AUC_C} = \frac{V_c}{V_m}\frac{T_{mel}}{T_m} + \frac{V_c}{V_m}\frac{1-F}{F}\frac{T_{mel}(T_m + T_{el})}{T_m T_{el}} \qquad (18.18)$$

The first pass effect can be estimated from the following equation, obtained by rearranging Equation (18.18):

$$\frac{1}{\text{First pass bioavailability } (F)} = \left(\frac{AUC_M}{AUC_C} + \frac{T_{mel}V_c}{T_{el}V_m}\right)\frac{T_{el,t}}{T_m} \qquad (18.19)$$

The renal clearance time can be determined from the cumulative urine recovery:

$$\text{Renal clearance time}\left(\frac{T_{el}}{V}\right) = \frac{AUC}{X_u} \qquad (18.20)$$

The above equation applies to both the parent drug and the metabolite. The hepatic clearance time can be determined as follows. First, Equation (18.a14) is integrated from 0 to time t to give

$$V_m M_t = \frac{V_1}{T_m}AUC_{C,0-t} - \frac{V_m}{T_{mel}}AUC_{M,0-t} + f(1 - F)X_0(1 - e^{-K_a t})$$

$$(18.21)$$

where K_a can be estimated from the curve-stripping methods, assuming no flip-flop occurs. Then a linear regression can be performed with $V_m/T_{mel} \cdot AUC_{M,0-t}$ as the dependent variable, and M_t, $AUC_{C,0-t}$ and $(1 - e^{-K_a t})$ as the independent variables. The values of T_m/V_1 and V_m can be estimated from the linear regression. The total clearance time can be estimated from the following equations:

$$\text{Apparent total clearance time}\left(\frac{T_{el,t}}{V_1}fF\right) = \frac{AUC_C}{X_0}$$

or

$$\frac{1}{\text{Total clearance time } (T_{el,t}/V_1)} = \frac{V_1}{T_{el}} + \frac{V_1}{T_m} \qquad (18.22)$$

The fraction absorbed can be estimated from the urine recovery, assuming renal excretion is the predominant eliminating route.

$$\text{Fraction absorbed } (f) = \frac{X_{uc} + X_{um}}{X_0} \qquad (18.23)$$

The apparent volume of distribution can be expressed in the following two ways:

$$\text{Apparent volume of distribution } (V_z) = T_z \frac{V_1}{T_{el,t}} \qquad (18.24)$$

$$\text{Steady-state volume of distribution } (V_{ss}) = \bar{t} \frac{V_1}{T_{el,t}} \qquad (18.25)$$

Following an intravenous dose, the mean residence times of the concentration curves of the drug and the metabolite are the sum of input and output times:

$$\text{Volume of distribution of C following iv dose } (\bar{t}_{C,iv}) = \frac{\text{AUMC}}{\text{AUC}}$$

$$= \text{Input time } (T_{c,iv,in}) + \text{Output time } (T_{c,iv,out}) = T_{el,t} + T_{el,t} \frac{T_{21}}{T_{12}}$$

$$(18.26)$$

$$\text{Mean residence time of M following iv dose } (\bar{t}_{M,iv})$$

$$= \text{Input time } (T_{m,iv,in}) + \text{Output time } (T_{m,iv,out}) = T_{el,t} + T_{el,t} \frac{T_{21}}{T_{12}} + T_{mel}$$

$$(18.27)$$

The mean residence time may be affected by hepatic impairment when the hepatic elimination time, the renal elimination time, or the distribution rate are altered by the disease. The absorption time constant can be estimated from the difference in the mean residence time following oral and intravenous doses:

$$\text{Absorption time } (T_a) = \bar{t}_{C,po} - \bar{t}_{C,iv} \qquad (18.28)$$

The oral bioavailability of the drug is equal to the ratio of the area under the drug concentration curve after the oral dose to that after the intravenous dose:

$$\text{Bioavailability } (fF) = \frac{\text{AUC}_{C,po}}{\text{AUC}_{C,iv}} \qquad (18.29)$$

However, the ratio of the area under the metabolite concentration curve after the oral dose to that after the intravenous dose also depends on the first pass effect. The ratio increases with a decrease in the first pass effect as shown in the following equation:

$$\frac{\text{AUC}_{M,po}}{\text{AUC}_{M,iv}} = fF + f(1 - F)\frac{T_{el} + T_m}{T_{el}} \qquad (18.30)$$

The ratio of the area under the metabolite concentration curve to the area under the drug concentration curve following an intravenous dose can be expressed as:

$$\frac{\text{AUC}_{M,iv}}{\text{AUC}_{C,iv}} = \frac{T_{mel}V_1}{T_m V_m} = \frac{\text{Elimination clearance time of metabolite}}{\text{Hepatic clearance time toward metabolite}} \qquad (18.31)$$

This is a simpler expression of the $\text{AUC}_M/\text{AUC}_C$ ratio than that for the oral dose [Equation (18.18)]. The renal clearance time and the hepatic clearance time can be estimated from the following equations:

$$\text{Renal clearance time of metabolite} \left(\frac{T_{mel}}{V_m}\right) = \frac{\text{AUC}_M}{X_{um}} \qquad (18.32)$$

$$\text{Hepatic clearance time} \left(\frac{T_m}{V_1}\right) = \frac{\text{AUC}_C}{X_{um}} \qquad (18.33)$$

CASE STUDIES

Case 1: Metabolism Is the Dominant Route of Elimination

The two major possible effects of hepatic impairment on the pharmacokinetics of drugs are a reduction in hepatic clearance and an increase in volume of distribution, due to deteriorated hepatic function and diminished protein binding. If a drug is eliminated primarily through hepatic metabolism in the normal subjects, liver diseases may cause an accumulation of the drug in the body by retarding the hepatic clearance. If the protein binding of the drug decreases during the disease, renal elimination may increase due to an increase in the free fraction of drug in the plasma. Such an increase in renal elimination will compensate for part of the decrease in the hepatic metabolism. As the protein binding drops in hepatic impairment, the extent of increase in the volume of distribution depends on the ability of the drug to penetrate into the tissue compartment. If the drug penetrates into the tissue compartment to a small extent, an increase in the unbound free fraction in the blood is likely to cause little change in the volume of distribution. On the other hand, if a drug penetrates well into and binds to the tissues, the reduced protein binding is likely to have significant effects on the volume of distribution. In this example, the drug has a dominating hepatic elimination and good penetration into the tissue compartment. This example can be described by Model 2. The plasma drug concentration profiles are simulated using the model and shown in Figure 18.1.

In the example, the hepatic metabolism significantly decreases, and the central compartment volume of distribution, the rate of distribution, and

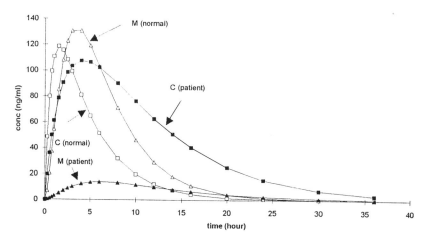

FIGURE 18.1. Simulated plasma drug concentration using Model 2 for normal and hepatic-impaired subjects. The hepatic elimination is the predominant route of elimination. The time constant plot comparing the healthy subject with the patient is shown in Figure 18.2. The parameters used in this simulation are normal: $X_0 = 10$ mg, $f = 0.7$, $F = 0.95$, $V_1 = 7$ L, $V_2 = 15$ L, $V_m = 10$ L, $K_a = 0.25$ hr^{-1}, $K_{12} = 0.1$ hr^{-1}, $K_{21} = 0.5$ hr^{-1}, $K_{el} = 0.1$ hr^{-1}, $K_m = 1.2$ hr^{-1}, $K_{mel} = 0.6$ hr^{-1}; patient: $X_0 = 10$ mg, $f = 0.7$, $F = 0.98$, $V_1 = 20$ L, $V_2 = 15$ L, $V_m = 25$ L, $K_a = 0.25$ hr^{-1}, $K_{12} = 0.25$ hr^{-1}, $K_{21} = 0.5$ hr^{-1}, $K_{el} = 0.12$ hr^{-1}1, $K_m = 0.1$ hr^{-1}, $K_{mel} = 0.6$ hr^{-1}.

TABLE 18.1. The Estimated Time Constants of Model 2 for the Example in Figure 18.1.

Parameter	Normal Subject		Patient		Equation
	Time Constant Analysis	Model Value	Time Constant Analysis	Model Value	
$\bar{t}_C$ (hr)	4.9	4.9	10.8	10.8	(18.17)
$\bar{t}_M$ (hr)	6.5	6.5	12.1	12.2	
$T_{z,c}$ (hr)	3.7	4 (T_a)	7.3	7.6 (T_z)	(18.3)
$T_{z,m}$ (hr)	3.3	4 (T_a)	7.5	7.6 (T_z)	(18.3)
T_{el}/V_1 (hr/L)	0.17	0.17	0.067	0.067	(18.20)
T_{mel}/V_m (hr/L)	6	6	15	15	(18.20)
T_m/V_1 (hr/L)	0.11	0.12	0.48	0.5	(18.21)
AUC_C (ng·hr/L)	734	730	1565	1559	
AUC_M (ng·hr/L)	1087	1081	218	217	
AUC_M/AUC_C	1.48	1.48	0.14	0.14	(18.18)
$X_{u,c}$ (μg)	514	511	3757	3741	
$X_{u,m}$ (μg)	6522	6488	3268	3258	
$X_{u,m}/(X_{u,c} + X_{u,m})$	0.93	0.93	0.47	0.47	
F	0.984	0.95	0.998	0.98	(18.19)
f	0.7	0.7	0.7	0.7	(18.23)
V_z (L)	34.3	36.4	34.9	33.6	(18.24)
V_{ss} (L)	45.8	44.6	48.4	47.6	(18.25)

the rate of renal elimination increase in the patient with liver disease. The maximum concentration is smaller in the hepatic-impaired than in the normal subject, indicating an increase in the volume of distribution in the patient. Since the hepatic metabolism is the primary route of elimination, the decrease in the hepatic function results in an increase in total clearance time and an increased mean residence time. The time to reach the maximum concentration, which depends on the total elimination time, is longer in the patient than the normal subject. The metabolite concentration is significantly reduced in the patient; however, the parent drug concentration does not show the same degree of increase. This occurs because a significant increase in the unbound fraction of the drug in the plasma causes a compensating increase in the renal elimination in the patient.

Since hepatic metabolism is the dominant route of elimination, the elimination of the drug is expected to be notably affected by hepatic disease. Therefore, the key time constant in this example is the hepatic elimination time. The estimated pharmacokinetic parameters of the above example using the time constant analysis are listed in Table 18.1, and the estimated time constants are presented in Figure 18.2. The area under the curve of the

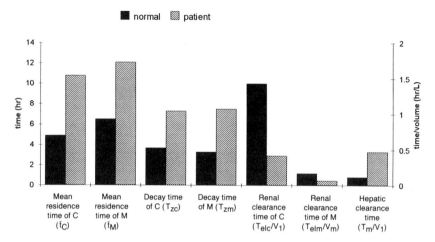

FIGURE 18.2. The time constant plot comparing the healthy subject and hepatic-impaired patient in the example shown in Figure 18.1. The renal clearance times of both parent drug (T_{el}/V_1) and metabolite (T_{mel}/V_m) in the patient decrease significantly due to the increase in the unbound free fraction in the plasma. The hepatic clearance time (T_m/V_1) of the parent drug increases fourfold in the patient.

parent drug is greater in the patient, while that of the metabolite drops significantly. The ratio of the area under the curve of the metabolite to the parent decreases almost tenfold in the patient, indicating severely impaired hepatic function.

Now let us examine the time constant plot (Figure 18.2). The mean residence time of the metabolite is longer than that of the parent drug, indicating that the metabolite elimination time is significantly longer than the parent drug elimination time. The mean residence time of the parent drug increases in the patient, indicating that the hepatic metabolism dominates the elimination, and the reduction in metabolism results in an increase in the total clearance time. Since the absorption time is longer than the elimination time in the healthy subject, the decay time T_zs for the parent drug and the metabolite are equal to the absorption time constant (flip-flop). As the elimination time increases in the patient and becomes longer than the absorption time, the flip-flop disappears and the decay time constant represents $1/\lambda_2$. Therefore, in this case the decay time constant is not a good indicator for comparing the total elimination time between the normal subject and the patient. The urine data show an increase in the excreted parent drug and a decrease in the excreted metabolite in the patient. The ratio of the excreted metabolite to the total drug drops from 0.93 in the normal subject to 0.47 in the patient.

The renal clearance time T_{el}/V of both parent drug and metabolite in the patient decreases significantly due to the increase in the unbound free fraction in the plasma. The hepatic clearance time of the parent drug increases fourfold in the patient, while the total clearance time only increases twofold because the increase in the renal clearance compensates for the decrease in the hepatic clearance. The apparent volumes of distribution, V_z and V_{ss}, do not differ between the normal subject and the patient. Therefore, the values of V_z and V_{ss} are not good indicators for comparing the volume of distribution between the subjects in this case. An intravenous administration of the drug to both subjects is a better way to determine the volume of distribution. Since a flip-flop is likely to occur in a hepatic impairment study because of the drastic change in the elimination rate, an intravenous, instead of an oral, study is recommended to avoid the confusion over the determination of elimination time and volume of distribution.

Case 2: Metabolism Is Not the Dominant Route of Elimination

If the hepatic metabolism does not dominate the elimination of a drug in the normal subject, the total clearance time will only be slightly affected by

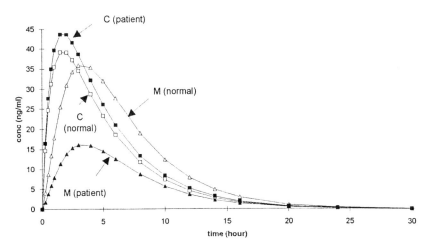

FIGURE 18.3. Simulated plasma drug concentration using Model 2 for normal and hepatic-impaired subjects, where the hepatic elimination is not the predominant route of elimination. The time constant plot comparing the normal subject and the patient is shown in Figure 18.4. The parameters used in this simulation are normal: $X_0 = 10$ mg, $f = 0.7$, $F = 0.8$, $V_1 = 20$ L, $V_2 = 25$ L, $V_m = 25$ L, $K_a = 0.25$ hr^{-1}, $K_{12} = 0.1$ hr^{-1}, $K_{21} = 0.5$ hr^{-1}, $K_{el} = 0.5$ hr^{-1}, $K_m = 0.6$ hr^{-1}, $K_{mel} = 0.6$ hr^{-1}; patient: $X_0 = 10$ mg, $f = 0.7$, $F = 0.9$, $V_1 = 20$ L, $V_2 = 25$ L, $V_m = 30$ L, $K_a = 0.25$ hr^{-1}, $K_{12} = 0.12$ hr^{-1}, $K_{21} = 0.5$ hr^{-1}, $K_{el} = 0.8$ hr^{-1}, $K_m = 0.3$ hr^{-1}, $K_{mel} = 0.6$ hr^{-1}.

TABLE 18.2. The Estimated Time Constants of Model 2
for the Example in Figure 18.3.

Parameter	Normal Subject		Patient		Equation
	Time Constant Analysis	Model Value	Time Constant Analysis	Model Value	
$\bar{t}_C$ (hr)	5.1	5.1	5.1	5.1	(18.17)
$\bar{t}_M$ (hr)	6.4	6.4	6.5	6.5	
$T_{z,c}$ (hr)	3.7	4 (T_a)	3.7	4 (T_a)	(18.3)
$T_{z,m}$ (hr)	3.3	4 (T_a)	3.3	4 (T_a)	(18.3)
T_{el}/V_1 (hr/L)	0.1	0.1	0.063	0.063	(18.20)
T_{mel}/V_m (hr/L)	0.067	0.067	0.056	0.056	(18.20)
T_m/V_1 (hr/L)	0.069	0.083	0.143	0.167	(18.21)
AUC_C (ng·hr/L)	255	254	287	286	
AUC_M (ng·hr/L)	298	296	135	134	
AUC_M/AUC_C	1.2	1.2	0.47	0.47	(18.18)
$X_{u,c}$ (μg)	2558	2545	4605	4581	
$X_{u,m}$ (μg)	4477	4454	2430	2418	
$X_{u,m}/(X_{u,c} + X_{u,m})$	0.64	0.64	0.35	0.35	
F	0.1	0.1	0.063	0.063	(18.19)
f	0.7	0.7	0.7	0.7	(18.23)
V_z (L)	90	88	85	88	(18.24)
V_{ss} (L)	124	112	118	113	(18.25)

the hepatic impairment. The increase in the renal clearance due to a reduction in the protein binding will compensate the decrease in the hepatic clearance. If a drug does not readily penetrate into the tissue compartment, the volume of distribution will not significantly change with a decreased protein binding in liver disease. An example is described by Model 2 and simulated plasma drug concentration profiles are shown in Figure 18.3. In this example, the hepatic elimination rate drops, the renal excretion rate increases, and the volume of distribution remains the same in the patient. The maximum concentration and the area under the curve are higher in the patient than those in the normal subject due to a reduction in the hepatic clearance by the disease. The time to reach the maximum concentration is not altered much in the patient, indicating that the decrease in hepatic clearance is not significant compared with the total clearance (i.e., hepatic clearance does not dominate the total clearance). The maximum concentration of the metabolite decreases substantially, indicating a deteriorated hepatic function.

The parent drug can be eliminated either by renal or hepatic route. Hepatic impairment will reduce the rate of elimination via the hepatic route (due to impaired liver function) but may offset this decrease by increasing the rate of elimination via the renal route (by reducing protein binding). Therefore, the key time constants in this example are the renal elimination time and the hepatic elimination time. The estimated pharmacokinetic parameters of the above example using the time constant analysis are listed in Table 18.2, and the estimated time constants are presented in Figure 18.4. The area under the concentration curve of the metabolite decreases twofold while that of the parent drug only slightly increases in the patient, indicating that the hepatic clearance does not dominate the total clearance and that the nonhepatic clearance may compensate for the decrease in the hepatic clearance. The ratio of the area under the curve of the metabolite to the parent drug drops significantly in the patient, indicating an increased hepatic clearance time.

Now let us examine the time constant plot (Figure 18.4). The mean residence times of both metabolite and the parent drug do not differ much between the normal subject and patient, another indication that the hepatic clearance does not dominate the total clearance. The decay times of both parent drug and metabolite do not change from the normal subject to patient due to a flip-flop, where the absorption time dominates the decay time in both subjects. The renal clearance time shortens substantially in the patient and compensates for the increase in the hepatic clearance time. The values of V_z and V_{ss} do not change from the normal subject to patient, and they are not good indicators for comparing the volume of distribution.

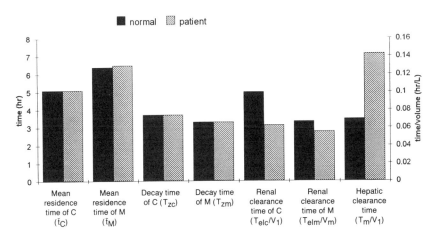

FIGURE 18.4. The time constant plot comparing the normal subject and the hepatic-impaired patient in the example shown in Figure 18.3. The renal clearance time (T_{elc}/V_1) shortens substantially in the patient and compensates for the increase in the hepatic clearance time (T_m/V_1).

Case 3: Hepatic Impairment Affects Protein Binding

The pharmacological effects of a drug may have a direct relationship with the concentration of the unbound drug in the plasma. Therefore, it is informative to measure the unbound fraction of the drug in cases such as the hepatic impairment study when the protein binding is expected to change. The unbound fraction concentration affects all the rate constants that originate from the central compartment, including distribution (K_{12}), renal elimination $(K_{el}$ and $K_{mel})$, and hepatic elimination (K_m). An example is described by Model 1, and the simulated plasma drug concentration profiles using the model are shown in Figures 18.5 and 18.6. In this example, the unbound fraction increases twofold in the patient. As a result, the distribution and renal elimination rate constants increase. The volume of the central compartment is not affected by the change in protein binding. The patient also has a mild concomitant renal failure. The plasma concentration in the patient only slightly elevates compared with the normal subject, indicating that the hepatic metabolism does not dominate the total elimination. The significantly low metabolite concentration indicates the deteriorated hepatic function in the patient. The difference in the unbound concentration

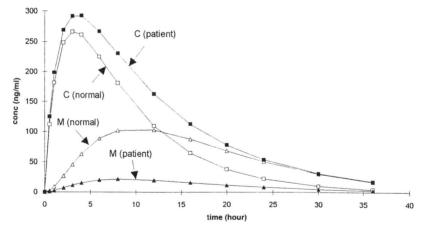

FIGURE 18.5. Simulated plasma drug concentration using Model 1 for normal and hepatic-impaired subjects, with the hepatic impairment affecting the protein binding. The time constant plot comparing the normal subject and the patient is shown in Figure 18.7. The parameters used in this simulation are normal: $X_0 = 10$ mg, $f = 1$, $F = 0.85$, $V_1 = 15$ L, $V_2 = 30$ L, $V_m = 15$ L, $K_a = 0.5$ hr^{-1}, $K_{12} = 0.3$ hr^{-1}, $K_{21} = 1$ hr^{-1}, $K_{el} = 0.09$ hr^{-1}, $K_m = 0.09$ hr^{-1}, $K_{mel} = 0.12$ hr^{-1}, $f_u = 0.15$; patient: $X_0 = 10$ mg, $f = 1$, $F = 0.98$, $V_1 = 15$ L, $V_2 = 30$ L, $V_m = 15$ L, $K_a = 0.5$ hr^{-1}, $K_{12} = 0.5$ hr^{-1}, $K_{21} = 1$ hr^{-1}, $K_{el} = 0.12$ hr^{-1}, $K_m = 0.024$ hr^{-1}, $K_{mel} = 0.24$ hr^{-1}, $f_u = 0.3$.

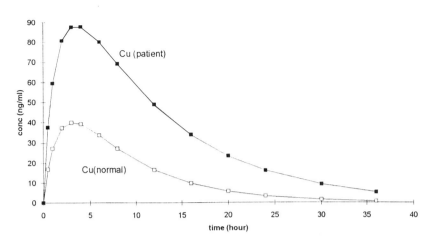

FIGURE 18.6. Simulated unbound drug concentration in the plasma using Model 1 for the normal subject and the patient in the example shown in Figure 18.3.

is greater than the difference in the total plasma concentration between the subjects. Therefore, a reduction of the dose may be necessary for the hepatic impairment patient, in spite of the similar total plasma concentration between the patient and the normal subject.

The concentration profiles in Figure 18.5 show a typical case of reduced protein binding: a combination of prolonged decay time and lower maximum concentration in the patient relative to the normal subject. Therefore, the key parameters in this example are the volume of distribution as well as the hepatic elimination time. The estimated pharmacokinetic parameters of the above example using the time constant analysis are listed in Table 18.3, and the estimated time constants are presented in Figure 18.7. The area under the curve of the parent drug increases only by 45%, while that of the metabolite decreases sixfold, indicating that the metabolism does not dominate the total clearance of parent drug.

Now let us examine the time constant plot (Figure 18.7). The increase in the hepatic clearance time is also reflected by the significant reduction in the ratio of the area under the curve of the metabolite to that of the parent drug. The mean residence time of both parent drug and metabolite increase in the patient as a result of an increased total elimination time. The decay time of the drug is longer in the patient than in the normal subject due to a greater distribution to the peripheral compartment and a longer total elimination time in the patient. The fraction of the metabolite in the urine decreases in the patient, reflecting a decrease in the hepatic metabolism. The renal clearance time of the drug decreases in the patient due to a significant in-

TABLE 18.3. The Estimated Time Constants of Model 1 for the Example in Figures 18.5 and 18.6.

Parameter	Normal Subject		Patient		Equation
	Time Constant Analysis	Model Value	Time Constant Analysis	Model Value	
$\bar{t}_C$ (hr)	9.2	9.2	12.4	12.4	(18.1)
$\bar{t}_M$ (hr)	18.2	17.5	17.1	16.6	(18.2)
$T_{z,c}$ (hr)	7.69	7.14	11.1	11.1	(18.3)
$T_{z,m}$ (hr)	12.5	8.33			
		(T_{mel})	11.1	11.1	(18.3)
T_{el}/V_1 (hr/L)	0.74	0.74	0.56	0.56	(18.5)
$T_{el,u}/V_1$ (hr/L)	0.11	0.11	0.17	0.17	(18.5)
T_m/V_1 (hr/L)	0.72	0.74	2.74	2.8	(18.6)
AUC_C (ng·hr/L)	3163	3148	4547	4537	
AUC_M (ng·hr/L)	2452	2361	459	453	
AUC_M/AUC_C	0.78	0.75	0.1	0.1	(18.4)
$X_{u,c}$ (μg)	4270	4250	8186	8166	
$X_{u,m}$ (μg)	4414	4250	1654	1633	
$X_{u,m}/(X_{u,c} + X_{u,m})$	0.51	0.5	0.17	0.17	
fF	0.87	0.85	0.98	0.98	(18.9)
V_z (L)	20	20	23	23	(18.10)
V_{zu} (L)	135	135	77	76	(18.10)

crease in the unbound fraction of the drug in the plasma, in spite of the fact that the intrinsic renal clearance time ($T_{el,u}/V_1$) of the unbound drug increases as a result of a concomitant renal failure. The apparent volume of distribution of the total drug V_z increases slightly, while the volume of distribution of the unbound drug decreases twofold.

EXAMPLES

Example 1: Liver Disease Affects Elimination

The pharmacokinetics of ximoprofen were investigated in healthy subjects and patients with chronic hepatic cirrhosis in two studies [10]. In study I, a 22.75-mg ximoprofen intravenous dose and a 30-mg ximoprofen oral dose were administered in twelve healthy male subjects. In study II, a 30-mg ximoprofen oral dose was administered to twelve healthy subjects and ten patients with chronic hepatic cirrhosis. The mean plasma concentration profiles of ximoprofen in the two studies are shown in Figure 18.8. The con-

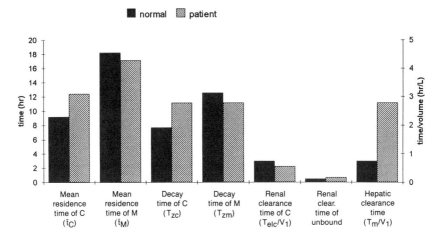

FIGURE 18.7. The time constant plot comparing the normal subject and the hepatic-impaired patient in the example shown in Figure 18.6. The renal clearance time (T_{el}/V_1) of the drug decreases in the patient due to a significant increase in the unbound fraction of the drug in the plasma, in spite of the fact that the intrinsic renal clearance time ($T_{el,u}/V_1$) of the unbound drug increases as a result of a concomitant renal failure.

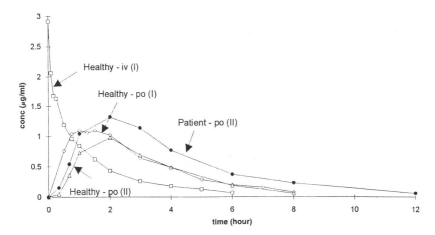

FIGURE 18.8. Mean concentration profiles of ximoprofen following (I) the intravenous administration of 22.75 mg ximoprofen and oral administration of 30 mg ximoprofen to twelve healthy subjects and (II) the oral administration of 30 mg ximoprofen to twelve healthy subjects and ten patients with chronic hepatic cirrhosis. (Reproduced from Reference [10] with permission.) The time constant plot comparing the healthy subject and hepatic-impaired patient is shown in Figure 18.9.

457

centration profiles following the intravenous administration in the healthy subjects show a very short initial distribution phase. The plasma concentrations of ximoprofen in the patients with cirrhosis are higher than those in the healthy subjects.

The protein binding of ximoprofen in healthy subjects is about 80–90% [10], but the drug has a short decay time and small volume of distribution, indicating little tissue distribution. Therefore, volume of distribution of the drug is not likely to change with hepatic impairment. The oral bioavailability is 98% with very little first pass effect; however, the drug is predominantly eliminated by metabolism with a very small extraction ratio. Therefore, elimination of the drug may potentially be affected by the hepatic disease, and the key time constant in this example is the hepatic elimination time. The pharmacokinetic parameters of ximoprofen are estimated using Model 1 since the first pass effect of the drug is relatively low. The estimated pharmacokinetic parameters are listed in Table 18.4, and the estimated time constants are presented in Figure 18.9.

Now let us examine the time constant plot (Figure 18.9). The decay time of the concentration profiles is similar between the intravenous and oral administrations in the healthy subjects, indicating that no flip-flop of the concentration curve occurs following the oral dose. The decay time of the concentration profile in study II is greater in the patients than in the healthy subjects, indicating an increase in the elimination time due to the hepatic cirrhosis. The area under the concentration curve increases in the patients compared with the healthy subjects, probably due to the increased elimination time. The mean residence time is prolonged in the patients, reflecting

TABLE 18.4. The Estimated Pharmacokinetic Parameters
of Ximoprofen Using Model 1.

Parameter*	Healthy iv (I)	Healthy po (I)	Healthy po (II)	Patient po (II)	Equation
T_z (hr)	2.30	2.41	2.13	2.89	(18.3)
$\bar{t}$ (hr)	2.1	3.1	3.5	4.1	(18.1, 18.2)
T_a (hr)		1.20			(18.14)
$T_{el,t}*f/V_1$ (hr/L)	0.149	0.148	0.118	0.204	(18.7)
AUC (μg·hr/L)	3.41	4.43	3.54	6.12	
f		0.98			(18.8)
f_u	0.07	0.11		0.18	measured
V_c (L)	7.4				(18.16)
V_z (L)	15.4	16.6	18.0	14.2	(18.10)
V_{ss} (L)	14.0	21.0	30.0	30.0	(18.11)

*Parameters estimated from the mean concentration profiles or the reported mean values.

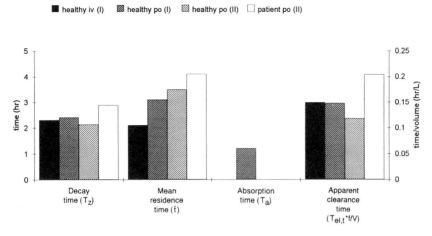

FIGURE 18.9. The time constant plot of ximoprofen comparing the healthy subject and the hepatic-impaired patient using Model 1. The total clearance time of ximoprofen increases in the patients ($T_{el,t}*f/V_1$), which is consistent with the increased decay time (T_z) of the concentration curve.

the increase in the elimination time. The total clearance times following the intravenous and oral administrations are similar because of the almost complete oral absorption ($f \rightarrow 1$). The total clearance time of ximoprofen increases in the patients, which is consistent with the increased decay time of the concentration curve. The fraction of the unbound drug increases in the patients, probably due to a decrease in the plasma protein concentration or an accumulation of protein binding inhibitors in the patients. The volume of the central compartment is small, only slightly greater than the blood volume, suggesting very little tissue penetration and weak tissue binding. Therefore, the volume of distribution is not likely to increase with the increased unbound fraction in the patient. Both V_z and V_{ss} do not indicate any increase in the volume of distribution in the patients. To summarize, liver disease does not cause major change in the concentration of ximoprofen probably because a decrease in hepatic blood flow with the disease has minimal effects on the hepatic clearance of a drug with small hepatic extraction ratio [10].

Example 2: Hepatic Impairment Affects Protein Binding

The pharmacokinetics of cefpiramide were investigated following the intravenous administration of 1 g cefpiramide in eleven healthy subjects and eleven patients with alcoholic cirrhosis [4]. The mean concentration profiles of cefpiramide in the healthy subjects and patients are shown in Figure 18.10. The decay time of the concentration curve clearly increases in the patients compared with the healthy subjects.

Cefpiramide is extensively bound to plasma proteins ($>97\%$) [4] and has a long decay time; therefore, the volume of distribution is likely to be affected by hepatic disease. The key parameters in this example are the volume of distribution, as well as the total elimination time. The pharmacokinetic parameters of cefpiramide are estimated using Model 2 and are listed in Table 18.5, and the estimated time constants are presented in Figure 18.11. The unbound fraction (f_u) of cefpiramide in the plasma increases fivefold in the patients compared with the normal subjects.

Now let us examine the time constant plot (Figure 18.11). The decay times of both total and unbound concentration curves increase in the patients, indicating that the intrinsic elimination rate (of the unbound fraction) as well as the apparent elimination rate (of the total drug) are modified by the alcoholic cirrhosis. The area under the total concentration curve increases 2.4-fold in the patients, while the area under the unbound concentration curve increases tenfold in the patients due to the large increase in the unbound fraction. The urine recovery of the unchanged drug increases in the patients, indicating a decrease in the hepatic elimination. The total renal clearance time decreases in the patients, probably due to an increase in the volume of distribution. On the other hand, the unbound renal clearance

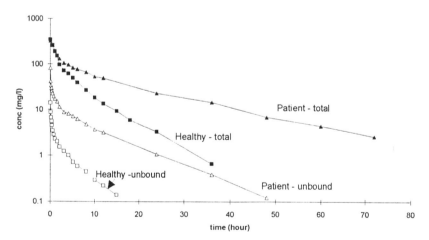

FIGURE 18.10. Mean concentration profiles of total and unbound cefpiramide in the plasma following the intravenous administration of 1 g cefpiramide in eleven healthy subjects and eleven patients with alcoholic cirrhosis. (Reproduced from Reference [4] with permission.) The time constant plot comparing the healthy subject and hepatic-impaired patient is shown in Figure 18.11.

TABLE 18.5. The Pharmacokinetic Parameters Estimated for the Total and Unbound Cefpiramide in the Plasma Using Model 2.

Parameter*	Subject Total	Patient Total	Subject Unbound	Patient Unbound	Equation
T_z (hr)	7.62	20	5.92	12.35	(18.3)
$\bar{t}$ (hr)	5.1	16.3	4.5	8.7	(18.17)
T_{el}/V_1 (min/ml)	0.25	0.106	0.0046	0.0096	(18.20)
$T_{el,t}/V_1$ (min/ml)	0.039	0.081	0.000712	0.000693	(18.22)
T_{nr}/V_1 (min/ml)	0.0456	0.345	0.000842	0.0214	$\dfrac{1}{V_c/T_{el,t} - V_c/T_{el}}$
AUC (mg·hr/L)	672	1598	12.8	130	
X_u (mg)	161	698			
V_z (L/kg)	0.17	0.22	7.0	1.7	(18.24)
V_{ss} (L/kg)	0.12	0.16	5.3	1.3	(18.25)
f_u (%)			1.9	10.4	measured

*Parameters estimated from the mean concentration profiles or the reported mean values.

time increases in the patients, indicating an impaired intrinsic renal clearance (of the unbound drug) in the patients. The nonrenal clearance times for the total and unbound drug increase in the patients, reflecting the impaired hepatic function. The volume of distribution of the total drug increases in the patients because the increase in the unbound fraction may result in an

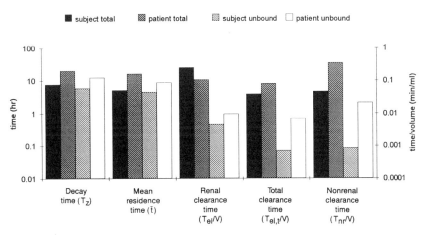

FIGURE 18.11. The time constant plot of cefpiramide comparing the healthy subject and hepatic-impaired patient using Model 2. The total renal clearance time (T_{el}/V) decreases in the patients, probably due to an increase in the volume of distribution. On the other hand, the unbound renal clearance time increases in the patients, indicating an impaired intrinsic renal clearance (of the unbound drug) in the patients.

increase in the tissue distribution. The decreased protein binding has a dual effect on the volume of distribution of the unbound drug in the patients: (1) it may decrease the volume of distribution by the increase in the unbound fraction, and (2) it may also increase by the increase in the tissue distribution. However, the former effect seems to outweigh the latter in this case, and the volume of distribution decreases in the patient.

To summarize, the renal clearance time of the total plasma cefpiramide decreases, probably due to a decreased protein binding, while the renal clearance time of the unbound drug increases, probably due to a generally concurrent renal impairment in the liver disease. The plasma concentration increases in the patients due to a significant increase in the nonrenal elimination time. Therefore, in patients with hepatic impairment, reduction in dosage or frequency of administration may be necessary to achieve the same level of plasma concentration of cefpiramide as in healthy subjects, as suggested in Reference [4].

Example 3: Hepatic Impairment Affects Renal and Hepatic Eliminations

The pharmacokinetics of clarithromycin and its metabolite were determined after a multiple-dose clarithromycin regimen (250 mg twice daily for five doses) in six healthy subjects and seven patients with hepatic impair-

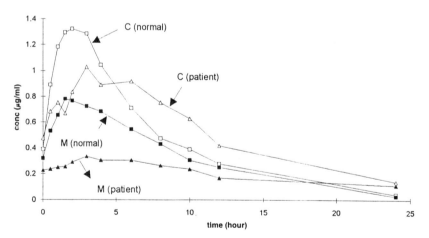

FIGURE 18.12. Mean plasma concentration profiles of clarithromycin and its metabolite following the last dose of a multiple-dose clarithromycin regimen (250 mg twice daily for five doses) in six healthy subjects and seven patients with hepatic impairment. (Reproduced from Reference [3] with permission.) The time constant plot comparing the healthy subject and the hepatic-impaired patient is shown in Figure 18.13.

TABLE 18.6. The Pharmacokinetic Parameters Estimated for
Clarithromycin and Its Metabolite in Healthy Subjects and
Hepatic-Impaired Patients Using Model 1.

Parameter*	Subject C	Patient C	Subject M	Patient M	Equation
T_z (hr)	4.76	7.14	7.14	11.11	(18.3)
$AUC_M/AUC_C =$					
$T_{mel}*V_1/(T_m*V_m)$	0.66	0.34			(8.4)
T_{el}/V_1 (min/ml)	0.0090	0.0059	0.0089	0.0075	(18.5)
T_m/V_1 (min/ml)	0.0135	0.0219			(8.6)
AUC (mg·hr/L)	9.29	9.29	6.1	3.17	
X_u (mg)	60.5	79	38.5	27.5	
V_z (L)	138	305			(18.10)

*Parameters estimated from the mean concentration profiles or the reported mean values.

ment [3]. The mean concentration profiles of clarithromycin and the metabolite after the last dose are shown in Figure 18.12. The decrease in the concentration in the hepatic-impaired patients a possible increase in the volume of distribution.

Clarithromycin has a moderate extraction ratio (0.4), and only 20–30% of the drug is excreted unchanged in the urine; therefore, elimination of the drug can be expected to be affected by hepatic impairment. The key time constant in this example is then the hepatic elimination time. The pharmacokinetic parameters of clarithromycin and the metabolite are estimated using Model 1 and are listed in Table 18.6, and the estimated time constants are presented in Figure 18.13. The area under the clarithromycin concentration curve does not change with the disease, while the area under the metabolite concentration curve decreases in the patients.

Now let us examine the time constant plot (Figure 18.13). The decay time of the clarithromycin concentration curve increases in the patients, indicating a prolongation in the elimination time. The renal clearance times of both clarithromycin and its metabolite decrease in the patients, probably due to an increased volume of distribution. The hepatic clearance time increases in the patients as a result of the impaired hepatic function. There is no evidence of an altered absorption by the disease, since the total urine recoveries are similar between the healthy subjects and the patients. To summarize, in patients with hepatic disease, the decrease in hepatic elimination seems to be partially offset by an increase in the renal elimination, causing little change in the area under the curve. However, the impaired hepatic function results in a reduction in the metabolite concentration; therefore, if the metabolite is the active component of the pharmacological

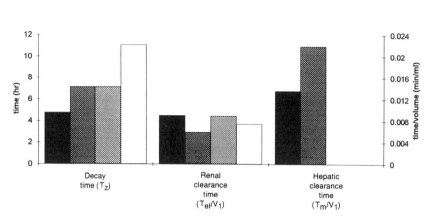

FIGURE 18.13. The time constant plot of clarithromycin comparing the healthy subject and the hepatic-impaired patient using Model 1. The renal clearance times (T_{el}/V_1) of both clarithromycin and its metabolite decrease in the patients, probably due to an increased volume of distribution. The hepatic clearance time (T_m/V_1) increases in the patients as a result of the impaired hepatic function.

effect, an increase in dosage may be necessary in hepatic impaired patients. Otherwise, no dosage adjustment in the patients is necessary to achieve the same level of clarithromycin as in the healthy subjects, as suggested in Reference [3].

REFERENCES

1. Blake J. C., Palmer J. L., Minton N. A., and Burroughs A. K., "The pharmacokinetics of intravenous ondansetron in patients with hepatic impairment," *Br. J. Clin. Pharmac.*, 1993; 35:441–443.

2. Brocks D. R., Jamali F., Russell A. S., and Skeith K. J., "The stereoselective pharmacokinetics of etodolac in young and elderly subjects, and after cholecystectomy," *J. Clin. Pharmacol.*, 1992; 32:982–989.

3. Chu, S. Y., Granneman G. R., Pichotta P. J., Decourt J., Girault J., and Fourtillan J. B., "Effect of moderate or severe hepatic impairment on clarithromycin pharmacokinetics," *J. Clin. Pharmacol.*, 1993; 33:480–485.

4. Demotes-Mainard F., Vincon G., Amouretti M., Dumas F., Necciari J., Kieffer G., and Begaud B., "Pharmacokinetics and protein binding of cefpiramide in patients with alcoholic cirrhosis," *Clin. Pharmacol. Ther.*, 1991; 49(3):263–269.

5. Kirch W., Nokhodian A., Halabi A., and Weidinger G., "Clinical pharmacokinetics of the nifedipine/co-dergocrine combination in impaired liver and renal function," *European Journal of Drug Metabolism and Pharmacokinetics*, 1992; 17(1):33–38.

6. Ko R. J., Sattler F. R., Nichols S., Akriviadis E., Runyon B., Appleman M., Cohen J. L., and Koda R. T., "Pharmacokinetics of cefotaxime and desacetylcefotaxime in patients with liver disease," *Antimicrobial Agents and Chemotherapy,* July 1991; 1376–1380.

7. Magueur E., Hagege H., Attali P., Singlas E., Etienne J. P., and Taburet A. M., "Pharmacokinetics of metoclopramide in patients with liver cirrhosis," *Br. J. Clin. Pharmac.,* 1991; 31:185–187.

8. Peter J. D., Jehl F., Pottecher T., Dupeyron J. P., and Monteil H., "Pharmacokinetics of intravenous fusidic acid in patients with cholestasis," *Antimicrobial Agents and Chemotherapy,* Mar. 1993; 501–506.

9. Shyu W. C., Wilber R. B., Pittman K. A., Garg D. C., and Barbhaiya R. H., "Pharmacokinetics of cefprozil in healthy subjects and patients with hepatic impairment," *J. Clin. Pharmacol.,* 1991; 31:372–376.

10. Taylor I. W., Taylor T., James I., Doyle G., Dorf G., Darragh A., and Chasseaud L. F., "Pharmacokinetics of the anti-inflammatory drug ximoprofen in healthy subjects and in disease states," *Eur. J. Clin. Pharmacol.,* 1991; 40:101–106.

11. Evans, W. E., Schentag J. J., and Jusko W. J., *Applied Pharmacokinetics,* Applied Therapeutics, Inc., 1992.

CHAPTER 19

Special Pharmacokinetic Considerations in Other Diseases

INTRODUCTION

Many diseases can affect the pharmacokinetics of drugs. As a result, dosing regimens must be modified in patients with disease to maintain the desired plasma drug concentration levels. Changes in protein binding due to diseases affect the half-life of drugs by changing the apparent volume of distribution, the distribution time, and the hepatic and renal elimination times. For example, the binding of many drugs to albumin decreases in renal and hepatic dysfunctions [1], and the binding of some basic drugs to α_1-acid glycoprotein rises in inflammatory diseases, such as arthritis and Crohn's disease [2–6]. The following changes may occur with congestive heart failure [12–22]: the hepatic blood flow decreases, and thus, the hepatic clearance of drugs may decline; α_1-acid glycoprotein binding increases, which may affect the apparent volume of distribution, and the rate and extent of absorption may be reduced. In hyperthyroidism [7–11], the gastrointestinal motility increases, which may result in a low bioavailability; the renal blood flow increases, which may raise the renal clearance; and the hepatic enzyme activity increases, which may raise the hepatic clearance. On the other hand, hypothyroidism has the opposite effect.

Three models are discussed in this chapter to describe the pharmacokinetics in inflammatory diseases, hyperthyroidism, and congestive heart failure: (1) the first model describes the pharmacokinetics in which the absorption, elimination, and protein binding may be affected by a disease; (2) the second model describes the pharmacokinetics in which the first pass effect and metabolism may be affected by a disease and the concentration profile exhibits a monoexponential terminal phase; and (3) the third model describes the pharmacokinetics in which the first pass effect and metabolism may be affected by a disease and the concentration profile exhibits a biexponential terminal phase. Three case studies and four literature examples are discussed to illustrate the utility of these models in pharmacokinetic studies in patients and healthy subjects. Additional examples of the comparison studies between patients and healthy subjects can be found in the literature [1–22].

PHARMACOKINETIC MODELS

This section presents three models that are useful in describing the pharmacokinetics in inflammatory diseases, hyperthyroidism, and congestive heart failure. The goal is to establish simple relationships between time constants and measurable parameters such as (1) mean residence time, which is the sum of input and output times, and (2) area under the curves. The derivations of these relationships are straightforward and are discussed in Chapter 2.

Model 1: Absorption, Elimination, and Protein Binding Affected by a Disease

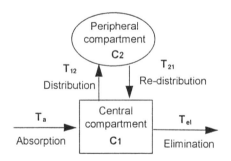

As the protein binding of a drug is affected by a disease, the volume of distribution and the distribution time constant may change. This can be described by Model 1, which accounts for the distribution of the drug.

The mean residence time is estimated from the ratio of the area under the first moment curve to the area under the curve. Following an oral administration, the mean residence time is simply the sum of input and output times (see Chapter 2):

$$\text{Mean residence time following oral administration } (\bar{t}_{po}) = \frac{\text{AUMC}}{\text{AUC}}$$

$$= \text{Input time } (T_{po,in}) + \text{Output time } (T_{po,out}) = T_a + T_{el} + T_{el}\frac{T_{21}}{T_{12}} \quad (19.1)$$

The mean residence time may be affected by a disease, if the absorption time, the elimination time, or the distribution time change in the disease. The accuracy of the estimated mean residence time relies on the accuracy of the estimated slope of the beta phase. This is because the area under the curve and the area under the first moment curve are extrapolated to infinity based on the slope of beta phase. Therefore, a sensitive analytical assay method and a long enough sampling time are necessary for an accurate estimation of λ_{z2} and the mean residence time for drug with long terminal decay time. The terminal decay time of alpha (T_{z1}) beta (T_{z2}) phases and the initial time constant (T_0) can be estimated from the partial area under the concentration curve using a curve-stripping technique (see Appendix 2):

$$\frac{1}{\text{Decay time } (T_z)} = \lambda_z = 2 \frac{(t_{\text{ref}} - t_{\text{last}}) \ln (C_{t_{\text{ref}}}) - \text{AUC} \ln C_{t_{\text{ref}}} - t_{\text{last}}}{(t_{\text{ref}} - t_{\text{last}})^2} \qquad (19.2)$$

The renal elimination time, the extent of absorption, and the absorption time are frequently affected by diseases such as celiac diseases, Crohn's disease, hypothyroidism, hyperthyroidism, and congestive heart failure, and these parameters can be characterized as follows:

$$\text{Renal clearance time } \left(\frac{T_{\text{el}}}{V_1}\right) = \frac{\text{AUC}_C}{X_{\text{uc}}} \qquad (19.3)$$

$$\text{Fraction absorbed } (f) = \frac{X_{\text{uc}}}{X_0} \qquad (19.4)$$

$$\text{Absorption time} \times \text{volume } (T_a V_1) = \frac{fFX_0}{A + B} \frac{\lambda_0 - K_{21}}{(\lambda_{z1} - \lambda_0)(\lambda_{z2} - \lambda_0)} \qquad (19.5)$$

where A and B are the intercepts of the alpha and beta phases with concentration axes respectively, λ_{z1} and λ_{z2} are the slopes of the alpha and beta phases, and λ_0 is the initial slope (see Chapter 6). These parameters can be obtained from the curve-stripping technique. If the two-compartment model collapses to a one-compartment model, Equation (19.5) becomes

$$\text{Absorption time} \times \text{volume } (T_a V_1) = \frac{fFX_0}{A} \frac{1}{(\lambda_0 - \lambda_{z1})} \qquad (19.6)$$

Following an intravenous dose, the mean residence time is equal to the output time:

$$\text{Mean residence time following iv dose } (\bar{t}_{iv}) = \frac{\text{AUMC}}{\text{AUC}}$$

$$= \text{Output time } (T_{iv,out}) = T_{el} + T_{el}\frac{T_{21}}{T_{12}} \qquad (19.7)$$

If the slope of the beta terminal phase can be accurately estimated, then the estimation of mean residence time is reliable and the absorption time constant can be determined as follows:

$$\text{Absorption time } (T_a) = \bar{t}_{po} - \bar{t}_{iv} \qquad (19.8)$$

The ratio of the area under the curve following the oral dose to that following the intravenous dose gives the bioavailability of the drug:

$$\text{Bioavailability } (f) = \frac{\text{AUC}_{po}}{\text{AUC}_{iv}} \qquad (19.9)$$

Model 2: Drug with Monoexponential Terminal Phase of Which the First Pass Effect and Metabolism Are Affected by a Disease

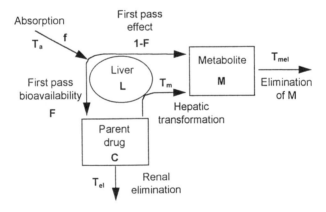

If a disease affects the first pass effect and the metabolism of a drug and if the drug exhibits a monoexponential elimination phase, Model 2 can be used to estimate the pharmacokinetic parameters of the drug. In the model, immediately after a drug is absorbed, the drug is subjected to the first pass effect, where a fraction of the drug $(1 - F)$ is metabolized in the liver and the rest of the drug (F) enters the systemic circulation. The drug in the circulating blood can further be metabolized with a first-order metabolic rate.

Because absorption and elimination of drugs can be altered by a disease, the extent of absorption, the absorption time, and the renal elimination time should be examined in a pharmacokinetic study in patients following an oral administration:

$$\text{Renal clearance time} \left(\frac{T_{el}}{V_1}\right) = \frac{\text{AUC}_C}{X_{uc}} \tag{19.10}$$

$$\text{Fraction absorbed } (f) = \frac{X_{uc}}{X_0} \tag{19.11}$$

$$\text{Absorption time} \times \text{volume } (T_a V_1) = \frac{fFX_0}{A + B} \frac{1}{(\lambda_0 - \lambda_z)} \tag{19.12}$$

The ratio of the area under the drug concentration curve after an oral dose to that after an intravenous dose is equal to the absolute bioavailability of the oral dose:

$$\text{Bioavailability } (fF) = \frac{\text{AUC}_{C,po}}{\text{AUC}_{C,iv}} \tag{19.13}$$

By comparison, the ratio of the area under the metabolite concentration curve after an oral dose to that after an intravenous dose is greater than the oral bioavailability because of the contribution of the first pass effect to the metabolite concentration (as shown in the following equation):

$$\frac{\text{AUC}_{M,po}}{\text{AUC}_{M,iv}} = fF + \frac{f(1 - F)(T_m + T_{el})}{T_{el}} \tag{19.14}$$

If an extensive first pass effect is involved, the hepatic elimination time and the renal elimination time of the metabolite can be estimated only from the intravenous data, but not from the oral data.

$$\text{Hepatic clearance time} \left(\frac{T_m}{V_1}\right) = \frac{\text{AUC}_{C,iv}}{X_{um,iv}} \tag{19.15}$$

$$\text{Elimination time of metabolite } (T_{mel}) = \bar{t}_{M,iv} - \bar{t}_{C,iv} \tag{19.16}$$

The absorption time can be estimated from the difference in the mean residence time after oral and intravenous administrations.

$$\text{Absorption time } (T_a) = \bar{t}_{C,po} - \bar{t}_{C,iv} \tag{19.17}$$

Model 3: Drug with Biexponential Terminal Phase of Which the First Pass Effect and Metabolism Are Affected by a Disease

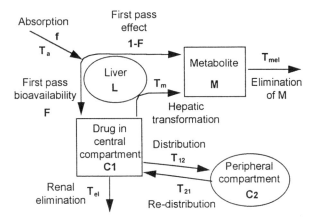

If a disease affects the metabolism of a drug that exhibits a biexponential terminal phase, Model 3 can be used to estimate the pharmacokinetic parameters. The model describes the first pass effect similarly to Model 2, with an additional peripheral compartment.

The mean residence time of the drug is equal to the ratio of the area under the first moment curve to the area under the curve. Following an oral dose, the mean residence time is the sum of input and output times (see Chapter 2):

$$\text{Mean residence time of C following oral dose } (\bar{t}_{C,po}) = \frac{\text{AUMC}_C}{\text{AUC}_C}$$

$$= \text{Input time } (T_{c,po,in}) + \text{Output time } (T_{c,po,out}) = T_a + T_{el,t} + T_{el,t}\frac{T_{21}}{T_{12}}$$

$$(19.18)$$

where $T_{el,t} = 1/(1/T_m + 1/T_{el})$. Therefore, the mean residence time may change in a disease, if the disease affects the hepatic elimination time or the distribution time (due to altered protein binding). The ratio of the area under the metabolite concentration curve to the area under the parent drug concentration curve gives

$$\frac{\text{AUC}_M}{\text{AUC}_C} = \frac{V_1}{V_m}\frac{T_{mel}}{T_m} + \frac{V_1}{V_m}\frac{1 - F}{F}\frac{T_{mel}(T_m + T_{el})}{T_m T_{el}} \qquad (19.19)$$

When the first pass effect is insignificant, the following equation can be used to estimate the hepatic elimination clearance time:

$$\text{Hepatic clearance time} \left(\frac{T_m}{V_1}\right) = \frac{\text{AUC}_C}{X_{um}} \qquad (19.20)$$

The absorption and elimination can be characterized by the following parameters:

$$\text{Renal clearance time} \left(\frac{T_{el}}{V_1}\right) = \frac{\text{AUC}_C}{X_{uc}} \qquad (19.21)$$

$$\text{Fraction absorbed } (f) = \frac{X_{uc} + X_{um}}{X_0} \qquad (19.22)$$

$$\text{Absorption time} \times \text{volume } (T_a V_1) = \frac{fFX_0}{A + B} \frac{\lambda_0 - K_{21}}{(\lambda_{z1} - \lambda_0)(\lambda_{z2} - \lambda_0)} \qquad (19.23)$$

Equation (19.23) applies when the first pass effect is negligible. When the slope of the beta phase (λ_{z2}) is insignificant compared with the slope of the alpha phase (λ_{z1}), the above equation collapses to

$$\text{Absorption time} \times \text{volume } (T_a V_1) = \frac{fFX_0}{A + B} \frac{1}{(\lambda_0 - \lambda_{z1})} \qquad (19.24)$$

They are usually large variabilities associated with the estimated λ_{z2} when its value is small. However, since the value of λ_{z2} does not appear in Equation (19.24), the variability of the estimated $T_a * V_1$ is not affected by the inaccuracy of λ_{z2} (Chapter 6).

Following an intravenous dose, the mean residence time of the drug concentration curve is the sum of input and output times:

$$\text{Mean residence time of C following iv dose } (\bar{t}_{C,iv}) = \frac{\text{AUMC}_C}{\text{AUC}_C}$$

$$= \text{Input time } (T_{c,iv,in}) + \text{Output time } (T_{c,iv,out}) = T_{el,t} + T_{el,t}\frac{T_{21}}{T_{12}} \qquad (19.25)$$

$$\text{Mean residence time of M following iv dose } (\bar{t}_{M,iv}) = \frac{\text{AUMC}_C}{\text{AUC}_C}$$

$$= \text{Input time } (T_{m,iv,in}) + \text{Output time } (T_{m,iv,out}) = T_{el,t} + T_{el,t}\frac{T_{21}}{T_{12}} + T_{mel} \qquad (19.26)$$

The accuracy of the estimated mean residence time depends on the accuracy of the estimated beta phase slope. The sampling time should be long enough for the accurate estimation by extrapolation of the area under the curve. The length of sampling time required to ensure an accurate estimation of area under the first moment curve is even longer than that for an accurate estimation of the area under the curve.

The absorption time and the extent of absorption can be estimated as follows:

$$\text{Absorption time } (T_a) = \bar{t}_{C,po} - \bar{t}_{C,iv} \tag{19.27}$$

$$\text{Bioavailability } (fF) = \frac{\text{AUC}_{C,po}}{\text{AUC}_{C,iv}} \tag{19.28}$$

$$\frac{\text{AUC}_{M,po}}{\text{AUC}_{M,iv}} = fF + f(1 - F)\frac{T_{el} + T_m}{T_{el}} \tag{19.29}$$

Therefore, the oral bioavailability of the metabolite is higher than the oral bioavailability of the parent drug, if the drug is subjected to the first pass effect. If a disease affects the first pass effect and metabolic rate, the oral bioavailability of the drug and the metabolite will be modified differently by the disease.

CASE STUDIES

Case 1: Inflammatory Diseases Affect Protein Binding

In inflammatory diseases [2–6], such at Crohn's disease and arthritis, plasma α_1-acid glycoprotein concentration increases, which may affect the pharmacokinetics of a drug. An elevated plasma protein concentration may result in a decrease in the unbound fraction of the drug in the plasma and, consequently, produce a decrease in the renal elimination rate, the hepatic elimination rate, and the distribution rate to the peripheral compartment. Model 1 can be used to describe the pharmacokinetics of drugs with altered protein binding. The plasma concentration profiles of a drug administered to a normal subject and a patient with inflammatory disease are simulated using Model 1 (Figure 19.1), assuming the increased protein binding with the disease results in a slower renal excretion rate and a slower distribution rate to the peripheral compartment in the patient than the normal subject.

Inflammatory diseases are known to increase the protein binding of drugs [2–6], which will consequently affect the elimination of the drugs and the

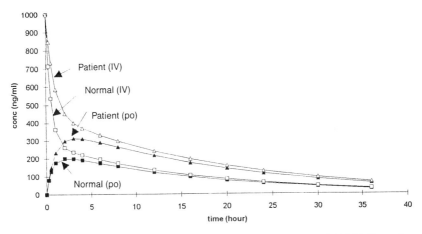

FIGURE 19.1. Simulated plasma drug concentration profiles for using Model 1, illustrating inflammatory disease affecting protein binding. The time constant plot comparing the normal subject and the patient is shown in Figure 19.2. The parameters used in this simulation are normal subject: $X_0 = 10$ mg, $f = 0.8$, $V_1 = 10$ L, $V_2 = 20$ L, $K_a = 0.5$ hr^{-1}, $K_{12} = 1.25$ hr^{-1}, $K_{21} = 0.6$ hr^{-1}, $K_{el} = 0.2$ hr^{-1}; patient: $X_0 = 10$ mg, $f = 0.8$, $V_1 = 10$ L, $V_2 = 20$ L, $K_a = 0.5$ hr^{-1}, $K_{12} = 0.6$ hr^{-1}, $K_{21} = 0.6$ hr^{-1}, $K_{el} = 0.1$ hr^{-1}.

apparent volume of distribution. Therefore the key time constant in this example is the elimination time and the volume of distribution. The estimated pharmacokinetic parameters are shown in Table 19.1, and the estimated time constants are presented in Figure 19.2.

Now let us examine the time constant plot (Figure 19.2). As a result of the increased protein binding and the decreased fraction of the unbound drug in

TABLE 19.1. *Estimated Time Constants of Model 1 for the Example Shown in Figure 19.1.*

	Normal Subject		Patient		
Parameter	Time Constant Analysis	Model Value	Time Constant Analysis	Model Value	Equation
T_{el} (hr)	5.0	5.0	10.0	10.0	(19.a8)
T_{z2} (hr)	16.3	16.6	20.6	20.9	(19.2)
$\bar{t}_{po}$ (hr)	17.2	17.4	21.8	22	(19.1)
$\bar{t}_{iv}$ (hr)	15.1	15.4	19.8	20	(19.7)
T_a (hr)	2.08	2.0	2.08	2.0	(19.8)
f	0.79	0.8	0.8	0.8	(19.9)
V_z (L)	32.6	33.2	20.6	20.9	$T_{z2}*X_0/$AUC

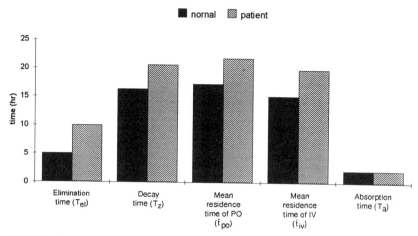

FIGURE 19.2. The time constant plot comparing the normal subject and the patient with inflammatory disease in the example shown in Figure 19.1. The renal elimination time (T_{el}) increases twofold. However, the decay time of the drug (T_z) increases in the patient only by 26%, not as significantly as the increase in the renal elimination time, due to a buffering capacity of the peripheral compartment.

the patient with the inflammatory disease, the renal elimination time T_{el} increases twofold. However, the decay time of the drug (T_z) increases in the patient only by 26%, not as significantly as the increase in the elimination time, due to a buffering capability of the peripheral compartment. On the other hand, the absorption time is not affected by the disease. The increased elimination time also results in an increase in the mean residence time in the patient, reflected by a broader concentration profile. Because of the increased elimination time and the increased protein binding, the plasma concentration of the drug is much higher in the patient than in the normal subject. However, the difference in the unbound drug concentration between the normal subject and the patient may not be as significant as the difference in the total plasma concentration (Figure 19.3). Therefore, the pharmacological effects may not be significantly different between the normal subject and the patient after a single dose, assuming the effects depend on the unbound drug concentration. On the other hand, the dose strength may need to be reduced when multiple doses are given to the patient chronically, because of (1) a possible accumulation of plasma concentration due to the decreased elimination and (2) a possible accumulation of the unbound drug due to a saturation of protein binding.

The decay time of the drug in the above example is only 26% greater in the patient than the normal subject, in spite of the fact that the elimination

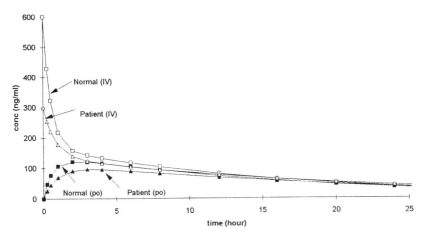

FIGURE 19.3. Unbound drug concentration in plasma from the example shown in Figure 19.1, assuming the unbound fraction is 60% in a normal subject and 30% in the patient.

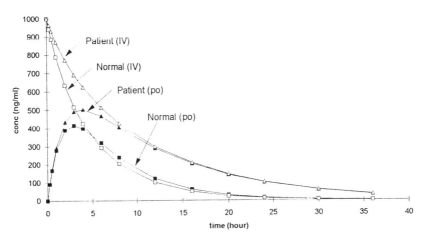

FIGURE 19.4. An example of Model 1, where distribution to the peripheral compartment is negligible. The time constant plot comparing the normal subject and the patient is shown in Figure 19.5. The parameters used in this simulation are normal subject: $X_0 = 10$ mg, $f = 0.8$, $V_1 = 10$ L, $V_2 = 20$ L, $K_a = 0.5$ hr^{-1}, $K_{12} = 0.05$ hr^{-1}, $K_{21} = 0.5$ hr^{-1}, $K_{el} = 0.2$ hr^{-1}; patient: $X_0 = 10$ mg, $f = 0.8$, $V_1 = 10$ L, $V_2 = 20$ L, $K_a = 0.5$ hr^{-1}, $K_{12} = 0.05$ hr^{-1}, $K_{21} = 0.5$ hr^{-1}, $K_{el} = 0.1$ hr^{-1}.

477

TABLE 19.2.   Estimated Time Constants of Model 1 for the Example Shown in Figure 19.4.

Parameter	Normal Subject		Patient		Equation
	Time Constant Analysis	Model Value	Time Constant Analysis	Model Value	
T_{el} (hr)	5.0	5.0	10.0	10.0	(19.a8)
T_z (hr)	5.2	5.8	10.8	11.2	(19.2)
$\bar{t}_{po}$ (hr)	7.4	7.5	12.9	13	(19.1)
$\bar{t}_{iv}$ (hr)	5.4	5.5	10.8	11	(19.7)
T_a (hr)	2.0	2.0	2.04	2.0	(19.8)
f	0.79	0.8	0.8	0.8	(19.9)
V_1 (L)	10	10	10	10	

time is much (100%) longer in the patient. This is due to the buffering capacity of the peripheral compartment. If a drug does not distribute to the tissue compartment, the increase in decay time should be proportional to the increase in elimination time in the patient with elevated protein binding, assuming no flip-flop of the concentration profile occurs. To illustrate this point, an example is provided, where the distribution to the peripheral compartment is negligible (Figure 19.4). The only difference in model parame-

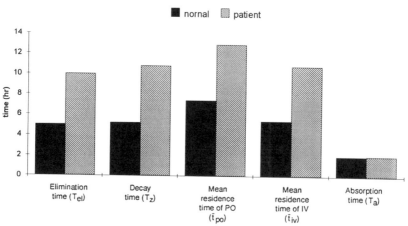

FIGURE 19.5.   The time constant plot comparing the normal subject and the patient with inflammatory disease in the example shown in Figure 19.4. The decay time (T_z) increases proportionally with the renal elimination time (T_{el}), and the mean residence times ($\bar{t}_{po}$ and $\bar{t}_{iv}$) are longer in the patient than in the normal subject.

ters between this example and the earlier one is that K_{12} is negligible in this example. The estimated time constants of this example are listed in Table 19.2, and the estimated time constants are presented in Figure 19.5. As a result of the increase in protein binding in the patient, the decay time increases proportionally with the renal elimination time; the mean residence time is longer in the patient than in the normal subject (as shown in the time constant plot, Figure 19.5); thus, the drug plasma concentration and the area under the concentration curve are greater in the patient.

Case 2: Thyroidism Affects Bioavailability, Renal and Hepatic Elimination

In the hyperthyroidism patient [7–11], the gastrointestinal motility increases, which may result in a reduced bioavailability; the renal blood flow increases, which may raise the renal clearance; and the hepatic enzyme activity increases, which may raise the hepatic clearance. Therefore, the key pharmacokinetic parameters in hyperthyroidism are bioavailability, the hepatic elimination time constant, and the renal elimination time constant. The pharmacokinetics in the hyperthyroidism patient can be described by Model 2. A simulated example using the model is shown in Figures 19.6 and

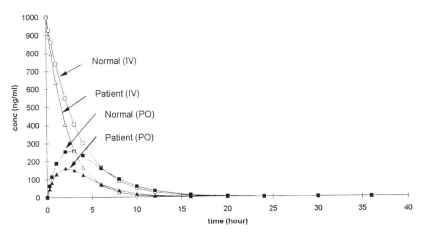

FIGURE 19.6. Concentration profiles of the parent drug in a simulated example of Model 2, illustrating thyroidism affecting bioavailability and renal and hepatic eliminations. The time constant plot comparing the normal subject and the patient is shown in Figure 19.8. The parameters used in this simulation are normal subject: $X_0 = 10$ mg, $f = 0.8$, $F = 0.7$, $V_c = 10$ L, $V_m = 15$ L, $K_a = 0.5$ hr^{-1}, $K_{el} = 0.2$ hr^{-1}, $K_m = 0.1$ hr^{-1}, $K_{mel} = 0.07$ hr^{-1}; patient: $X_0 = 10$ mg, $f = 0.6$, $F = 0.7$, $V_c = 10$ L, $V_m = 15$ L, $K_a = 0.5$ hr^{-1}, $K_{el} = 0.3$ hr^{-1}, $K_m = 0.15$ hr^{-1}, $K_{mel} = 0.07$ hr^{-1}.

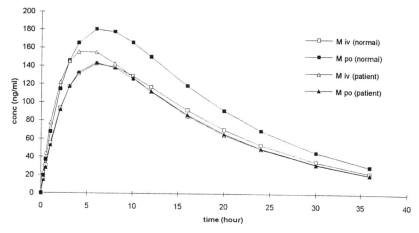

FIGURE 19.7. Concentration profiles of the metabolite in the example of Figure 19.5.

19.7, where the comparison between a normal subject and a patient is made. In this example, the oral bioavailability decreases, and the renal and hepatic elimination rates increase in the patient. It is shown from the parent drug concentration profiles (Figure 19.6) that the elimination time is shorter and the bioavailability is smaller in the patient. On the other hand, the decay

TABLE 19.3. Estimated Time Constants of Model 2 for the
Example Shown in Figures 19.6 and 19.7.

| Parameter | Normal Subject | | Patient | | |
	Time Constant Analysis	Model Value	Time Constant Analysis	Model Value	Equation
$T_{el,t}$ (hr)	3.13	3.33	1.96	2.22	(19.a14)
T_{mel} (hr)	14.7	14.3	14.3	14.3	(19.16)
T_{mel}/V_m (hr/L)	0.95	0.95	0.95	0.95	(19.10)
T_m (hr)	10.0	10.0	6.67	6.67	(19.15)
T_a (hr)	2.04	2.0	2.04	2.0	(19.17)
T_{el} (hr)	5.0	5.0	3.33	3.33	(19.10), V_c
$AUC_{C,po}/AUC_{C,iv}$	0.55	0.56	0.41	0.42	(19.13)
$AUC_{M,po}/AUC_{M,iv}$	1.28	1.28	0.96	0.96	(19.14)
$AUC_{M,iv}/AUC_{C,iv}$	0.94	0.95	1.40	1.42	
$AUC_{M,po}/AUC_{C,po}$	2.18	2.18	3.26	3.27	
V_c (L)	10	10	10	10	X_0/C_0
V_m (L)	15.7	15	15.0	15	(19.10, 19.16)
f	0.78	0.8	0.57	0.6	(19.13, 19.14)
F	0.71	0.7	0.72	0.7	T_m, T_{el} (19.13), f

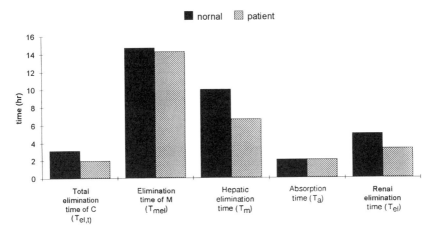

FIGURE 19.8. The time constant plot comparing the normal subject and the patient with thyroidism in the examples shown in Figure 19.7. The renal elimination time (T_{el}) and hepatic elimination time (T_m) are shorter in the patient, which results in a shorter total elimination time ($T_{el,t}$).

time of the metabolite is not affected by the disease (Figure 19.7). The reasons are that (1) T_{mel} is much longer than T_{el} and thus T_{mel} dominates the decay time of the metabolite concentration profile, and (2) T_{mel} of the patient and the normal subject is the same.

The key pharmacokinetic parameters in hyperthyroidism are bioavailability ($f*F$), the renal elimination time constant (T_{el}), and the hepatic elimination time constant (T_m), and they are estimated using the time constant analysis and listed in Table 19.3. The estimated time constants are also presented in Figure 19.8. The fraction absorbed (f) is smaller in the patient (57%) than the normal subject (78%), which results in a smaller systemic bioavailability ($AUC_{C,po}/AUC_{C,iv}$) in the patient (41% vs. 55%). The metabolite bioavailability ($AUC_{M,po}/AUC_{M,iv}$) is smaller in the patient (96% vs. 128%). Due to the first pass effects, the metabolite to parent drug ratio is higher after the oral dose than after the intravenous dose for both normal subject and patient. As shown in the time constant plot (Figure 19.8), the renal elimination time (T_{el}) and hepatic elimination time (T_m) are shorter in the patient, which results in a shorter total elimination time ($T_{el,t}$). The drug is absorbed less and eliminated faster in the patient; therefore, a higher dose may be required for the patient.

Case 3: Congestive Heart Failure Affects Absorption, First Pass Metabolism, and Hepatic and Renal Eliminations

In congestive heart failure [23], the hepatic blood flow decreases, and thus, the hepatic clearance of a drug may decline; α_1-acid glycoprotein binding increases, which may reduce the apparent volume of distribution, and the rate and extent of absorption may reduce. Therefore, the key pharmacokinetic parameters in congestive heart failure are the fraction absorbed, the absorption time constant, the distribution time constant, the renal elimination time constant, and the hepatic elimination time constant. The pharmacokinetics in this case can be described by Model 3. A simulated example of plasma concentration profiles in a normal subject and a patient is shown in Figures 19.9 and 19.10. In this example, as a result of congestive heart failure, the rate and extent of absorption decrease; the first pass effect decreases due to a declined metabolic rate; the renal elimination, the hepatic elimination, and the distribution rate drop due to an increased protein binding.

The key time constants in the congestive heart failure patients of this example are the absorption time, the renal elimination time, and the hepatic elimination time. The pharmacokinetic parameters of the above example are estimated and listed in Table 19.4. The estimated time constants are presented in Figure 19.11. The time constant analysis shows that the normal subject has a higher bioavailability (64%) than the patient (51%). The meta-

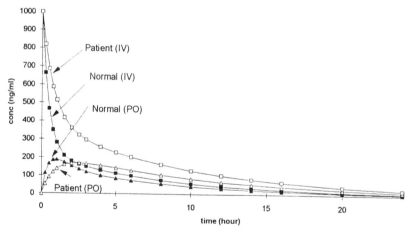

FIGURE 19.9. Concentration profiles of the parent drug in a simulated example of Model 3, illustrating congestive heart failure affecting absorption, first pass metabolism, and hepatic and renal eliminations. The time constant plot comparing the normal subject and the patient is shown in Figure 19.11. The parameters used in this simulation are normal subject: $X_0 = 10$ mg, $f = 0.8$, $F = 0.8$, $V_1 = 10$ L, $V_2 = 20$ L, $V_m = 9$ L, $K_a = 1$ hr^{-1}, $K_{12} = 1.25$ hr^{-1}, $K_{21} = 0.6$ hr^{-1}, $K_{el} = 0.2$ hr^{-1}, $K_m = 0.3$ hr^{-1}, $K_{mel} = 0.1$ hr^{-1}; patient: $X_0 = 10$ mg, $f = 0.6$, $F = 0.85$, $V_1 = 10$ L, $V_2 = 20$ L, $V_m = 9$ L, $K_a = 0.5$ hr^{-1}, $K_{12} = 0.6$ hr^{-1}, $K_{21} = 0.6$ hr^{-1}, $K_{el} = 0.1$ hr^{-1}, $K_m = 0.15$ hr^{-1}, $K_{mel} = 0.1$ hr^{-1}.

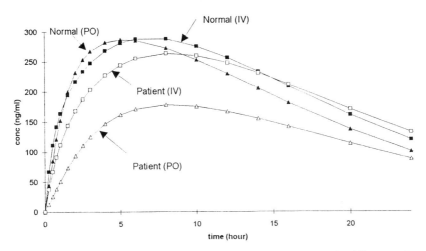

FIGURE 19.10. Concentration profiles of the metabolite in the example of Figure 19.6.

bolite to parent drug ratio is higher after the oral dose than the intravenous dose for both normal subject and patient as a result of the first pass effect. The metabolite to parent drug ratio decreases in the patient due to the declined metabolite rate. As shown in the time constant (Figure 19.11), the renal elimination time T_{el} and hepatic elimination time T_m increase in the

TABLE 19.4. Estimated Time Constants of Model 2 for the
Example Shown in Figures 19.9 and 19.10.

Parameter	Normal Subject		Patient		
	Time Constant Analysis	Model Value	Time Constant Analysis	Model Value	Equation
T_z (hr)	7.1	7.4	8.6	8.9	(19.2)
$T_{el,t}$ (hr)	2.04	2.0	4.0	4.0	(19.a25)
T_{mel}/V_m (hr/L)	1.11	1.1	1.1	1.1	(19.21)
T_m (hr)	3.33	3.33	6.67	6.67	(19.20), V_1
T_a (hr)	1.04	1.0	2.0	2.0	(19.27)
T_{el} (hr)	5.0	5.0	10.0	10.0	(19.21), V_1
$AUC_{C,po}/AUC_{C,iv}$	0.64	0.64	0.51	0.51	(19.28)
$AUC_{M,po}/AUC_{M,iv}$	0.90	0.91	0.66	0.66	(19.29)
$AUC_{M,iv}/AUC_{C,iv}$	3.35	3.33	1.70	1.66	
$AUC_{M,po}/AUC_{C,po}$	4.77	4.72	2.21	2.36	
V_1 (L)	10.0	10.0	10.0	10.0	X_0/C_0
f	0.8	0.8	0.6	0.6	(19.22)
F	0.8	0.8	0.84	0.85	(19.28), f

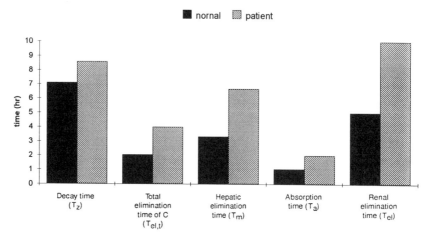

FIGURE 19.11. The time constant plot comparing the normal subject and the patient with congestive heart failure in the example shown in Figure 19.10. The renal elimination time (T_{el}) and hepatic elimination time (T_m) increase in the patient, resulting in a longer total elimination time ($T_{el,t}$).

patient, resulting in a longer total elimination time ($T_{el,t}$). The prolonged decay time T_z in the patient is due to the increased elimination and distribution times.

EXAMPLES

Example 1: Celiac Disease and Crohn's Disease Affect Volume of Distribution

The pharmacokinetics of propranolol in eight patients with celiac disease and ten patients with Crohn's disease were compared with those in twelve healthy subjects [6]. In both celiac disease and Crohn's disease, the patients suffer malabsorption and their serum α-acid glycoprotein concentration rises. Therefore, pharmacokinetics of propranolol may be affected in terms of absorption and distribution. The mean plasma concentration of propranolol in the patients and normal subjects is shown in Figure 19.12. The plasma concentrations of propranolol are much higher in patients with the diseases, especially Crohn's disease, than the healthy subjects.

The concentration of propranolol in the patients shows typical profiles of increased protein binding: a combination of increased maximum concentration and decreased decay time. The volume of distribution is a key pa-

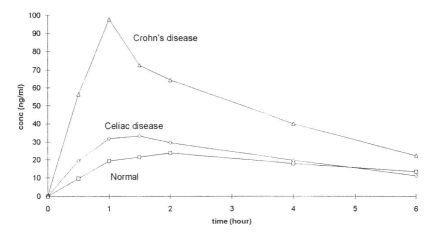

FIGURE 19.12. Mean plasma concentrations of propranolol following oral administration of 40 mg propranolol to eight patients with celiac disease, ten patients with Crohn's disease, and twelve healthy subjects. (Reproduced from Reference [6] with permission.) The time constant plot comparing the normal subjects and the patients is shown in Figure 19.13.

rameter in this example, since it may be affected by the change in protein binding. The pharmacokinetic parameters of propranolol are estimated using Model 1. The estimated pharmacokinetic parameters are listed in Table 19.5, and the estimated time constants are presented in Figure 19.13. The drug is known to have a large volume of distribution and to distribute well into the peripheral compartment. However, the pharmacokinetics of the drug in this example show a monoexponential terminal phase, probably due to the short sampling time, which does not capture the terminal beta phase.

TABLE 19.5. The Pharmacokinetic Parameters of Propranolol Estimated for the Example in Figure 19.8 Using the Time Constant Analysis, Model 1.

Parameter*	Normal	Celiac	Crohn's	Equation
T_z (hr)	7.14	4.35	4.0	(19.2)
T_0 (hr)	0.79	0.56	0.48	(19.2) stripping
$\bar{t}$ (hr)	7.7	4.9	4.5	AUMC/AUC
$\bar{t}$ (hr)	7.93	4.91	4.48	$T_0 + T_z$
$T_a*V/f/F$ (hr·L)	1123.6	540.5	204.5	(19.6)
AUC_{0-6} (ng·hr/ml)	103	129	296	
AUC (ng·hr/ml)	196.4	178.1	385.2	
$V/f/F$ (L)	1427	975	430	(19.6)

*Estimated from the mean concentration profile or the reported mean values.

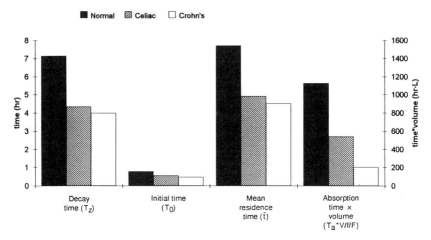

FIGURE 19.13. The time constant plot of propranolol using Model 1, comparing the normal subjects and the patients with celiac disease and Crohn's disease. The value of $T_a*V/f/F$ decreases by half in celiac disease and by fivefold in Crohn's disease.

The area under the plasma concentration curve in the patients with Crohn's disease is much higher than that in the normal subjects, while the difference in area under the curve between the patients with celiac disease and the normal subjects is less substantial. The two most likely causes of the change in area under the concentration curve in this example are a change in volume of distribution and a change in the extent of absorption.

Propranolol has a large volume of distribution, and it is a basic drug that binds to α-acid glycoprotein. In both celiac and Crohn's diseases, serum concentration of α-acid glycoprotein increases, which may reduce the free fraction of the drug and the volume of distribution. These changes could account for the increase in the area under the plasma concentration curve. The absorption of other drugs in celiac and Crohn's disease has been known to increase or decrease compared with the normal subjects [5].

Now let us examine the time constant plot (Figure 19.13). In this example, both decay time T_z and initial time constant T_0 decrease in the celiac and Crohn's diseases. However, it is uncertain which one (T_0 or T_z) represents the absorption time constant because of the possibility of flip-flop. Therefore, parameter $T_a*V/f/F$ is estimated to characterize the absorption kinetics. The value of $T_a*V/f/F$ decreases by half in celiac disease and by fivefold in Crohn's disease. This decrease in $T_a*V/f/F$ cannot be explained by the decrease in T_a alone, since neither T_z or T_0 decrease by more than twofold in the diseases. The fraction absorbed, f, may not increase much in the diseases since propranolol is well absorbed (90%) in the normal subjects. The first pass effect $(1 - F)$ of propranolol is known to be significant ($>50\%$). However, it is also not likely that the change in first pass effect alone is responsible for the fivefold decrease in $T_z^* V/f/F$ in the Crohn's disease. The extent to which the diseases affect the first pass effect cannot be determined since the metabolite concentrations are not available. Assuming the initial time constant T_0 represents the absorption time T_a, then $V/f/F$ can be estimated. The value of $V/f/F$ so estimated decreases significantly in both celiac and Crohn's disease. It is difficult to explain the decrease in the elimination time constants (T_2 or T_0) in the diseases. One of the possibilities is that the ratio of the blood volume to the central compartment volume increases in the diseases, so that the apparent hepatic extraction ratio ($ER_{app} = ER_{int} V_b/V_c$, where V_b is the blood volume and V_c is the central compartment volume) is elevated and causes a faster apparent hepatic elimination.

Example 2: Celiac and Crohn's Diseases Affect Absorption

Pharmacokinetics of cephalexin were studied in twenty-two patients with celiac disease, ten patients with Crohn's disease, and fourteen normal subjects following the oral administration of 500 mg of cephalexin [5]. The mean concentration profiles of cephalexin in the patients and the normal subjects are shown in Figures 19.14 and 19.15. The change in the area under

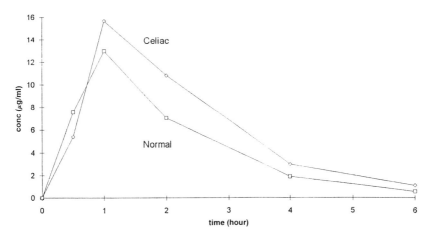

FIGURE 19.14. Mean plasma concentrations of cephalexin following oral administration of 500 mg cephalexin to twenty-two patients with celiac disease and twelve healthy subjects. (Reproduced from Reference [5] with permission.) The time constant plots comparing the normal subjects and the patients is shown in Figures 19.16 and 19.17.

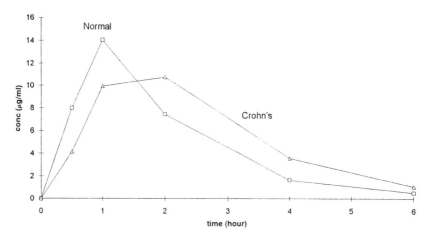

FIGURE 19.15. Mean plasma concentrations of cephalexin following oral administration of 500 mg cephalexin to eight patients with Crohn's disease and twelve healthy subjects. (Reproduced from Reference [5] with permission.)

the cephalexin concentration curve in the patients with diseases is not as significant as in the previous example of propranolol. There is a slight delay in the peak cephalexin concentration in the patients with Crohn's disease compared with the normal subjects.

Cephalexin is an acidic drug, of which the volume of distribution is not likely to be affected by a change in α-acid glycoprotein. Alteration of absorption of drugs in celiac disease and Crohn's disease have been noted [2,3,5]; therefore, the key time constant in this example is the absorption time. The pharmacokinetic parameters of cephalexin are estimated using Model 1, a one-compartment model. The estimated pharmacokinetic parameters are listed in Table 19.6, and the estimated time constants are presented in Figures 19.16 and 19.17. The area under the concentration increases by 25% in celiac disease and by 23% in Crohn's disease. The increase in the area under the concentration curve may be due to an increase in the fraction absorbed, a decrease in the elimination rate, or a decrease in the volume of distribution.

Now let us examine the time constant plots (Figures 19.16 and 19.17). Both the initial time constant (T_0) and the decay time constant (T_z) of the concentration profiles increase in the diseases, indicating the absorption time is likely to increase in the diseases. The mean residence time increases in both diseases, indicating an increase in absorption time, elimination time, or distribution rate. An increase in T_a*V/f provides additional evidence of an increase in the absorption time. However, the changes in T_a (T_z

TABLE 19.6. The Pharmacokinetic Parameters of Cephalexin Estimated
for the Example in Figures 19.14 and 19.15 Using
the Time Constant Analysis, Model 1.

Parameter*	Normal	Celiac	Normal	Crohn's	Equation
T_z (hr)	1.56	1.92	1.47	1.79	(19.2)
T_0 (hr)	0.57	0.88	0.58	0.89	(19.2)
$\bar{t}$ (hr)	1.97	2.32	1.89	1.85	(19.1)
T_a*V/f (hr·L)	10.9	25.6	11.2	22.7	(19.6)
T_{el}/V (hr/L)	0.1	0.093	0.093	0.088	(19.3)
AUC (μg·hr/ml)	29.2	39.8	30.4	37.3	
X_u (mg)	293	426	327	425	
f	0.59	0.85	0.65	0.85	(19.4)

*Estimated from the mean concentration profile or the reported mean values.

or T_0) alone cannot account for the change in $T_a*V/f/F$, and there may be a
slight decrease in the volume of distribution. Compared with propranolol in
the previous example, the possible change in the volume of distribution of
cephalexin is relatively small since the cephalexin is an acidic drug and may
not bind to α-acid glycoprotein as extensively as propranolol, which is a
basic drug.

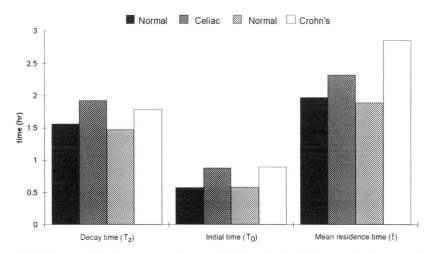

FIGURE 19.16. The time constant plot of cephalexin using Model 1, comparing the normal
subjects and the patients with celiac and Crohn's diseases. Both the initial time constant
(T_0) and the decay time constant (T_z) of the concentration profiles increase in the diseases,
indicating the absorption time is likely to increase in the diseases.

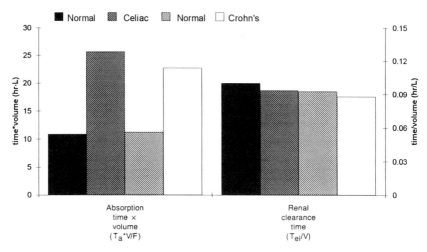

FIGURE 19.17. The estimated absorption and elimination time constants of cephalexin using Model 1, comparing the normal subjects and the patients with celiac and Crohn's diseases. An increase in T_a^*V/f provides additional evidence of an increase in the absorption time.

Example 3: Thyroidism Affects Elimination

The pharmacokinetics of digoxin were compared between hyperthyroid, hypothyroid, and euthyroid patients following the intravenous dose of 0.75 to 1 mg and the oral dose of 1.0 to 1.5 mg of digoxin to these patients [7]. Tritiated digoxin was given in all cases. The total radioactivity of digoxin, which represents the total amount of digoxin and its metabolites, in the plasma following the oral and intravenous administrations is shown in Figures 19.18 and 19.19. The plasma concentration of digoxin decreases in the hyperthyroid patients and increases in the hypothyroid patients compared with the euthyroid patients.

Digoxin is eliminated through both renal and hepatic routes at about the same rates, and thyroidism is known to affect both elimination routes. However, the metabolite concentrations are not available in this example. Therefore, the key time constant in this example is the renal elimination time. The plasma concentration of digoxin follows a two-compartment model and digoxin is metabolized through the liver; therefore, the pharmacokinetic parameters can be estimated using Model 3. The estimated pharmacokinetic parameters are listed in Table 19.7, and the estimated time constants are presented in Figure 19.20. The number of patients in the oral study is small (two with hyperthyroid and two with hypothyroid), and the estimated parameters may not represent the population values. The area

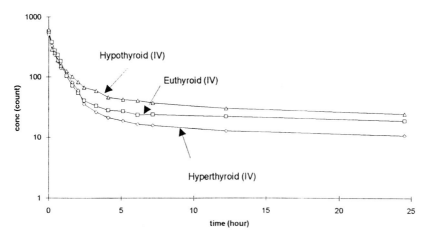

FIGURE 19.18. Mean plasma concentrations of digoxin (total radioactivity) following intravenous administration of 0.75 to 1 mg digoxin to thirteen euthyroid patients, ten hyperthyroid patients, and seven hypothyroid patients. (Reproduced from Reference [7] with permission.) The time constant plot comparing the normal subjects and the patients is shown in Figure 19.20.

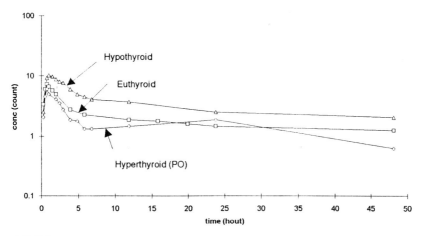

FIGURE 19.19. Mean plasma concentrations of digoxin (total radioactivity) following oral administration of 1 to 1.5 mg digoxin to twelve euthyroid patients, two hyperthyroid patients, and two hypothyroid patients. (Reproduced from Reference [7] with permission.)

491

TABLE 19.7. The Pharmacokinetic Parameters of Digoxin Estimated for the Example in Figures 19.11 and 19.12 Using the Time Constant Analysis, Model 3.

Parameter*	Euthyroid (iv)	Hyperthyroid (iv)	Hypothyroid (iv)	Euthyroid (po)	Hyperthyroid (po)	Hypothyroid (po)	Equation
T_{z1} (hr)	0.72	0.46	0.92	1.20	1.64	2.04	(19.2)
T_{z2}	47.6	52.6	62.5	45.5	43.5	66.7	(19.2)
T_{el}/V_c (min/ml)	0.011	0.0063	0.012				(19.10)
AUC_{0-24}	907	680	1138	55	45	99	
X_u (%)	0.8	0.71	0.7	0.42	0.54	0.46	
X_s (%)	0.12	0.14	0.08	0.2	0.15	0.6	
f				0.62	0.69	0.52	(19.11)

*Estimated from the mean concentration profiles or reported mean values.

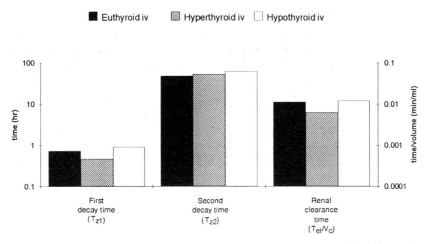

FIGURE 19.20. The time constant plot of digoxin using Model 3, comparing the normal subjects and the patients with hyper- and hypothyroidism. The renal clearance time (T_{el}/V_c) decreases in the hyperthyroid patient and increases in the hypothyroid patient.

under the concentration curve decreases in the hyperthyroid patient and increases in the hypothyroid patient.

Now let us examine the time constant plot (Figure 19.20). The change in the area under the curve is consistent with the change in the renal clearance time, which decreases in the hyperthyroid patient and increases in the hypothyroid patient. The influence of the diseases on the elimination time is probably due to a change in the renal and hepatic blood flow. The change in the first decay time T_{z1} corresponds to the change in the renal elimination time; therefore, it is likely that a flip-flop occurs and the alpha phase represents the elimination and the beta phase represents the distribution. This hypothesis is supported by the fact that digoxin has a large volume of distribution and the redistribution of the drug from tissues to the blood may be the rate limiting step. To summarize, digoxin concentration increases in hypothyroidism and decreases in hyperthyroidism, probably corresponding to the change in hepatic and renal elimination time in these conditions. Therefore, it may be necessary to administer higher doses of digoxin to patients with hyperthyroidism and lower doses to those with hypothyroidism, as suggested in Reference [7].

Example 4: Congestive Heart Failure Affects Absorption, Renal Elimination, and Hepatic Elimination

The pharmacokinetics of enalapril were studied in twelve patients with congestive heart failure and ten healthy subjects following the oral administration of 10 mg enalapril maleate and the intravenous admininstration of 5 mg enalapril maleate [14]. The mean plasma concentration profiles of enalapril and its metabolite enalaprilat, following the oral and intravenous doses to the patients and the normal subjects, are shown in Figures 19.21–19.23. The peak concentration of enalapril is delayed, and the concentration profile is broader in the patients with congestive heart failure, indicating a slower absorption or, more likely, a slower elimination in the patients.

Congestive heart failure results in decreases in blood flow through the gastrointestinal tract, liver, and kidney, which may affect absorption and elimination. Therefore, the key time constants in this example are absorption time, hepatic elimination time, and renal elimination time. The concentration profile of enalapril follows a two-compartment model, and, therefore, the pharmacokinetic parameters of enalpril and enalaprilat are estimated using Model 3. The estimated pharmacokinetic parameters are listed in Table 19.8, and the estimated time constants are presented in Figure 19.24. The area under the concentration curve of both enalapril and enalaprilat is greater in the patients than the normal subjects.

Now let us examine the time constant plot (Figure 19.24). Both initial time constant (T_0) and the first decay time (T_{z1}) are longer in the patients, indicating a possible increase in the absorption time or the elimination time as a result of the disease. The urine recovery of the drug does not change with the disease, suggesting that an increase in bioavailability may not be responsible for the increase in the area under the curve. Both the hepatic

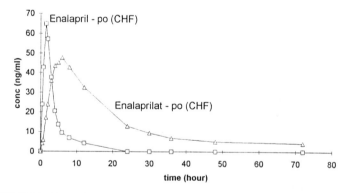

FIGURE 19.21. Mean plasma concentrations of enalapril and enalaprilat following oral administration of 10 mg enalapril maleate to twelve patients with congestive heart failure. (Reproduced from Reference [14] with permission from Blackwell Science Ltd.) The time constant plot comparing the normal subject and the patient is shown in Figure 19.24.

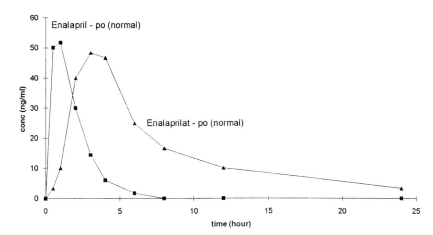

FIGURE 19.22. Mean plasma concentrations of enalapril and enalaprilat following oral administration of 10 mg enalapril maleate to ten healthy subjects. (Reproduced from Reference [14] with permission from Blackwell Science Ltd.)

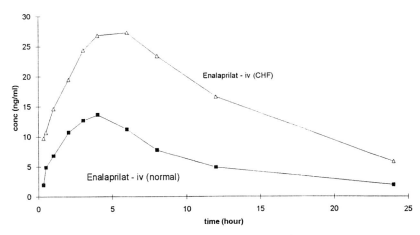

FIGURE 19.23. Mean plasma concentrations of enalaprilat following intravenous administration of 5 mg enalapril maleate to patients with congestive heart failure and healthy subjects. (Reproduced from Reference [14] with permission from Blackwell Science Ltd.)

TABLE 19.8. The Pharmacokinetic Parameters of Enalapril Estimated for the Example in Figures 19.21–19.23 Using the Time Constant Analysis, Model 3.

Parameter*	CHF E (po)	CHF ET (po)	Normal E (po)	Normal ET (po)	CHF ET (iv)	Normal ET (iv)	Equation
T_{z1} (hr)	2.99	20.83	1.47	6.62	11.76	9.09	(19.2)
T_0 (hr)	0.94		0.33				(19.2)
T_m/V_c (hr/L)	0.076		0.034				(19.20)
T_{el}/V_c (hr/L)	0.128	0.294	0.062	0.103	0.192	0.079	(19.21)
T_a*V_c (hr·L)	66.7		23.3				(19.24)
AUC (ng·hr/ml)	254	993	120	367	392	147	(19.19)
AUC_M/AUC_C		3.9		3.05	2.05	1.85	
X_u (mg)	1.97	3.34	1.95	3.55			(19.22)
f	0.53		0.55				

*Estimated from the mean concentration profiles or the reported mean values.
E: enalapril, ET: enalaprilat.

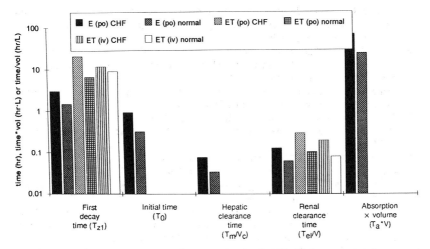

FIGURE 19.24. The time constant plot of enalapril using Model 3, comparing the normal subject and the patient with congestive heart failure. Both the hepatic (T_m/V_c) and the renal (T_m/V_c) clearance times increase by 100% in the patients, probably due to decreases in hepatic and renal blood flows.

and the renal clearance times increase by 100% in the patients, probably due to decreases in hepatic and renal blood flows. In the process of estimating T_a*V_c using Equation (19.23), the terms containing λ_{z2} in the denominator and the numerator cancel out each other because of the relatively small λ_{z2} [giving Equation (19.24)]. Therefore, the large variability of λ_{z2} does not affect the accuracy of the estimated T_a*V_c. The value of T_a*V_c increases in the patients, suggesting an increase in the absorption time, probably due to a decrease in the gastrointestinal blood flow associated with the disease.

REFERENCES

1. Reidenberg M. M., "The binding of drugs to plasma proteins and the interpretation of measurements of plasma concentrations of drugs in patients with poor renal functions," *Am. J. Med.*, 1977:62:466.
2. Holt S., Heading R. C., Clements J. A., Tothill P., and Prescott F. P., "Acetaminophen absorption and metabolism in celiac disease and Crohn's disease," *Clinical Pharmacol. Ther.*, 1982; 30(2):232–238.
3. Parson R. L., "Drug absorption in gastrointestinal disease with particular reference to malabsorption syndromes," *Clinical Pharmacokinetics*, 1977; 2:45–60.
4. Parson R. L., Kaye C. M., and Raymond K., "Pharmacokinetics of salicylate and indomethacin in coeliac disease," *Europ. J. Clin. Pharmacol.*, 1977; 11:473–477.

5. Parsons R. L. and Paddock G. M., "Absorption of two antibacterial drugs, cephalexin and co-trimoxazole, in malabsorption syndromes," *Journal of Antimicrobial Chemotherapy*, 1975; 1(Suppl):59–67.

6. Schneider R. E., Babb J., Bishop H., Hoare A. M., and Hawkins C. F., "Plasma levels of propranolol in treated patients with coeliac disease and patients with Crohn's disease," *British Medical Journal*, 1976; 794–795.

7. Doherty J. E. and Perkins W. H., "Digoxin metabolism in hypo- and hyperthyroidism," *Annals of Internal Medicine*, 1966; 64(3):489–507.

8. Forfar J. C., Pottage A., Toft A. D., Irvine W. J., Clements J. A., and Prescott L. F., "Paracetamol pharmacokinetics in thyroid disease," *Eur. J. Clin. Pharmacol.*, 1980; 18:269–273.

9. O'Connor P. and Feely J., "Clinical pharmacokinetics and endocrine disorders therapeutic implication," *Clinical Pharmacokinetics*, 1987; 13:345–364.

10. Shenfield G. M., "Influence of thyroid dysfunction on drug pharmacokinetics," *Clinical Pharmacokinetics*, 1981; 6:275–297.

11. Vesell E. S., Shapiro J. R. Passanati G. T., Jorgensen H., and Shively C. A., "Altered plasma half-lives of antipyrine, propylthiouracil, and methimazole in thyroid dysfunction," *Clinical Pharmacology and Therapeutics*, 1974; (17)1:48–56.

12. Applefeld M. M., Adir J., Crouthamel W. G., and Roffman D. S., "Digoxin pharmacokinetics in congestive heart failure," *J. Clin. Pharmacol.*, 1981; 21:114–120.

13. Baughman R. A., Arnold S., Benet L. Z., Lin E. T., Chatterjee K., and Williams R. L., "Altered prazosin pharmacokinetics in congestive heart failure," *Eur. J. Clin. Pharmacol.*, 1980, 17:425–428.

14. Dickstein K., Till A. E., Aarsland T., Tjelta K., Abrahamsen A. M., Kristianson K., Gomez H. J., Gregg H., and Hichens M., "The pharmacokinetics of enalapril in hospitalized patients with congestive heart failure," *Br. J. Clin. Pharmac.*, 1987; 23:403–410.

15. Jaillon P., Rubin P., Yee Y., Ball R., Kates R., Harrison D., and Blaschke T., "Influence of congestive heart failure on prazosin kinetics," *Clin. Pharmacol. Ther.*, 1979; 25(6):790–794.

16. Motwani J. G., Lang C. C., Allen M. J., Johnson H. F., and Struthers A. D., "Dose ranging effects of candoxatril on elimination of exogenous atrial natriuretic peptide in chronic heart failure," *Clinical Pharmacology & Therapeutics*, 1993; 54(6):661n–669.

17. Prescott L. F., Adjepon-Yamoan K. K. and Talbot R. G., "Impaired lignocaine metabolism in patients with myocardial infarction and cardiac failure," *British Medical Journal*, 1976; 939–941.

18. Ruder M. A., Lebsack C., Winkle R. A. Mead R. H., Smith N., and Kates R., "Disposition kinetics of orally administered enoximone in patients with moderate to severe heart failure," *J. Clin. Pharmacol.*, 1991; 31:702–708.

19. Shammas F. V. and Dickstein K., "Clinical pharmacokinetics in heart failure," *Clinical Pharmacokinetics*, 1988; 15:94–113.

20. Ueda C. T. and Dzindzio B. S., "Pharmacokinetics of dihydroquinidine in congestive heart failure patients after intravenous quinidine administration," *Eur. J. Clin. Pharmacol.*, 1979; 16:101–105.

21. Ueda C. T. and Dzindzio B. S., "Quinidine kinetics in congestive heart failure," *Clin. Pharmacol. Ther.*, 1978; 23(2):158–164.

22. Weiss Y. A., Safer M. E., Chevillard C., Frydman A., Simon A., Lemaire P., and Alexandre J. M., "Comparison of the pharmacokinetics of intravenous dl-propranolol in borderline and permanent hypertension," *Europ. J. Clin. Pharmacol.*, 1976; 10:387–393.

23. Benet L. Z., Massoud N., and Gambertoglio J. G., *Pharmacokinetic Basis for Drug Treatment*, Raven Press, 1984.

Evaluation of Mean Residence Times from Input and Output Times

As discussed in Chapter 2, the mean residence time is equal to the summation of mean input time and mean output time. Here, the derivations of relationship between mean residence time and time constants for several complicated models are presented. A schematic plot illustrating a compartment with multiple inputs and outputs is shown below:

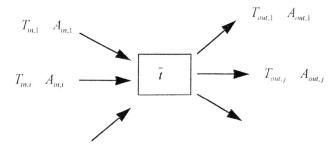

In this model, $T_{in,i}$ and $A_{in,i}$ represent the input time and amount of input from the i-th input process, while $T_{out,j}$ and $A_{out,j}$ represent the output time and amount of output from the j-th output process. A $T_{in,i}$ is either the mean residence time of the prior compartment or the mean input time when the drug is administered directly into the compartment. On the other hand, each of $T_{out,j}$ is the mean time that is required for the process "alone" to transfer drug from one compartment to another. The mean residence time of drug molecules in a compartment is equal to the sum of mean input time and the mean output time:

$$\bar{t} = T_{in} + T_{out} \tag{1.a1}$$

For a system with linear kinetics,

$$T_{in} = \sum_i \frac{T_{in,i} \cdot A_{in,i}}{A_{in,tot}} \tag{1.a2}$$

$$T_{out} = \sum_i \frac{T_{out,j} \cdot A_{iout,j}^2}{A_{out,tot}^2} \tag{1.a3}$$

where $A_{in,tot}$ and $A_{out,tot}$ are the total amounts of inputs and outputs respectively. Equation (1.a2) defines an amount-average input time. Equation (1.a3) defines an amount-average output time based on the following derivation. The output time of the j-th process, $T_{out,j}$, is the time required for the process "alone" to remove the total amount of the drug from the compartment. Then for the j-process to remove an amount of $A_{out,j}$, , the time required is proportional to the amount removed, $T_{out,j}(A_{iout,j}/A_{out,tot})$. Consequently, the amount-average input time of all the input processes becomes Equation (1.a3). For a linear system with first-order kinetics, the amount removed by the j-th process is proportional to the rate constants $K_{out,j} = 1/T_{out,j}$:

$$\frac{A_{j,out}}{A_{out,tot}} = \frac{1/T_{out,j}}{\sum_j 1/T_{out,j}} \tag{1.a4}$$

Substituting Equation (1.a4) into (1.a3) gives

$$T_{out} = \frac{1}{\sum_j 1/T_{out,j}} \tag{1.a5}$$

The following are the derivations of the relationship between time constants and mean residence times for several frequently used models.

MODEL 1

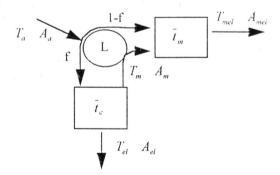

From Equations (1.a1) and (1.a5), it can be derived that

$$\bar{t}_C = T_{c,in} + T_{c,out}$$

$$= T_a + \frac{1}{1/T_m + 1/T_{el}} = T_a + T_{el,t} \tag{1.a6}$$

$$\bar{t}_M = T_{m,in} + T_{m,out}$$

$$= T_a \frac{(1-f)A_a}{(1-f)A_a + A_m} + \bar{t}_C \frac{A_m}{(1-f)A_a + A_m} + T_{mel} \tag{1.a7}$$

The values of A_a and A_m must be determined next, so that the mean residence time can be estimated. By assuming the amount absorbed is FD, where F is fraction absorbed and D is dose,

$$A_a = FD \tag{1.a8}$$

it can be deduced from Equation (1.a4) that

$$A_m = fFD \frac{1/T_m}{1/T_{el} + 1/T_m} = fFD \frac{T_{el}}{T_m + T_{el}} \tag{1.a9}$$

From Equation (1.a7), knowing A_a and A_m from Equations (1.a8) and (1.a9), it can be derived that

$$\bar{t}_M = T_a \frac{(1-f)FD}{(1-f)FD + \dfrac{T_{el}}{T_m + T_{el}} fFD} + \bar{t}_C \frac{\dfrac{T_{el}}{T_m + T_{el}} fFD}{(1-f)FD + \dfrac{T_{el}}{T_m + T_{el}} fFD} + T_{mel}$$

$$\tag{1.a10}$$

Substituting Equation (1.a6) into (1.a10) gives

$$\bar{t}_M = T_a + \frac{1}{1/T_m + 1/T_{el}} \frac{\dfrac{T_{el}}{T_m + T_{el}} f}{(1-f) + \dfrac{T_{el}}{T_m + T_{el}} f} + T_{mel}$$

$$= T_a + T_{el,t} \frac{fT_{el}}{(1-f)T_m + fT_{el}} + T_{mel} \tag{1.a11}$$

MODEL 2

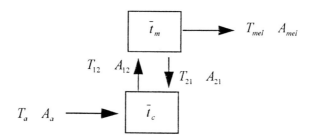

From Equations (l.al) and (1.a5), it can be derived that

$$\bar{t}_C = T_{c,in} + T_{c,out}$$

$$= T_a \frac{A_a}{A_a + A_{21}} + \bar{t}_M \frac{A_{21}}{A_a + A_{21}} + T_{12} \qquad (1.a12)$$

$$\bar{t}_M = T_{m,in} + T_{m,out}$$

$$= \bar{t}_C + \frac{1}{1/T_{21} + 1/T_{mel}} = \bar{t}_C + T_{mel,t} \qquad (1.a13)$$

The values of A_a and A_{21} must be determined next, so that the mean residence time can be estimated. By assuming the amounts absorbed and eliminated are known,

$$A_a = A_{mel} = FD \qquad (1.a14)$$

it can be deduced from Equation (1.a4) that

$$A_{21} = FD \frac{T_{mel}}{T_{21}} \qquad (1.a15)$$

From Equations (l.al2), (1.al4), and (1.al5), it can be derived that

$$\bar{t}_C = T_a \frac{FD}{FD + FD \cdot T_{mel}/T_{21}} + \bar{t}_M \frac{FD \cdot T_{mel}/T_{21}}{FD + FD \cdot T_{mel}/T_{21}} + T_{12}$$

$$(1.a16)$$

Substituting Equation (1.a13) into Equation (1.al6) obtains

$$\bar{t}_C = T_a \frac{T_{21}}{T_{21} + T_{mel}} + (\bar{t}_C + T_{mel,t}) \frac{T_{mel}}{T_{21} + T_{mel}} + T_{12} \qquad (1.a17)$$

Multiplying both sides of Equation (1.a17) by $T_{21} + T_{mel}$ and rearranging terms gives

$$\bar{t}_C = T_a + T_{mel,t}\frac{T_{mel}}{T_{21}} + T_{12} + T_{12}\frac{T_{mel}}{T_{21}} \tag{1.a18}$$

MODEL 3

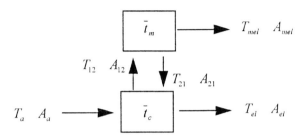

From Equations (1.a1) and (1.a5), it can be derived that

$$\bar{t}_C = T_{c,in} + T_{c,out}$$

$$= T_a\frac{A_a}{A_a + A_{21}} + \bar{t}_M\frac{A_{21}}{A_a + A_{21}} + \frac{1}{1/T_{12} + 1/T_{el}} \tag{1.a19}$$

$$\bar{t}_M = T_{m,in} + T_{m,out}$$

$$= \bar{t}_C + \frac{1}{1/T_{21} + 1/T_{mel}} = \bar{t}_C + T_{mel,t} \tag{1.a20}$$

The values of A_a and A_{21} must be determined next, so that the mean residence time can be estimated. By assuming the amount absorbed is equal to the total amount eliminated,

$$A_a = FD = A_{mel} + A_{el} \tag{1.a21}$$

It can be deduced from Equation (1.a4) that

$$A_{12} = A_{el}\frac{T_{el}}{T_{12}} \tag{1.a22}$$

$$A_{21} = A_{12}\frac{T_{mel}}{T_{21} + T_{mel}} \tag{1.a23}$$

$$A_{mel} = A_{12}\frac{T_{21}}{T_{21} + T_{mel}} = A_{el}\frac{T_{el}}{T_{12}}\frac{T_{21}}{T_{21} + T_{mel}} \tag{1.a24}$$

Substituting Equation (1.a24) into (1.a21) gives

$$FD = A_{el}\frac{T_{el}}{T_{12}}\frac{T_{21}}{T_{21} + T_{mel}} + A_{el} = A_{el}\frac{1}{T_{12}}\frac{T_{el}T_{21} + T_{21}T_{12} + T_{mel}T_{12}}{T_{21} + T_{mel}} \tag{1.a25}$$

Then A_{el} can be solved from Equation (1.a25)

$$A_{el} = FD\frac{T_{12}(T_{21} + T_{mel})}{T_{el}T_{21} + T_{21}T_{12} + T_{mel}T_{12}} \tag{1.a26}$$

Substituting Equation (1.a26) into (1.a23) gives

$$A_{21} = FD\frac{T_{12}(T_{21} + T_{mel})}{T_{el}T_{21} + T_{21}T_{12} + T_{mel}T_{12}}\frac{T_{el}}{T_{12}}\frac{T_{mel}}{T_{21} + T_{mel}}$$

$$= FD\frac{T_{el}T_{mel}}{T_{el}T_{21} + T_{21}T_{12} + T_{mel}T_{12}} \tag{1.a27}$$

From Equations (1.a19) and (1.a27), it can be derived that

$$\bar{t}_C = T_a\frac{T_{el}T_{21} + T_{21}T_{12} + T_{mel}T_{12}}{T_{el}T_{21} + T_{21}T_{12} + T_{mel}T_{12} + T_{el}T_{mel}}$$

$$+ \bar{t}_M\frac{T_{el}T_{mel}}{T_{el}T_{21} + T_{21}T_{12} + T_{mel}T_{12} + T_{el}T_{mel}} + T_{el,t} \tag{1.a28}$$

Substituting Equation (1.a20) into Equation (1.a28) gives

$$\bar{t}_C = T_a\frac{T_{el}T_{21} + T_{21}T_{12} + T_{mel}T_{12}}{T_{el}T_{21} + T_{21}T_{12} + T_{mel}T_{12} + T_{el}T_{mel}}$$

$$+ (\bar{t}_C + T_{mel,t})\frac{T_{el}T_{mel}}{T_{el}T_{21} + T_{21}T_{12} + T_{mel}T_{12} + T_{el}T_{mel}} + T_{el,t}$$

$$\tag{1.a29}$$

Multiplying both sides of Equation (1.a29) by $T_{el}T_{21} + T_{21}T_{12} + T_{mel}T_{12} + T_{el}T_{mel}$ and rearranging terms gives

$$\bar{t}_C = T_a + T_{mel,t}\frac{T_{el}T_{mel}}{T_{el}T_{21} + T_{21}T_{12} + T_{mel}T_{12}} + T_{el,t} + T_{el,t}\frac{T_{el}T_{mel}}{T_{el}T_{21} + T_{21}T_{12} + T_{mel}T_{12}}$$

$$\tag{1.a30}$$

Derivation of AUC and AUMC Using Laplace Transformation

Here, we like to derive the relationships among the time constants and the concentration time curve for the single-compartment model. In the Time Constant Approach, these relationships can be stated in terms of the AUC and AUMC. The derivation is most simply done by applying the Laplace transform. Fortunately, familiarity with the Laplace transform is not necessary since the necessary steps can be reduced to substitutions, algebraic manipulations, and one differentiation. In general, the steps are as follows:

(1) Construct a kinetic model diagram.
(2) Set up the differential equations of the model.
(3) Transform (i.e., make substitutions) from the time domain, t, to the frequency domain, s (this is known as the Laplace transform).
(4) Solve algebraically for the concentration (in the frequency domain).
(5) To obtain the AUC, evaluate the solution of Step (4) at $s = 0$.
(6) To obtain the AUMC, take the negative derivative $(-d/ds)$ of the solution of Step (4) and evaluate at $s = 0$.

Once the relationship between and AUC and AUMC is established through steps (1) to (6), the time constants can be estimated from AUC and AUMC of concentration profiles accordingly. We apply these steps to the single-compartment model.

Step (1): The diagram of the simple compartment model is given below:

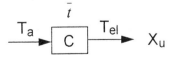

Step (2): The model is described by two differential equations – one for X, the amount of drug administered and the other for C, the concentration of the drug in the compartment (note that the amount of drug in the compartment $V \cdot C$, where V is the volume of distribution, is needed to match the units of X).

$$\frac{dX(t)}{dt} = -\frac{1}{T_a}X(t) \tag{2.a1}$$

$$V\frac{dC(t)}{dt} = -\frac{V}{T_{el}}C(t) + \frac{1}{T_a}X(t) \tag{2.a2}$$

Step (3): The transformation to the frequency domain involves simple substitutions when the drug is administered as a bolus. Any time function, $F(t)$, is replaced by its Laplace transform, $\mathscr{F}(s)$. Any time derivation, $dF(t)/dt$, is replaced by $s\mathscr{F}(s) - F(0)$, and if the initial value $F(0)$ is zero, this will reduce to $s\mathscr{F}(s)$. The caveat here is that Laplace transforms only apply to linear differential equations so if nonlinear terms like $F(t)G(t)$ or $F(t)dF(t)/dt$ are present, the substitutions are not permitted. In the single-compartment model, let us assume that the drug is administered as an oral bolus ($X(0) = X_0$) and that, initially, there is no drug in the compartment ($C(0) = 0$). In this case, the differential equations are replaced with the following equations:

$$s\mathscr{X}(s) - X_0 = -\frac{1}{T_a}\mathscr{X}(s) \tag{2.a3}$$

$$V_s\mathscr{C}(s) = -\frac{V}{T_{el}}\mathscr{C}(s) + \frac{1}{T_a}\mathscr{X}(s) \tag{2.a4}$$

Step (4): We can now solve for $\mathscr{C}(s)$ in the frequency domain:

$$\mathscr{C}(s) = \frac{1}{VT_a}\frac{\mathscr{X}(s)}{s + 1/T_{el}} \tag{2.a5}$$

but $\mathscr{X}(s) = X_0/\{s + (1/T_a)\}$ so

$$\mathscr{C}(s) = \frac{1}{VT_a}\frac{X_0}{(s + 1/T_{el})(s + 1/T_a)} \tag{2.a6}$$

Step (5):

$$\text{AUC} = \mathscr{C}(s = 0) = T_{el}X_0/V \tag{2.a7}$$

Since, for this model, Cl_{tot} (the total clearance) is given by V/T_{el}, this formula is expected.

Step (6): We now solve for $-d\mathscr{C}(s)/ds$

$$-\frac{d\mathscr{C}(s)}{ds} = \frac{1}{VT_a}\frac{X_0}{(s + 1/T_{el})(s + 1/T_a)}\left(\frac{1}{s + 1/T_{el}} + \frac{1}{s + 1/T_a}\right) \tag{2.a8}$$

and AUMC is equal to $-d\mathcal{C}(s = 0)/ds$

$$\text{AUMC} = -\frac{d\mathcal{C}(s = 0)}{ds} = \frac{T_{el}X_0}{V}(T_a + T_{el}) \tag{2.a9}$$

Once the linear differential equations are set down, this straightforward procedure can be used to calculate the AUCs and AUMCs of the drug or any of its metabolites. In the appendices of following chapters, the results of such derivations will be provided without going into the details of the algebraic manipulations.

Let's continue to derive for each time constant in the one-compartmental model. The mean residence time can be estimated from AUMC and AUC:

$$\bar{t} = \frac{\text{AUMC}}{\text{AUC}} = T_a + T_{el} \tag{2.a10}$$

The decay time constant T_z can be estimated from a partial area under the curve

$$\frac{1}{T_z} = \lambda_z = 2\frac{(t - t_{last})\ln(C_t) - \text{AU}\ln C_{t-t_{last}}}{(t - t_{last})^2} \tag{2.a11}$$

where t_{last} is the last time point of concentration profile, and t is a reference time point that the terminal phase starts. The rule of choosing t is that it must be long enough so that either the absorption time or the elimination time dominates the concentration profile after time t; however, there should also be enough time points between t and t_{last} for the estimation of T_z. A good choice of t is $2 \cdot \bar{t}$, which is about three times the half-life of either absorption or elimination. The initial time constant T_0 can be estimated as follows: $T_0 = \bar{t} - T_z$.

In the one-compartmental model, the assignment of T_z and T_0 to T_a and T_{el} is dependent on the relationship between T_a and T_{el}. If $T_{el} > T_a$, then $T_a = T_0$ and $T_{el} = T_z$. If $T_a > T_{el}$, then $T_a = T_z$ and $T_{el} = T_0$. In the case of $T_a > T_{el}$, it is referred to as a flip-flop. Because of this uncertainty of assigning values to T_a and T_{el}, a less ambiguous time constant T_aV is devised to describe the absorption process. The time constant T_aV can be estimated as follows (the details are described in Chapter 6):

$$T_aV = \frac{fFX_0}{A(1/T_0 - 1/T_1)} \tag{2.a12}$$

where $fFX_0 = X_u$, assuming the drug is eliminated predominantly through the kidney, and A is the intercept of the extrapolation of the terminal phase with $t = 0$ axis. This estimation of T_aV applies to both situations, with or without flip-flop of concentration profiles. Another useful time constant is the renal clearance time $T_{el}V$, which can be estimated from AUC and the cumulative amount of the drug in the urine, X_u:

$$\frac{T_{el}}{V} = \frac{\text{AUC}}{X_u} \tag{2.a13}$$

This illustrates that, in theory, the Time Constant Approach works. In the following chapters (Chapters 5-19), we will examine more closely various types of pharmacokinetic studies. In these chapters the validity of the Time Constant Approach will be demonstrated by applying it to simulated models where the answers are known. The utility of the method will be illustrated by applying it to data from the literature.

Does the Time Constant Approach offer a desirable alternative to methods currently in wide use? In Chapter 2, distinct advantages of the Time Constant Approach are given: (1) it yields a more robust parameter estimate than does compartmental modeling, and (2) compared with compartmental modeling and the more widely used noncompartmental approach (which measures clearance times and decay times), the Time Constant Approach optimizes the (information extracted)/(computational complexity) ratio.

Derivation of AUC and AUMC

CHAPTER 5

Model 1

For drugs with linear absorption kinetics, the ordinary differential equation describing the change in the amount of drugs in the intestine after an oral administration is

$$\frac{dX}{dt} = -K_a X \qquad (5.a1)$$

By assuming a linear elimination kinetics, the equation describing the change in plasma drug concentrations with time is

$$\frac{dC}{dt} = \frac{fF}{V} K_a X - K_{el} C \qquad (5.a2)$$

There are two rate constants involved in Equation (5.a2): the absorption rate constant K_a and the elimination rate constant K_{el}. Both constants determine the level of plasma concentrations of the drug. However, only the elimination rate constant affects the area under the plasma concentration curve, as shown below:

$$\text{AUC}_{po} = \frac{fF}{V} \frac{X_0}{K_{el}} \qquad (5.a3)$$

In a bioavailability study, the fraction absorbed (f) and first pass effect ($1 - F$) after an oral dose will affect the area under the concentration curve. On the other hand, the area under the first moment of the concentration curve is a function of both absorption and elimination constants.

$$\text{AUMC}_{\text{po}} = \frac{fF}{V}\left[\frac{X_0}{K_a}\frac{1}{K_{\text{el}}} + \frac{X_0}{K_{\text{el}}^2}\right] \qquad (5.a4)$$

The area under the concentration curve and the area under the first moment of the concentration curve after an intravenous administration are slightly different from those after the oral dosing, since the absorption is not involved following the intravenous administration

$$\text{AUC}_{\text{iv}} = \frac{1}{V}\frac{X_0}{K_{\text{el}}} \qquad (5.a5)$$

$$\text{AUMC}_{\text{iv}} = \frac{1}{V}\frac{X_0}{K_{\text{el}}^2} \qquad (5.a6)$$

When an intravenous infusion is administered, the drug is slowly presented to the blood. Assume the infusion time is T and total dose is X_0, then the constant infusion rate is $R = X_0/T$. The area under the concentration curve and the area under the first moment of the concentration curve become

$$\text{AUC}_{\text{infu}} = \frac{R}{V}\frac{T}{K_{\text{el}}} \qquad (5.a7)$$

$$\text{AUMC}_{\text{infu}} = \frac{R}{V}\frac{2T + T^2 K_{\text{el}}}{2K_{\text{el}}^2} \qquad (5.a8)$$

Model 2

The ordinary differential equation describing the temporal change in the amount of a drug in the intestine after an oral administration is

$$\frac{dX}{dt} = -K_a X \qquad (5.a9)$$

The equations describing the concentration time profiles in the central and peripheral compartments are

$$\frac{dC_1}{dt} = \frac{fF}{V_1}K_a X - (K_{\text{el}} + K_{12})C_1 + \frac{V_2}{V_1}K_{21}C_2 \qquad (5.a10)$$

$$\frac{dC_2}{dt} = \frac{V_1}{V_2}K_{12}C_1 - K_{21}C_2 \qquad (5.a11)$$

The area under the concentration curve and the area under the first moment of the concentration curve can be derived from Laplace transform:

$$\text{AUC}_{\text{po}} = \frac{fFX_0}{V_1}\frac{K_{21}}{\lambda_1 \lambda_2} \qquad (5.a12)$$

$$\text{AUMC}_{\text{po}} = \frac{fFX_0}{V_1} \frac{K_{21}}{\lambda_1\lambda_2} \left[-\frac{1}{K_{21}} + \frac{1}{K_a} + \frac{1}{\lambda_1} + \frac{1}{\lambda_2} \right] \tag{5.a13}$$

where λ_1 and λ_2 are the slopes of the two exponential phases, and their relationship with the rate constants are

$$\lambda_1 + \lambda_2 = K_{\text{el}} + K_{12} + K_{21} \tag{5.a14}$$

$$\lambda_1\lambda_2 = K_{\text{el}}K_{21} \tag{5.a15}$$

After an intravenous administration, the area under the concentration curve and the area under the first moment of the concentration curve for Model 2 are expressed as

$$\text{AUC}_{\text{iv}} = \frac{X_0}{V_1} \frac{K_{21}}{\lambda_1\lambda_2} \tag{5.a16}$$

$$\text{AUMC}_{\text{iv}} = \frac{X_0}{V_1} \frac{K_{21}}{\lambda_1\lambda_2} \left[-\frac{1}{K_{21}} + \frac{1}{\lambda_1} + \frac{1}{\lambda_2} \right] \tag{5.a17}$$

Model 3

The ordinary differential equations describing the temporal change in the amount of unabsorbed drug and drug concentration in the plasma and the liver are

$$\frac{dX}{dt} = -K_a X \tag{5.a18}$$

$$\frac{dC_L}{dt} = \frac{1}{V_L} K_a X - (K_{\text{el}} + K_{21}) C_L + \frac{V_1}{V_L} K_{12} C_1 \tag{5.a19}$$

$$\frac{dC_1}{dt} = \frac{V_L}{V_1} K_{21} C_L - K_{12} C_1 \tag{5.a20}$$

After an oral administration, the area under the concentration curve and the area under the first moment of the concentration curve are expressed as

$$\text{AUC} = \frac{X_0}{V_1} \frac{K_{21}}{\lambda_1\lambda_2} \tag{5.a21}$$

$$\text{AUMC} = \frac{X_0}{V_1} \frac{K_{21}}{\lambda_1\lambda_2} \left[\frac{1}{K_a} + \frac{1}{\lambda_1} + \frac{1}{\lambda_2} \right] \tag{5.a22}$$

where λs are related to the rate constants

$$\lambda_1 + \lambda_2 = K_{\text{el}} + K_{12} + K_{21} \tag{5.a23}$$

$$\lambda_1\lambda_2 = K_{\text{el}}K_{12} \tag{5.a24}$$

After an intravenous dose, the area under the concentration curve and the area under the first moment of the concentration curve become

$$\text{AUC} = \frac{X_0}{V_1} \frac{K_{21} + K_{el}}{\lambda_1 \lambda_2} \tag{5.a25}$$

$$\text{AUMC} = \frac{X_0}{V_1} \frac{K_{21} + K_{el}}{\lambda_1 \lambda_2} \left[-\frac{1}{K_{21} + K_{el}} + \frac{1}{\lambda_1} + \frac{1}{\lambda_2} \right] \tag{5.a26}$$

The area under the concentration curve derived from Model 3 depends not only on the elimination rate, but also on the distribution rate between the central compartment and the liver. This is a more complicated expression for the area under the curve than those in Models 1 and 2, and the distribution rate constants between the liver and the blood compartments are not always estimable, depending on whether the concentration profile shows biexponential elimination phase.

Model 4

The ordinary differential equations describing the temporal change in the plasma concentration of the parent drug and metabolites are

$$\frac{dC}{dt} = \frac{fF}{V_c} K_a X - (K_{m1} + K_{m2} + K_{el})C \tag{5.a27}$$

$$\frac{dM_1}{dt} = \frac{V_c}{V_{m1}} K_{m1} C - K_{mel1} M_1 + \frac{f(1 - F)}{V_{m1}} K_a X \tag{5.a28}$$

$$\frac{dM_2}{dt} = \frac{V_c}{V_{m2}} K_{m2} C - K_{mel2} M_2 \tag{5.a29}$$

After an oral dose the area under the concentration curve is as follows

$$\text{AUC}_C = \frac{fFX_0}{V_c} \frac{1}{K_{m1} + K_{m2} + K_{el}} \tag{5.a30}$$

$$\text{AUC}_{M1} = \frac{fFX_0}{V_{m1}} \frac{K_{m1}}{(K_{m1} + K_{m2} + K_{el})K_{mel1}} + \frac{f(1 - F)X_0}{V_{m1} K_{mel1}} \tag{5.a31}$$

$$\text{AUC}_{M2} = \frac{fFK_{m2}X_0}{V_{m2}} \frac{1}{(K_{m1} + K_{m2} + K_{el})K_{mel2}} \tag{5.a32}$$

The first pass effect also contributes to the area under the concentration curve of metabolite M1.

After an intravenous dose, the drug is not subjected to the first pass effect and the area under the curve becomes

$$\text{AUC}_C = \frac{X_0}{V_c} \frac{1}{K_{m1} + K_{m2} + K_{el}} \tag{5.a33}$$

$$\text{AUC}_{M1} = \frac{X_0}{V_{m1}} \frac{K_{m1}}{(K_{m1} + K_{m2} + K_{el})K_{mel1}} \tag{5.a34}$$

$$\text{AUC}_{M2} = \frac{K_{m2}X_0}{V_{m2}} \frac{1}{(K_{m1} + K_{m2} + K_{el})K_{mel2}} \tag{5.a35}$$

CHAPTER 6

Model 1

The ordinary differential equations describing the model are

$$\frac{dX}{dt} = -K_a X \tag{6.a1}$$

$$\frac{dC}{dt} = \frac{fF}{V} K_a X - K_{el} C \tag{6.a2}$$

In this model, flip-flops of the concentration curves may occur when the absorption time constant is longer than the elimination time constant. As a result, the initial time constant T_0 ($1/\lambda_0$) of the plasma concentration curve is governed by the elimination time, and the decay time constant T_z ($1/\lambda_z$) is governed by the absorption time. The area under the concentration curve and the area under the first moment of the concentration curve can be obtained by Laplace transform:

$$\text{AUC} = \frac{fF}{V} \frac{X_0}{K_{el}} \tag{6.a3}$$

$$\text{AUMC} = \frac{fF}{V} \left[\frac{X_0}{K_a} \frac{1}{K_{el}} + \frac{X_0}{K_{el}^2} \right] \tag{6.a4}$$

The area under the curve of different formulations in a bioequivalence study may be affected by different extents of absorption between formulations.

Model 2

The ordinary differential equations derived for the model are

$$\frac{dX}{dt} = -K_a X \tag{6.a5}$$

$$\frac{dC_1}{dt} = \frac{fF}{V_1} K_a X - (K_{el} + K_{12})C_1 + \frac{V_2}{V_1} K_{21} C_2 \tag{6.a6}$$

$$\frac{dC_2}{dt} = \frac{V_1}{V_2} K_{12} C_1 - K_{21} C_2 \tag{6.a7}$$

The area under the concentration curve and the area under the first moment of the concentration curve can be expressed as

$$\text{AUC} = \frac{fFX_0}{V_1} \frac{K_{21}}{\lambda_1 \lambda_2} \tag{6.a8}$$

$$\text{AUMC} = \frac{fFX_0}{V_1} \frac{K_{21}}{\lambda_1 \lambda_2} \left[-\frac{1}{K_{21}} + \frac{1}{K_a} + \frac{1}{\lambda_1} + \frac{1}{\lambda_2} \right] \tag{6.a9}$$

where λs can be related to the rate constants:

$$\lambda_1 + \lambda_2 = K_{el} + K_{12} + K_{21} \tag{6.a10}$$

$$\lambda_1 \lambda_2 = K_{el} K_{21} \tag{6.a11}$$

The objective of the following derivation is to estimate $T_a \cdot V$.

First, the first and second decay phases of the terminal portion of the concentration curve can be fitted to two exponential terms:

$$C = Ae^{-\lambda_{z1}t} + Be^{-\lambda_{z2}t} \tag{6.a12}$$

where the intercepts of the first and second terminal phases can be expressed as:

$$A = \frac{K_a fFX_0}{V_1} \frac{K_{21} - \lambda_{z1}}{(\lambda_0 - \lambda_{z1})(\lambda_{z2} - \lambda_{z1})} \tag{6.a13}$$

$$B = \frac{K_a fFX_0}{V_1} \frac{K_{21} - \lambda_{z2}}{(\lambda_0 - \lambda_{z2})(\lambda_{z1} - \lambda_{z2})} \tag{6.a14}$$

Dividing the above two equations can eliminate f, F, K_a and V_1.

$$\frac{K_{21} - \lambda_{z1}}{K_{21} - \lambda_{z2}} = -\frac{A(\lambda_0 - \lambda_{z1})}{B(\lambda_0 - \lambda_{z2})} = -D \tag{6.a15}$$

Then K_{21} can be estimated from the exponentials of the first and second terminal phases.

$$K_{21} = -\frac{\lambda_{z1} + D\lambda_{z2}}{D + 1} \tag{6.a16}$$

Subsequently, the value of $T_a \cdot V$ can be obtained from the following expression, derived from Equations (6.a13), (6.a14) and (6.a16):

$$\frac{1}{T_a V_1} = \frac{K_a}{V_1} = \frac{A + B}{fFX_0} \frac{(\lambda_{z1} - \lambda_0)(\lambda_{z2} - \lambda_0)}{\lambda_0 - K_{21}} \tag{6.a17}$$

Another method for estimating T_a*V can be derived as follows. First, rearranging Equations (6.a13) and (6.a14) obtains

$$\frac{AT_a V_1}{fFX_0}(\lambda_0 - \lambda_{z1})(\lambda_{z2} - \lambda_{z1}) = K_{21} - \lambda_{z1} \tag{6.a18}$$

$$\frac{BT_a V_1}{fFX_0}(\lambda_0 - \lambda_{z2})(\lambda_{z1} - \lambda_{z2}) = K_{21} - \lambda_{z2} \tag{6.a19}$$

Subtracting Equation (6.a18) and (6.a19) gives

$$\frac{T_a V_1}{fF} = \frac{X_0}{A(\lambda_0 - \lambda_{z1}) + B(\lambda_0 - \lambda_{z2})} \tag{6.a20}$$

CHAPTER 7

Model 1

The area under the curve and the area under the first moment curve can be expressed as

$$AUC = \frac{fF}{V}\frac{X_0}{K_{el}} \tag{7.a1}$$

$$AUMC = \frac{fF}{V}\left[\frac{X_0}{K_a}\frac{1}{K_{el}} + \frac{X_0}{K_{el}^2}\right] \tag{7.a2}$$

The area under the concentration curve can be disproportional with dose as a result of a nonlinear elimination K_{el} (either renal or hepatic).

Model 2

Assuming first-order absorption and elimination kinetics, the ordinary differential equations governing the temporal change in the parent drug and the metabolite concentrations are

$$\frac{dX}{dt} = -K_a X \tag{7.a3}$$

$$\frac{dC}{dt} = \frac{fF}{V} K_a X - (K_{el} + K_m) C \tag{7.a4}$$

$$\frac{dM_i}{dt} = \frac{K_{mi} V}{V_{mi}} C - K_{meli} M_i \tag{7.a5}$$

where i represents the i-th metabolite, and K_m is a sum of all K_{mi}:

$$K_m = \sum_i K_{mi} \tag{7.a6}$$

Equations (7.a3) and (7.a6) can be expanded to any number of metabolites. The area under the concentration curve and the area under the first moment curve of the parent drug and the metabolites can be expressed in terms of rate constants using Laplace transform as follows:

$$AUC_C = \frac{fF}{V} \frac{X_0}{K_{el} + K_m} \tag{7.a7}$$

$$AUMC_C = \frac{fF}{V} \left[\frac{X_0}{K_a} \frac{1}{K_{el} + K_m} + \frac{X_0}{(K_{el} + K_m)^2} \right] \tag{7.a8}$$

$$AUC_{Mi} = \frac{fF K_{mi}}{V_{mi}} \frac{X_0}{K_{el} + K_m} \frac{1}{K_{meli}} \tag{7.a9}$$

$$AUMC_{Mi} = \frac{fF K_{mi} X_0}{V_{mi}} \frac{1}{K_{el} + K_m} \frac{1}{K_{meli}} \left(\frac{1}{K_a} + \frac{1}{K_{el} + K_m} + \frac{1}{K_{meli}} \right) \tag{7.a10}$$

The area under the drug concentration curve can be disproportional with dose as a result of nonlinear renal or hepatic elimination (K_{el} and K_m, respectively). The area under the metabolite concentration curve can be disproportional with dose due to nonlinear elimination kinetics of either metabolite (K_{meli}) or the parent drug (K_{el}) (or due to nonlinearities in hepatic metabolism K_m).

CHAPTER 8

Model 1

The ordinary differential equations describing the model are

$$\frac{dX_2}{dt} = K_r X_1 - K_a X_2 \tag{8.a1}$$

$$\frac{dC}{dt} = \frac{fF K_a}{V_c} X_2 - (K_{el} + K_m) C \tag{8.a2}$$

$$\frac{dM}{dt} = \frac{V_c}{V_m} K_m C - K_{mel} M \tag{8.a3}$$

The area under the concentration curve of a sustained release formulation may be smaller than that of an immediate release formulation due to a lesser extent of absorption. The portion of the drug released in the distal part of the intestine has a shorter transit time in the intestine and may be absorbed to a lesser degree than the portion released in the proximal part of the intestine. The area under the concentration curve and the area under the first moment of the concentration can be expressed as follows:

$$\text{AUC}_C = \frac{fF}{V_c} \frac{X_0}{K_{el} + K_m} \tag{8.a4}$$

$$\text{AUC}_M = \frac{fF}{V_m} \frac{X_0}{K_{el} + K_m} \frac{K_m}{K_{mel}} \tag{8.a5}$$

$$\text{AUMC}_C = \frac{fF}{V_c} \frac{X_0}{K_{el} + K_m} \left(\frac{1}{K_r} + \frac{1}{K_a} + \frac{1}{K_{el} + K_m} \right) \tag{8.a6}$$

$$\text{AUMC}_M = \frac{fF}{V_m} \frac{X_0}{K_{el} + K_m} \frac{K_m}{K_{mel}} \left(\frac{1}{K_r} + \frac{1}{K_a} + \frac{1}{K_{el} + K_m} + \frac{1}{K_{mel}} \right) \tag{8.a7}$$

Model 2

The ordinary differential equations describing the model are

$$\frac{dX}{dt} = -K_a X + u(t) \tag{8.a8}$$

$$\frac{dC}{dt} = \frac{fF}{V} K_a X - K_{el} C \tag{8.a9}$$

The area under the concentration curve and the area under the first moment of the concentration curve can be expressed as follows:

$$\text{AUC} = \frac{fFRT}{VK_{el}} \tag{8.a10}$$

$$\text{AUMC} = \frac{fFK_a R}{V} \frac{2(K_a + K_{el}) + T^2 K_a K_{el}}{2K_a^2 K_{el}^2} \tag{8.a11}$$

The area under the curve is affected by the extent of absorption, which may be less for a sustained release formulation than an immediate release formulation.

Model 3

The ordinary differential equations describing the model are

$$\frac{dX}{dt} = -K_a X + u(t) \qquad \text{with } X(0) = X_{ir} \tag{8.a12}$$

$$\frac{dC}{dt} = \frac{fF}{V} K_a X - K_{el} C \tag{8.a13}$$

The area under the concentration curve and the area under the first moment of the concentration curve can be expressed in terms of the rate constants:

$$AUC = \frac{fFRT}{VK_{el}} + \frac{fFX_{ir}}{VK_{el}} \tag{8.a14}$$

$$AUMC = \frac{fFK_a R}{V} \frac{2(K_a + K_{el}) + T^2 K_a K_{el}}{2K_a^2 K_{el}^2} + \frac{fF}{V} \frac{X_{ir}}{K_{el}} \left(\frac{1}{K_a} + \frac{1}{K_{el}} \right) \tag{8.a15}$$

where X_{ir} is the dose of the immediate release layer, and $R*T$ is the dose of the sustained release tablet.

CHAPTER 9

Model 1

The ordinary differential equations governing the temporal change in the amount of the drug in the intestine and the concentration of the drug in the plasma are

$$\frac{dX_2}{dt} = K_{emp} X_1 - K_a X_2 \tag{9.a1}$$

$$\frac{dC}{dt} = \frac{fFK_a}{V} X_2 - K_{el} C \tag{9.a2}$$

The area under the plasma concentration curve and the area under the first moment of the concentration curve can be expressed as follows:

$$AUC = \frac{fF}{V} \frac{X_0}{K_{el}} \tag{9.a3}$$

$$AUMC = \frac{fF}{V} \frac{X_0}{K_{el}} \left(\frac{1}{K_{emp}} + \frac{1}{K_a} + \frac{1}{K_{el}} \right) \tag{9.a4}$$

The area under the curve following the administration at different gastrointestinal sites can be different due to a different extent of absorption or a different first pass effect.

Model 2

The ordinary differential equations describing the model are

$$\frac{dX}{dt} = -K_a X + u(t) \tag{9.a5}$$

$$\frac{dC}{dt} = \frac{fF}{V} K_a X - K_{el} C \tag{9.a6}$$

The area under the curve and the area under the first moment curve can be expressed in terms of the rate constants:

$$\text{AUC} = \frac{fFRT}{VK_{el}} \tag{9.a7}$$

$$\text{AUMC} = \frac{fFK_a R}{V} \frac{2(K_a + K_{el}) + T^2 K_a K_{el}}{2K_a^2 K_{el}^2} \tag{9.a8}$$

The area under the concentration curve after the administration at various gastrointestinal sites can be different due to a change in the extent of absorption (f) or in the first pass effect (F).

Model 3

The ordinary differential equations governing the model are

$$\frac{dC}{dt} = \frac{fF}{V_c} K_a X - (K_m + K_{el}) C \tag{9.a9}$$

$$\frac{dM}{dt} = \frac{V_c}{V_m} K_M C - K_{mel} M + \frac{f(1 - F)}{V_m} K_a X \tag{9.a10}$$

The area under the drug and metabolite concentration curve can be expressed as follows:

$$\text{AUC}_C = \frac{fFX_0}{V_c} \frac{1}{K_m + K_{el}} \tag{9.a11}$$

$$\text{AUC}_M = \frac{fFX_0}{V_m} \frac{K_m}{(K_m + K_{el})K_{mel1}} + \frac{f(1 - F)X_0}{V_m K_{mel}} \tag{9.a12}$$

CHAPTER 10

Model 1

The ordinary differential equations describing the model are

$$\frac{dX}{dt} = -K_a X \tag{10.a1}$$

$$\frac{dC}{dt} = \frac{fF}{V} K_a X - (K_{el} + K_{lp})C \tag{10.a2}$$

$$\frac{dC_p}{dt} = \frac{V_c}{V_p} K_{lp} C - K_{pel} C_p \tag{10.a3}$$

The area under the concentration curve in the peripheral compartment is a good indicator for the degree of penetration. The area under the concentration curve and the area under the first moment of the concentration curve can be expressed in terms of the rate constants:

$$\mathrm{AUC_C} = \frac{fF}{V_c} \frac{X_0}{K_{el} + K_{lp}} \tag{10.a4}$$

$$\mathrm{AUMC_C} = \frac{fF}{V_c} \left[\frac{X_0}{K_a} \frac{1}{K_{el} + K_{le}} + \frac{X_0}{(K_{el} + K_{lp})^2} \right] \tag{10.a5}$$

$$\mathrm{AUC_P} = \frac{fF K_{le}}{V_p} \frac{X_0}{K_{el} + K_{lp}} \frac{1}{K_{pel}} \tag{10.a6}$$

$$\mathrm{AUMC_P} = \frac{fF K_{le} X_0}{V_p} \frac{1}{K_{el} + K_{lp}} \frac{1}{K_{pel}} \left(\frac{1}{K_a} + \frac{1}{K_{el} + K_{lp}} + \frac{1}{K_{pel}} \right) \tag{10.a7}$$

Model 2

The ordinary differential equations describing the model are

$$\frac{dX}{dt} = -K_a X \tag{10.a8}$$

$$\frac{dC_1}{dt} = \frac{fF}{V_1} K_a X - (K_{el} + K_{12})C_1 + \frac{V_2}{V_1} K_{21} C_2 \tag{10.a9}$$

$$\frac{dC_2}{dt} = \frac{V_1}{V_2} K_{12} C_1 - K_{21} C_2 \tag{10.a10}$$

The area under the concentration curve and the area under the first moment of the concentration curve can be expressed as follows:

$$\text{AUC}_1 = \frac{fFX_0}{V_1} \frac{K_{21}}{\lambda_1 \lambda_2} \tag{10.a11}$$

$$\text{AUMC}_1 = \frac{fFX_0}{V_1} \frac{K_{21}}{\lambda_1 \lambda_2} \left[-\frac{1}{K_{21}} + \frac{1}{K_a} + \frac{1}{\lambda_1} + \frac{1}{\lambda_2} \right] \tag{10.a12}$$

$$\text{AUC}_2 = \frac{K_{12} fFX_0}{V_2} \frac{1}{\lambda_1 \lambda_2} \tag{10.a13}$$

$$\text{AUMC}_2 = \frac{K_{12} fFX_0}{V_2} \frac{1}{\lambda_1 \lambda_2} \left[\frac{1}{K_a} + \frac{1}{\lambda_1} + \frac{1}{\lambda_2} \right] \tag{10.a14}$$

where the terminal slopes λs can be expressed in terms of the rate constants

$$\lambda_1 + \lambda_2 = K_{el} + K_{12} + K_{21} \tag{10.a15}$$

$$\lambda_1 \lambda_2 = K_{el} K_{21} \tag{10.a16}$$

Model 3

For irreversible distribution kinetics, the ordinary differential equation describing the concentration curve in the peripheral compartment is

$$\frac{dC_p}{dt} = \frac{V_c}{V_p} K_{1p} C - K_{pel} C_p \tag{10.a17}$$

Model 4

The ordinary differential equation describing the concentration profile in the peripheral compartment is

$$\frac{dC_p}{dt} = \frac{V_c}{V_p} K_{12} C - K_{21} C_p \tag{10.a18}$$

CHAPTER 11

Model 1

The ordinary differential equations governing the model are

$$\frac{dX}{dt} = -K_a X \tag{11.a1}$$

$$\frac{dC}{dt} = \frac{fF}{V} K_a X - (K_{el} + K_m)C \tag{11.a2}$$

$$\frac{dM_i}{dt} = \frac{V_c}{V_{mi}} K_{mi} C - K_{meli} M_i \tag{11.a3}$$

where K_m is the sum of all metabolic rate constants K_{mi}:

$$K_m = \sum_i K_{mi} \tag{11.a4}$$

The area under the plasma concentration curve and the area under the first moment of the concentration curve can be expressed in terms of the rate constants:

$$\text{AUC}_C = \frac{fF}{V} \frac{X_0}{K_{el} + K_m} \tag{11.a5}$$

$$\text{AUMC}_C = \frac{fF}{V} \left[\frac{X_0}{K_a} \frac{1}{K_{el} + K_m} + \frac{X_0}{(K_{el} + K_m)^2} \right] \tag{11.a6}$$

$$\text{AUC}_{mi} = \frac{fFK_{mi}}{V_{mi}} \frac{X_0}{K_{el} + K_m} \frac{1}{K_{meli}} \tag{11.a7}$$

$$\text{AUMC}_{mi} = \frac{fFK_{mi}X_0}{V_{mi}} \frac{1}{K_{el} + K_m} \frac{1}{K_{meli}} \left(\frac{1}{K_a} + \frac{1}{K_{el} + K_m} + \frac{1}{K_{meli}} \right) \tag{11.a8}$$

The area under the parent drug concentration depends only on the elimination rate of the drug and not on the formation rate of the drug. On the other hand, the area under the metabolite concentration curve depends not only on the elimination rate of the metabolite, but also on the formation rate of the metabolite.

Model 2

The ordinary differential equations describing the model are

$$\frac{dX}{dt} = -K_a X \tag{11.a9}$$

$$\frac{dC}{dt} = \frac{fF}{V_c} K_a X - (K_{el} + K_{m1})C \tag{11.a10}$$

$$\frac{dM_1}{dt} = \frac{K_{m1} V_c}{V_{m1}} C - (K_{mel1} + K_{m2})M_1 \tag{11.a11}$$

$$\frac{dM_2}{dt} = \frac{K_{m2} V_{m1}}{V_{m2}} M_1 - K_{mel2} M_2 \tag{11.a12}$$

The area under the concentration curve and the area under the first moment of the concentration curve can be expressed as

$$\text{AUC}_C = \frac{fF}{V_c} \frac{X_0}{K_{el} + K_{m1}} \tag{11.a13}$$

$$\text{AUMC}_C = \frac{fF}{V_c} \left[\frac{X_0}{K_a} \frac{1}{K_{el} + K_{m1}} + \frac{X_0}{(K_{el} + K_{m1})^2} \right] \tag{11.a14}$$

$$\text{AUC}_{M1} = \frac{fF K_{m1}}{V_{m1}} \frac{X_0}{K_{el} + K_{m1}} \frac{1}{K_{mel1} + K_{m2}} \tag{11.a15}$$

$$\text{AUMC}_{M1} = \frac{fF K_{m1} X_0}{V_{m1}} \frac{1}{K_{el} + K_{m1}} \frac{1}{K_{mel1} + K_{m2}} \left(\frac{1}{K_a} + \frac{1}{K_{el} + K_{m1}} + \frac{1}{K_{mel1} + K_{m2}} \right) \tag{11.a16}$$

$$\text{AUC}_{M2} = \frac{fF K_{m1} K_{m2}}{V_{m2}} \frac{X_0}{K_{el} + K_{m1}} \frac{1}{K_{mel1} + K_{m2}} \frac{1}{K_{mel2}} \tag{11.a17}$$

$$\text{AUMC}_{M2} = \frac{fF K_{m1} K_{m2} X_0}{V_{m2}} \frac{1}{K_{el} + K_{m1}} \frac{1}{K_{mel1} + K_{m2}} \frac{1}{K_{mel2}}$$

$$\times \left(\frac{1}{K_a} + \frac{1}{K_{el} + K_{m1}} + \frac{1}{K_{mel1} + K_{m2}} + \frac{1}{K_{mel2}} \right) \tag{11.a18}$$

Model 3

The area under the curve and the area under the first moment curve can be expressed as

$$\text{AUC}_C = \frac{fF X_0}{V K_{el}} \tag{11.a19}$$

$$\text{AUC}_M = \frac{K_{12} fF X_0}{V_m K_{21} K_{el}} \tag{11.a20}$$

Model 4

The area under the curve and the area under the first moment curve can be expressed as

$$\text{AUC}_C = \frac{fF X_0}{V_c} \frac{K_{21} + K_{mel}}{K_{mel} K_{12}} \tag{11.a21}$$

$$\text{AUC}_M = \frac{fF X_0}{V_m K_{mel}} \tag{11.a22}$$

Model 5

The area under the concentration curve can be expressed in terms of the rate constants:

$$\text{AUC}_C = \frac{fFX_0}{V_c} \frac{K_{21} + K_{mel}}{K_{mel}K_{12} + K_{el}K_{21} + K_{mel}K_{el}} \tag{11.a23}$$

$$\text{AUC}_M = \frac{K_{12}fFX_0}{V_M} \frac{1}{K_{mel}K_{12} + K_{el}K_{21} + K_{mel}K_{el}} \tag{11.a24}$$

The area under the drug concentration curve depends on the elimination rate constant of both the drug and the metabolite. The same is true for the area under the metabolite concentration curve.

Model 6

The area under the concentration curve can be expressed as follows:

$$\text{AUC}_C = \frac{fFX_0}{V_c} \frac{K_{1c} + K_{mel1}}{\lambda_1 \lambda_2} \tag{11.a25}$$

$$\text{AUC}_{M1} = \frac{K_{c1}fFX_0}{V_{m1}} \frac{1}{\lambda_1 \lambda_2} \tag{11.a26}$$

$$\text{AUC}_{M2} = \frac{fFX_0}{V_{m2}} \frac{K_{1c} + K_{mel1}}{\lambda_1 \lambda_2} \frac{K_{c2}}{K_{mel2}} \tag{11.a27}$$

Where the terminal slopes can be expressed in terms of the rate constants:

$$\lambda_1 + \lambda_2 = K_{el} + K_{mel1} + K_{c1} + K_{1c} + K_{c2} \tag{11.a28}$$

$$\lambda_1 \lambda_2 = K_{mel1}K_{c1} + (K_{el} + K_{2c})K_{1c} + K_{mel1}(K_{el} + K_{2c}) \tag{11.a29}$$

CHAPTER 12

Model 1

The ordinary differential equations governing the temporal change in the concentrations in the central and effect compartment are

$$\frac{dX}{dt} = -K_a X \tag{12.a1}$$

$$\frac{dC}{dt} = \frac{fF}{V} K_a X - (K_{el} + K_{1e})C \tag{12.a2}$$

$$\frac{dC_e}{dt} = \frac{V_c}{V_e} K_{1e} C - K_{eo} C_e \tag{12.a3}$$

The area under the concentration curve and the area under the first moment of the concentration curve are expressed as

$$AUC_C = \frac{fF}{V_c} \frac{X_0}{K_{el} + K_{1e}} \tag{12.a4}$$

$$AUMC_C = \frac{fF}{V_c}\left[\frac{X_0}{K_a} \frac{1}{K_{el} + K_{1e}} + \frac{X_0}{(K_{el} + K_{1e})^2}\right] \tag{12.a5}$$

$$AUC_E = \frac{fFK_{1e}}{V_e} \frac{X_0}{K_{el} + K_{1e}} \frac{1}{K_{eo}} \tag{12.a6}$$

$$AUMC_E = \frac{fFK_{1e}X_0}{V_e} \frac{1}{K_{el} + K_{1e}} \frac{1}{K_{eo}}\left(\frac{1}{K_a} + \frac{1}{K_{el} + K_{1e}} + \frac{1}{K_{eo}}\right) \tag{12.a7}$$

However, the effect instead of the effect site concentration is measured in pharmacokinetic/pharmacodynamic studies. Therefore, the area under the effect is estimated and assumed to be proportional with the effect concentration.

Model 2

The ordinary differential equations describing the model are

$$\frac{dX}{dt} = -K_a X \tag{12.a8}$$

$$\frac{dC}{dt} = \frac{fF}{V_c} K_a X - (K_{el} + K_{12})C + \frac{K_{21} V_e}{V_c} C_e \tag{12.a9}$$

$$\frac{dC_e}{dt} = \frac{V_c}{V_e} K_{12} C - K_{21} C_e \tag{12.a10}$$

The area under the concentration curve and the area under the first moment of the effect curve can be expressed as follows:

$$AUC_C = \frac{fFX_0}{V_c} \frac{K_{21}}{\lambda_1 \lambda_2} \tag{12.a11}$$

$$\text{AUMC}_\text{C} = \frac{fFX_0}{V_\text{c}} \frac{K_{21}}{\lambda_1 \lambda_2} \left[-\frac{1}{K_{21}} + \frac{1}{K_\text{a}} + \frac{1}{\lambda_1} + \frac{1}{\lambda_2} \right] \qquad (12.\text{a}12)$$

$$\text{AUC}_\text{E} = \frac{K_{12} fFX_0}{V_\text{e}} \frac{1}{\lambda_1 \lambda_2} \qquad (12.\text{a}13)$$

$$\text{AUMC}_\text{E} = \frac{K_{12} fFX_0}{V_\text{e}} \frac{1}{\lambda_1 \lambda_2} \left[\frac{1}{K_\text{a}} + \frac{1}{\lambda_1} + \frac{1}{\lambda_2} \right] \qquad (12.\text{a}14)$$

where the terminal slopes λs can be expressed in terms of the rate constants:

$$\lambda_1 + \lambda_2 = K_\text{el} + K_{12} + K_{21} \qquad (12.\text{a}15)$$

$$\lambda_1 \lambda_2 = K_\text{el} K_{21} \qquad (12.\text{a}16)$$

Model 3

The ordinary differential equations governing the model are

$$\frac{dX}{dt} = -K_\text{a} X \qquad (12.\text{a}17)$$

$$\frac{dC}{dt} = \frac{fF}{V_\text{c}} K_\text{a} X - (K_\text{el} + K_{12} + K_\text{1e})C + \frac{K_{21} V_2}{V_\text{c}} C_2 \qquad (12.\text{a}18)$$

$$\frac{dC_\text{e}}{dt} = \frac{V_\text{c}}{V_\text{e}} K_\text{1e} C - K_\text{eo} C_\text{e} \qquad (12.\text{a}19)$$

The area under the concentration curve and the area under the first moment of the concentration curve can be expressed as

$$\text{AUC}_\text{C} = \frac{fFX_0}{V_\text{c}} \frac{K_{21}}{\lambda_1 \lambda_2} \qquad (12.\text{a}20)$$

$$\text{AUMC}_\text{C} = \frac{fFX_0}{V_\text{c}} \frac{K_{21}}{\lambda_1 \lambda_2} \left[-\frac{1}{K_{21}} + \frac{1}{K_\text{a}} + \frac{1}{\lambda_1} + \frac{1}{\lambda_2} \right] \qquad (12.\text{a}21)$$

$$\text{AUC}_\text{E} = \frac{fFX_0}{V_\text{e}} \frac{K_\text{1e}}{(K_\text{el} + K_\text{1e})K_\text{eo}} \qquad (12.\text{a}22)$$

$$\text{AUMC}_\text{E} = \frac{fFX_0}{V_\text{e}} \frac{K_\text{1e}}{(K_\text{el} + K_\text{1e})K_\text{eo}} \left[\frac{1}{K_\text{a}} + \frac{1}{\lambda_1} + \frac{1}{\lambda_2} + \frac{1}{K_\text{eo}} - \frac{1}{K_{21}} \right] \qquad (12.\text{a}23)$$

where the terminal slopes can be expressed in terms of the rate constants:

$$\lambda_1 + \lambda_2 = K_{el} + K_{12} + K_{21} + K_{le} \tag{12.a24}$$

$$\lambda_1 \lambda_2 = (K_{el} + K_{le})K_{21} \tag{12.a25}$$

Model 4

The ordinary differential equations describing the model are

$$\frac{dX}{dt} = -K_a X \tag{12.a26}$$

$$\frac{dC}{dt} = \frac{fF}{V_c} K_a X - (K_{el} + K_{1r})C \tag{12.a27}$$

$$\frac{dR}{dt} = \frac{K_{1r}}{V_r} C - (K_{rel} + K_{re})R \tag{12.a28}$$

$$\frac{dC_e}{dt} = \frac{K_{re}}{V_e} R - K_{eo} C_e \tag{12.a29}$$

The area under the concentration curve and the area under the first moment of the concentration curve can be expressed in terms of the rate constants:

$$\text{AUC}_C = \frac{fF}{V_c} \frac{X_0}{K_{el} + K_{1r}} \tag{12.a30}$$

$$\text{AUMC}_C = \frac{fF}{V_c} \left[\frac{X_0}{K_a} \frac{1}{K_{el} + K_{1r}} + \frac{X_0}{(K_{el} + K_{1r})^2} \right] \tag{12.a31}$$

$$\text{AUC}_E = \frac{fFK_{1r}K_{m2}}{V_e} \frac{X_0}{K_{el} + K_{1r}} \frac{1}{K_{rel} + K_{re}} \frac{1}{K_{eo}} \tag{12.a32}$$

$$\text{AUMC}_E = \frac{fFK_{1r}K_{re}X_0}{V_e} \frac{1}{K_{el} + K_{1r}} \frac{1}{K_{rel} + K_{re}} \frac{1}{K_{eo}}$$

$$\times \left(\frac{1}{K_a} + \frac{1}{K_{el} + K_{1r}} + \frac{1}{K_{rel} + K_{re}} + \frac{1}{K_{eo}} \right) \tag{12.a33}$$

Model 5

The equation describing the temporal change of the effect concentration is

$$\frac{dC_e}{dt} = \frac{V_c}{V_e} K_{1e} C - K_{eo} C_e \tag{12.a34}$$

Model 6

The equation describing Model 6 is

$$\frac{dC_e}{dt} = \frac{V_c}{V_e} K_{12} C - K_{21} C_e \tag{12.a35}$$

CHAPTER 13

Model 1

The ordinary differential equations describing the temporal change of the drug concentration in the intestine and the blood are

$$\frac{dX_2}{dt} = K_{emp} X_1 - K_a X_2 \tag{13.a1}$$

$$\frac{dC}{dt} = \frac{fFK_a}{V} X_2 - K_{el} C \tag{13.a2}$$

where X_1 and X_2 are the amount of the drug in the stomach and the intestine, respectively, and C is the concentration of the drug in the blood. The area under the concentration curve and the area under the first moment of the concentration curve can be expressed as follows:

$$AUC = \frac{fF}{V} \frac{X_0}{K_{el}} \tag{13.a3}$$

$$AUMC = \frac{fF}{V} \frac{X_0}{K_{el}} \left(\frac{1}{K_{emp}} + \frac{1}{K_a} + \frac{1}{K_{el}} \right) \tag{13.a4}$$

Model 2

The ordinary differential equations describing the change in the amount of drug in the intestine and the change in the plasma concentration are as follows:

$$\frac{dX}{dt} = -K_a X + u(t) \qquad \text{and} \qquad X_0 = 0 \tag{13.a5}$$

$$\frac{dC}{dt} = \frac{fF}{V} K_a X - K_{el} C \tag{13.a6}$$

The area under the concentration curve is expressed in terms of rate constants:

$$\text{AUC} = \frac{fFRT}{VK_{el}} \tag{13.a7}$$

In the above equation, food is most likely to affect the fraction absorbed and the first pass effect and is not likely to affect volume of distribution and the elimination rate. The area under the first moment of the concentration curve is

$$\text{AUMC} = \frac{fFK_a R}{V} \frac{2(K_a + K_{el}) + T^2 K_a K_{el}}{2K_a^2 K_{el}^2} \tag{13.a8}$$

Model 3

The ordinary differential equations for the temporal change in plasma drug and metabolite concentrations derived from this model are

$$\frac{dC}{dt} = \frac{fF}{V_c} K_a X - (K_m + K_{el})C \tag{13.a9}$$

$$\frac{dM}{dt} = \frac{V_c}{V_m} K_m C - K_{mel}M + \frac{f(1 - F)}{V_m} K_a X \tag{13.a10}$$

The area under the concentration curve of the drug and metabolite can be expressed as

$$\text{AUC}_C = \frac{fFX_0}{V_c} \frac{1}{K_m + K_{el}} \tag{13.a11}$$

$$\text{AUC}_M = \frac{fFX_0}{V_m} \frac{K_m}{(K_m + K_{el})K_{mel1}} + \frac{f(1 - F)X_0}{V_m K_{mel}} \tag{13.a12}$$

In the above equations, food can affect the area under the curve of the drug and the metabolite differently.

The area under the first moment of the drug and metabolite concentration curves can also be expressed in terms of the rate constants:

$$\text{AUMC}_C = \frac{fFX_0}{V_c} \frac{1}{K_m + K_{el}} \left(\frac{1}{K_a} + \frac{1}{K_m + K_{el}} \right) \tag{13.a13}$$

$$\text{AUMC}_M = \frac{fFX_0}{V_m} \frac{K_m}{(K_m + K_{el})K_{mel}} \left(\frac{1}{K_a} + \frac{1}{K_m + K_{el}} + \frac{1}{K_{mel}} \right)$$

$$+ \frac{f(1 - F)X_0}{V_m} \frac{1}{K_{mel}} \left(\frac{1}{K_a} + \frac{1}{K_{mel}} \right) \tag{13.a14}$$

Model 4

The ordinary differential equations describing the temporal change in the plasma drug concentrations are

$$\frac{dC}{dt} = \frac{fF}{V_c} K_a X - (K_m + K_{el})C \tag{13.a15}$$

$$\frac{dM}{dt} = \frac{V_c}{V_m} K_M C - K_{mel} M + \frac{f(1 - F)}{V_m} K_a X \tag{13.a16}$$

The area under the concentration curve of the drug and the metabolite can be expressed as

$$\text{AUC}_C = \frac{fFRT}{V_c} \frac{1}{K_m + K_{el}} \tag{13.a17}$$

$$\text{AUC}_M = \frac{fFRT}{V_m} \frac{K_m}{(K_m + K_{el})K_{mel1}} + \frac{f(1 - F)RT}{V_m K_{mel}} \tag{13.a18}$$

The area under the first moment of the concentration curve can also be expressed in terms of rate constants:

$$\text{AUMC}_C = \frac{fFX_0}{V_c} \frac{1}{K_m + K_{el}} \left(\frac{1}{K_a} + \frac{1}{K_m + K_{el}} + \frac{T}{2} \right) \tag{13.a19}$$

$$\text{AUMC}_M = \frac{fFX_0}{V_m} \frac{K_m}{(K_m + K_{el})K_{mel}} \left(\frac{1}{K_a} + \frac{1}{K_m + K_{el}} + \frac{1}{K_{mel}} + \frac{T}{2} \right)$$

$$+ \frac{f(1 - F)X_0}{V_m} \frac{1}{K_{mel}} \left(\frac{1}{K_a} + \frac{1}{K_{mel}} + \frac{T}{2} \right) \tag{13.a20}$$

CHAPTER 14

Model 1

The area under the curve and the area under the first moment curve can be expressed as

$$\text{AUC} = \frac{fF}{V} \frac{X_0}{K_{el}} \tag{14.a1}$$

$$\text{AUMC} = \frac{fF}{V} \left[\frac{X_0}{K_a} \frac{1}{K_{el}} + \frac{X_0}{K_{el}^2} \right] \tag{14.a2}$$

The area under the curve of a drug may be affected by another drug due to a change in the fraction absorbed or the elimination time after the coadministration.

Model 2

The area under the curve and the area under the first moment curve for this model can be expressed as

$$\text{AUC} = \frac{fFX_0}{V} \frac{K_{21}}{\lambda_1 \lambda_2} = \frac{fFX_0}{V} \frac{1}{K_{el}} \tag{14.a3}$$

$$\text{AUMC} = \frac{fFX_0}{V} \frac{K_{21}}{\lambda_1 \lambda_2} \left[-\frac{1}{K_{21}} + \frac{1}{K_a} + \frac{1}{\lambda_1} + \frac{1}{\lambda_2} \right] \tag{14.a4}$$

where

$$\lambda_1 + \lambda_2 = K_{el} + K_{12} + K_{21} \tag{14.a5}$$

$$\lambda_1 \lambda_2 = K_{el} K_{21} \tag{14.a6}$$

Since a change in protein binding may affect the volume of distribution and elimination time constant, the area under the concentration curve may change if a drug interaction involves an altered protein building.

Model 3

The ordinary differential equations describing the model are as follows:

$$\frac{dX}{dt} = -K_a X \tag{14.a7}$$

$$\frac{dC}{dt} = \frac{fF}{V_c} K_a X - (K_{el} + K_m) C \tag{14.a8}$$

$$\frac{dM}{dt} = \frac{V_c}{V_m} K_m C - K_{mel} M \tag{14.a9}$$

The metabolic rate constant K_m is the summation of rate constants of all metabolic reactions, if more than one metabolic pathways are involved. According to this model, the area under the concentration curve and the area under the first moment of the concentration curve of the drug can be expressed in terms of rate constants:

$$\text{AUC}_C = \frac{fF}{V} \frac{X_0}{K_{el} + K_m} \tag{14.a10}$$

$$\text{AUMC}_\text{C} = \frac{fF}{V}\left[\frac{X_0}{K_\text{a}}\frac{1}{K_\text{el} + K_\text{m}} + \frac{X_0}{(K_\text{el} + K_\text{m})^2}\right] \qquad (14.\text{a}11)$$

Similarly, the area under the concentration curve and the area under the first moment of the concentration curve of the metabolite can be expressed as

$$\text{AUC}_\text{M} = \frac{fFK_\text{m}}{V_\text{m}}\frac{X_0}{K_\text{el} + K_\text{m}}\frac{1}{K_\text{mel}} \qquad (14.\text{a}12)$$

$$\text{AUMC}_\text{M} = \frac{fFK_\text{m}X_0}{V_\text{m}}\frac{1}{K_\text{el} + K_\text{m}}\frac{1}{K_\text{mel}}\left(\frac{1}{K_\text{a}} + \frac{1}{K_\text{el} + K_\text{m}} + \frac{1}{K_\text{mel}}\right) \qquad (14.\text{a}13)$$

CHAPTER 15

Model 1

The area under the concentration curve may be different in different age groups, due to a change in the extent of absorption, the first pass effect, the volume of distribution, or elimination rate:

$$\text{AUC} = \frac{fF}{V}\frac{X_0}{K_\text{el}} \qquad (15.\text{a}1)$$

An unambiguous method to characterize the absorption time is described as follows. First, the terminal portion of the concentration curve is fitted to a monoexponential function and the intercept between this monoexponential function and the y axis is

$$A = \frac{fFX_0}{V}\frac{K_\text{a}}{\lambda_0 - \lambda_z} \qquad (15.\text{a}2)$$

The ratio of area under the curve to the intercept gives an expression containing only the initial (λ_0) and terminal slope (λ_z):

$$\frac{\text{AUC}}{A} = \frac{1}{\lambda_z} - \frac{1}{\lambda_0} \qquad (15.\text{a}3)$$

Then the initial slope λ_0 can be estimated directly by a curve-stripping technique or from the following equation:

$$\lambda_0 = 2\left/\left(\bar{t} - \frac{\text{AUC}}{A}\right)\right. \qquad (15.\text{a}4)$$

The accuracy of the stripping method may be improved with a large number of data points along the rising phase of the concentration curve. With known values of λs and $f*F$, the value of T_a*V can be expressed as follows:

$$\frac{1}{T_a*V} = \frac{K_a}{V} = \frac{A(\lambda_0 - \lambda_z)}{fFX_0} \tag{15.a5}$$

Model 2

The area under the curve can be expressed as

$$\mathrm{AUC} = \frac{fFX_0}{V_1 K_{el}} \tag{15.a6}$$

The following derivation provides the procedure to estimate this parameter.

First, the α and β phases of the terminal portion of the concentration curve can be fitted to two exponential terms:

$$C = Ae^{-\lambda_{z1}} + Be^{-\lambda_{z2}} \tag{15.a7}$$

Then the intercepts of α and β phases can be expressed as

$$A = \frac{K_a fFX_0}{V_1} \frac{K_{21} - \lambda_{z1}}{(\lambda_0 - \lambda_{z1})(\lambda_{z2} - \lambda_{z1})} \tag{15.a8}$$

$$B = \frac{K_a fFX_0}{V_1} \frac{K_{21} - \lambda_{z2}}{(\lambda_0 - \lambda_{z2})(\lambda_{z1} - \lambda_{z2})} \tag{15.a9}$$

Dividing the above two equations can eliminate f, F, K_a and V_1.

$$\frac{K_{21} - \lambda_{z1}}{K_{21} - \lambda_{z2}} = -\frac{A(\lambda_0 - \lambda_{z1})}{B(\lambda_0 - \lambda_{z2})} = -D \tag{15.a10}$$

Then K_{21} can be estimated from the exponentials of the alpha and beta phases.

$$K_{21} = -\frac{\lambda_{z1} + D\lambda_{z2}}{D + 1} \tag{15.a11}$$

Subsequently, the value of T_a*V_1 can be obtained from the following expression:

$$\frac{1}{T_a*V_1} = \frac{K_a}{V_1} = \frac{A + B}{fFX_0} \frac{(\lambda_{z1} - \lambda_0)(\lambda_{z2} - \lambda_0)}{\lambda_0 - K_{21}} \tag{15.a12}$$

Model 3

The area under the metabolite concentration curve can be expressed as

$$AUC_M = \frac{fFX_0 K_m}{V_m K_{el} K_{mel}} \tag{15.a13}$$

CHAPTER 16

Model 1

The ordinary differential equations describing the model are as follows:

$$\frac{dX}{dt} = -K_a X \tag{16.a1}$$

$$\frac{dC_1}{dt} = \frac{fF}{V_1} K_a X - (K_{el} + K_{12} + K_m)C_1 + \frac{K_{21} V_2}{V_1} C_2 \tag{16.a2}$$

$$\frac{dC_2}{dt} = \frac{V_1}{V_2} K_{12} C_1 - K_{21} C_2 \tag{16.a3}$$

$$\frac{dM}{dt} = \frac{V_I}{V_m} K_m C_1 - K_{mel} M \tag{16.a4}$$

Following an oral administration of a drug, the area under the concentration curve and the area under the first moment curve can be expressed in terms of the rate constants:

$$AUC_C = \frac{fFX_0}{V} \frac{K_{21}}{\lambda_1 \lambda_2} \tag{16.a5}$$

$$AUC_M = \frac{fFX_0 K_m}{V_1 K_{mel} K_{el}} \tag{16.a6}$$

$$AUMC_C = \frac{fFX_0}{V} \frac{K_{21}}{\lambda_1 \lambda_2} \left[-\frac{1}{K_{21}} + \frac{1}{K_a} + \frac{1}{\lambda_1} + \frac{1}{\lambda_2} \right] \tag{16.a7}$$

The area under the curve in a male versus female study is frequently affected by the volume of distribution and the elimination rate constant. In studies comparing pharmacokinetics between pregnant and nonpregnant women, the area under the concentration curve can be affected by the extent of absorption, the volume of distribution, and the elimination rate constant. The terminal slopes λs can be expressed in terms of the rate constants:

$$\lambda_1 + \lambda_2 = K_{el} + K_{12} + K_{21} \tag{16.a8}$$

$$\lambda_1\lambda_2 = K_{el}K_{21} \tag{16.a9}$$

CHAPTER 17

Model 1

The ordinary differential equations describing the model are

$$\frac{dX}{dt} = -K_aX \tag{17.a1}$$

$$\frac{dC}{dt} = \frac{fF}{V_c} K_aX - (K_{el} + K_m + K_b)C \tag{17.a2}$$

$$\frac{dM}{dt} = \frac{K_mV_c}{V_m} C - (K_{mel} + K_{mb})M \tag{17.a3}$$

The area under the concentration curve and the area under the first moment of the concentration curve can be expressed in terms of the rate constants:

$$AUC_C = \frac{fF}{V} \frac{X_0}{K_{el} + K_m + K_b} \tag{17.a4}$$

$$AUMC_C = \frac{fF}{V}\left[\frac{X_0}{K_a}\frac{1}{K_{el} + K_m + K_b} + \frac{X_0}{(K_{el} + K_m + K_b)^2}\right] \tag{17.a5}$$

$$AUC_M = \frac{fFK_m}{V_m} \frac{X_0}{K_{el} + K_m + K_b} \frac{1}{K_{mel} + K_{mb}} \tag{17.a6}$$

$$AUMC_M = \frac{fFK_mX_0}{V_m} \frac{1}{K_{el} + K_m + K_b} \frac{1}{K_{mel} + K_{mb}}$$

$$\left(\frac{1}{K_a} + \frac{1}{K_{el} + K_m + K_b} + \frac{1}{K_{mel} + K_{mb}}\right) \tag{17.a7}$$

Renal diseases can affect the area under the concentration curve by decreasing the renal and hepatic elimination rate constants.

Model 2

The ordinary differential equations governing the model are

$$\frac{dX}{dt} = -K_a X \tag{17.a8}$$

$$\frac{dC}{dt} = \frac{fF}{V_c} K_a X - (K_{el} + K_m + K_b + K_{12})C + \frac{V_p}{V_c} K_{21} P \tag{17.a9}$$

$$\frac{dM}{dt} = \frac{V_c}{V_m} K_m C - (K_{mel} + K_{mb})M \tag{17.a10}$$

The area under the concentration curve and the area under the first moment of the concentration curve can be expressed as

$$AUC_C = \frac{fFX_0}{V} \frac{K_{21}}{\lambda_1 \lambda_2} \tag{17.a11}$$

$$AUMC_C = \frac{fFX_0}{V} \frac{K_{21}}{\lambda_1 \lambda_2} \left[-\frac{1}{K_{21}} + \frac{1}{K_a} + \frac{1}{\lambda_1} + \frac{1}{\lambda_2} \right] \tag{17.a12}$$

$$AUC_M = \frac{fFX_0 K_m}{V_m(K_{mel} + K_{mb})(K_{el} + K_m + K_b)} \tag{17.a13}$$

where the terminal slopes can be expressed in terms of the rate constants:

$$\lambda_1 + \lambda_2 = K_{el} + K_m + K_b + K_{12} + K_{21} \tag{17.a14}$$

$$\lambda_1 \lambda_2 = (K_{el} + K_m + K_b)K_{21} \tag{17.a15}$$

The area under the drug concentration curve in renal diseases can be affected by a change in the volume of distribution and the renal and hepatic elimination rate constants.

CHAPTER 18

Model 1

The ordinary differential equations governing the temporal change in the drug concentrations are

$$\frac{dX}{dt} = -K_a X \tag{18.a1}$$

$$\frac{dC_1}{dt} = \frac{fF}{V_1} K_a X - (K_{el} + K_m + K_{12})C_1 + \frac{V_2}{V_1} K_{21} C_2 \tag{18.a2}$$

$$\frac{dC_2}{dt} = \frac{V_1}{V_2} K_{12} C_1 - K_{21} C_2 \tag{18.a3}$$

$$\frac{dM}{dt} = \frac{V_1}{V_m} K_m C - K_{mel} M \tag{18.a4}$$

Following an oral administration, the area under the concentration curve and the area under the first moment curve can be expressed as follows:

$$AUC = \frac{fFX_0}{V_1} \frac{K_{21}}{\lambda_1 \lambda_2} \tag{18.a5}$$

$$AUMC = \frac{fFX_0}{V_1} \frac{K_{21}}{\lambda_1 \lambda_2}\left[-\frac{1}{K_{21}} + \frac{1}{K_a} + \frac{1}{\lambda_1} + \frac{1}{\lambda_2} \right] \tag{18.a6}$$

where the exponents can be expressed in terms of the rate constants:

$$\lambda_1 + \lambda_2 = K_{el} + K_m + K_{12} + K_{21} \tag{18.a7}$$

$$\lambda_1 \lambda_2 = (K_{el} + K_m)K_{21} \tag{18.a8}$$

Liver diseases can affect the area under the concentration by altering the volume of distribution and the rate of metabolism.

Following an intravenous administration, the area under the concentration curve and the area under the first moment curve can be expressed in terms of the rate constants:

$$AUC_C = \frac{X_0}{V_1} \frac{K_{21}}{\lambda_1 \lambda_2} \tag{18.a9}$$

$$AUC_M = \frac{fFX_0 K_m}{V_m K_{mel} K_{el}} \tag{18.a10}$$

$$AUMC_C = \frac{X_0}{V_1} \frac{K_{21}}{\lambda_1 \lambda_2}\left[-\frac{1}{K_{21}} + \frac{1}{\lambda_1} + \frac{1}{\lambda_2} \right] \tag{18.a11}$$

Model 2

The ordinary differential equations governing the temporal change in the concentrations are

$$\frac{dX}{dt} = -K_a X \tag{18.a12}$$

$$\frac{dC_1}{dt} = \frac{fF}{V_1} K_a X - (K_m + K_{el} + K_{12})C_1 + \frac{V_2}{V_1} K_{21} C_2 \qquad (18.a13)$$

$$\frac{dM}{dt} = \frac{V_1}{V_m} K_m C_1 - K_{mel} M + \frac{f(1 - F)}{V_m} K_a X \qquad (18.a14)$$

Following an oral administration of the drug, the area under the curve and the area under the first moment curve can be expressed as follows:

$$AUC_C = \frac{fFX_0}{V_1} \frac{K_{21}}{\lambda_1 \lambda_2} \qquad (18.a15)$$

$$AUC_M = \frac{fFX_0}{V_m} \frac{K_m K_{21}}{\lambda_1 \lambda_2 K_{mel}} + \frac{f(1 - F)X_0}{V_m} \frac{1}{K_{mel}} \qquad (18.a16)$$

$$AUMC_C = \frac{fFX_0}{V_1} \frac{K_{21}}{\lambda_1 \lambda_2} \left[-\frac{1}{K_{21}} + \frac{1}{K_a} + \frac{1}{\lambda_1} + \frac{1}{\lambda_2} \right] \qquad (18.a17)$$

$$AUMC_M = \frac{fFX_0}{V_m} \frac{K_m K_{21}}{\lambda_1 \lambda_2 K_{mel}} \left[-\frac{1}{K_{21}} + \frac{1}{K_a} + \frac{1}{\lambda_1} + \frac{1}{\lambda_2} + \frac{1}{K_{mel}} \right]$$

$$+ \frac{f(1 - F)X_0}{V_m} \frac{1}{K_{mel}} \left[\frac{1}{K_a} + \frac{1}{K_{mel}} \right] \qquad (18.a18)$$

where the terminal slopes can be expressed as

$$\lambda_1 + \lambda_2 = K_{el} + K_m + K_{12} + K_{21} \qquad (18.a19)$$

$$\lambda_1 \lambda_2 = (K_{el} + K_m)K_{21} \qquad (18.a20)$$

Liver diseases can affect the area under the curve by altering the first pass effect F, the volume of distribution V_1, and the metabolic elimination K_m. A decrease in the first pass effect will increase the area under the drug concentration curve but decrease the area under the metabolite concentration curve.

Following an intravenous administration, the area under the concentration curve and the area under the first moment curve become

$$AUC_C = \frac{X_0}{V_1} \frac{K_{21}}{\lambda_1 \lambda_2} \qquad (18.a21)$$

$$AUC_M = \frac{X_0}{V_m} \frac{K_m K_{21}}{\lambda_1 \lambda_2 K_{mel}} = \frac{X_0}{V_m} \frac{K_m}{(K_{el} + K_m)K_{mel}} \qquad (18.a22)$$

$$AUMC_C = \frac{X_0}{V_1} \frac{K_{21}}{\lambda_1 \lambda_2} \left[-\frac{1}{K_{21}} + \frac{1}{\lambda_1} + \frac{1}{\lambda_2} \right] \qquad (18.a23)$$

$$\text{AUMC}_M = \frac{X_0}{V_m} \frac{K_m K_{21}}{\lambda_1 \lambda_2 K_{mel}} \left[-\frac{1}{K_{21}} + \frac{1}{\lambda_1} + \frac{1}{\lambda_2} + \frac{1}{K_{mel}} \right] \quad (18.a24)$$

Liver diseases may affect the area under the curve by altering the volume of distribution and the metabolic rate constant.

CHAPTER 19

Model 1

The ordinary differential equations governing the model are

$$\frac{dX}{dt} = -K_a X \quad (19.a1)$$

$$\frac{dC_1}{dt} = \frac{fF}{V_1} K_a X - (K_{el} + K_{12})C_1 + \frac{V_2}{V_1} K_{21} C_2 \quad (19.a2)$$

$$\frac{dC_2}{dt} = \frac{V_1}{V_2} K_{12} C_1 - K_{21} C_2 \quad (19.a3)$$

The area under the concentration curve and the area under the first moment of the concentration curve following an oral administration can be expressed as follows:

$$\text{AUC} = \frac{fFX_0}{V_1} \frac{K_{21}}{\lambda_1 \lambda_2} = \frac{fFX_0}{V_1 K_{el}} \quad (19.a4)$$

$$\text{AUMC} = \frac{fFX_0}{V_1} \frac{K_{21}}{\lambda_1 \lambda_2} \left[-\frac{1}{K_{21}} + \frac{1}{K_a} + \frac{1}{\lambda_1} + \frac{1}{\lambda_2} \right] \quad (19.a5)$$

where

$$\lambda_1 + \lambda_2 = K_{el} + K_{12} + K_{21} \quad (19.a6)$$

$$\lambda_1 \lambda_2 = K_{el} K_{21} \quad (19.a7)$$

The area under the curve may change in diseases that affect the protein binding, if the change in protein binding results in a change in the volume of distribution and the elimination rate.

Following an intravenous dose, the area under the curve and the area under the first moment curve are estimated as follows:

$$\text{AUC} = \frac{X_0}{V_1} \frac{K_{21}}{\lambda_1 \lambda_2} = \frac{X_0}{V_1} T_{el} \quad (19.a8)$$

$$AUMC = \frac{X_0}{V_1} \frac{K_{21}}{\lambda_1 \lambda_2} \left[-\frac{1}{K_{21}} + \frac{1}{\lambda_1} + \frac{1}{\lambda_2} \right] \tag{19.a9}$$

Model 2

The ordinary differential equations used to describe the temporal change in the drug concentrations are

$$\frac{dC}{dt} = \frac{fF}{V_c} K_a X - (K_m + K_{el})C \tag{19.a10}$$

$$\frac{dM}{dt} = \frac{V_c}{V_m} K_m C - K_{mel} M + \frac{f(1-F)}{V_m} K_a X \tag{19.a11}$$

Following an oral administration of a drug, the area under the curve of the drug and its metabolite can be expressed as follows:

$$AUC_C = \frac{fFX_0}{V_c} \frac{1}{K_m + K_{el}} \tag{19.a12}$$

$$AUC_M = \frac{fFX_0}{V_m} \frac{K_m}{(K_m + K_{el})K_{mel}} + \frac{f(1-F)X_0}{V_m K_{mel}} \tag{19.a13}$$

The area under the curve can be affected by a disease if the hepatic or renal elimination time changes in the disease.

Following an intravenous administration of a drug, the area under the curve does not depend on the first pass effect as in the oral administration:

$$AUC_C = \frac{X_0}{V_c} \frac{1}{K_m + K_{el}} \tag{19.a14}$$

$$AUC_M = \frac{X_0}{V_m} \frac{K_m}{(K_m + K_{el})K_{mel}} \tag{19.a15}$$

The volume of the central compartment can be estimated from the ratio of dose to the initial concentration ($V_c = X_0/C_0$).

Model 3

The ordinary differential equations governing the model are

$$\frac{dX}{dt} = -K_a X \tag{19.a16}$$

$$\frac{dC_1}{dt} = \frac{fF}{V_1} K_a X - (K_m + K_{el} + K_{12})C_1 + \frac{V_2}{V_1} K_{21} C_2 \tag{19.a17}$$

$$\frac{dM}{dt} = \frac{V_1}{V_m} K_m C_1 - K_{mel} M + \frac{f(1 - F)}{V_m} K_a X \qquad (19.a18)$$

After an oral administration of a drug, the area under the curve and the area under the first moment curve can be expressed in terms of the rate constants:

$$\text{AUC}_C = \frac{fFX_0}{V_1(K_{el} + K_m)} \qquad (19.a19)$$

$$\text{AUC}_M = \frac{fFX_0}{V_m} \frac{K_m K_{21}}{\lambda_1 \lambda_2 K_{mel}} + \frac{f(1 - F)X_0}{V_m} \frac{1}{K_{mel}} \qquad (19.a20)$$

$$\text{AUMC}_C = \frac{fFX_0}{V_1} \frac{K_{21}}{\lambda_1 \lambda_2} \left[-\frac{1}{K_{21}} + \frac{1}{K_a} + \frac{1}{\lambda_1} + \frac{1}{\lambda_2} \right] \qquad (19.a21)$$

$$\text{AUMC}_M = \frac{fFX_0}{V_m} \frac{K_m K_{21}}{\lambda_1 \lambda_2 K_{mel}} \left[-\frac{1}{K_{21}} + \frac{1}{K_a} + \frac{1}{\lambda_1} + \frac{1}{\lambda_2} + \frac{1}{K_{mel}} \right]$$

$$+ \frac{f(1 - F)X_0}{V_m} \frac{1}{K_{mel}} \left[\frac{1}{K_a} + \frac{1}{K_{mel}} \right] \qquad (19.a22)$$

where

$$\lambda_1 + \lambda_2 = K_{el} + K_m + K_{12} + K_{21} \qquad (19.a23)$$

$$\lambda_1 \lambda_2 = (K_{el} + K_m)K_{21} \qquad (19.a24)$$

The area under the curve may change in a disease if the disease affects the first pass effect, the volume of distribution, or the metabolism.

Following an intravenous administration of a drug, the area under the curve and the area under the first moment curve can be expressed in terms of the rate constants:

$$\text{AUC}_C = \frac{X_0}{V_1} \frac{1}{K_{el} + K_m} \qquad (19.a25)$$

$$\text{AUC}_M = \frac{X_0}{V_m} \frac{K_m K_{21}}{\lambda_1 \lambda_2 K_{mel}} = \frac{X_0}{V_m} \frac{K_m}{(K_{el} + K_m)K_{mel}} \qquad (19.a26)$$

$$\text{AUMC} = \frac{X_0}{V_1} \frac{K_{21}}{\lambda_1 \lambda_2} \left[-\frac{1}{K_{21}} + \frac{1}{\lambda_1} + \frac{1}{\lambda_2} \right] \qquad (19.a27)$$

$$\text{AUMC}_M = \frac{X_0}{V_m} \frac{K_m K_{21}}{\lambda_1 \lambda_2 K_{mel}} \left[-\frac{1}{K_{21}} + \frac{1}{\lambda_1} + \frac{1}{\lambda_2} + \frac{1}{K_{mel}} \right] \qquad (19.a28)$$